W9-DEU-299

WOMEN, GENDER, AND HEALTH

Susan L. Smith and Nancy Tomes, Series Editors

# Nurse-Midwifery

## The Birth of a New American Profession

LAURA E. ETTINGER

THE OHIO STATE UNIVERSITY PRESS
COLUMBUS

Library of Congress Cataloging-in-Publication Data
Ettinger, Laura Elizabeth, 1968–
Nurse-midwifery : the birth of a new American profession / Laura E. Ettinger.
p. cm.—(Women, gender, and health)
Includes bibliographical references and index.
ISBN-13: 978–0-8142–1023–9 (cloth : alk. paper)
ISBN-13: 978–0-8142–5150–8 (pbk. : alk. paper)
ISBN-13: 978–0-8142–9100–9 (cd-rom)
1. Midwifery—United States—History. 2. Midwives—United States—History.
I. Title. II. Series.
RG950.E77 2006
618.2—dc22
2006003984

Cover design by Laurence Nozik.
Text design by Jennifer Shoffey Forsythe.
Type set in Adobe Caslon.
Printed by Thomson-Shore, Inc.

Portions of chapter 2 from "Mary Breckinridge," *American National Biography,* edited by John Garraty, copyright © 1999 by the American Council of Learned Societies. Used by permission of Oxford University Press, Inc.

Portions of chapters 2 and 3 from "Nurse-Midwives, the Mass Media, and the Politics of Maternal Health Care in the United States, 1925–1955," Laura E. Ettinger, *Nursing History Review* 7 (1999), copyright © 1999, Springer Publishing Company, Inc., New York 10036. Used by permission.

Portions of chapter 5 from "Mission to Mothers: Nuns, Latino Families, and the Founding of Santa Fe's Catholic Maternity Institute," *Women, Health, and Nation: Canada and the United States Since 1945,* edited by Georgina Feldberg, Molly Ladd-Taylor, Alison Li, and Kathryn McPherson, copyright © 2003 by McGill-Queen's University Press. Used by permission.

The paper used in this publication meets the minimum requirements of the American National Standard for Information Sciences—Permanence of Paper for Printed Library Materials. ANSI Z39.48–1992.

9 8 7 6 5 4 3 2 1

For Phyllis and David Ettinger
and
Jondavid DeLong

With love and gratitude

# CONTENTS

# ILLUSTRATIONS

## Figures

## Tables

## Illustrations

# ACKNOWLEDGMENTS

I AM filled with gratitude as I think about the many people who have helped and supported me throughout the writing of this book.

My book has benefited greatly from the comments and suggestions of a number of scholars and editors. Theodore Brown and Lynn Gordon were instrumental in getting this project—and its author—off the ground when the book was in its earliest stages. I am very thankful for all of their comments on my work, as well as their warm support while I was a graduate student at the University of Rochester. I also thank Molly Ladd-Taylor and Joan Lynaugh for their comments on my articles on the history of nurse-midwives, and Kathleen Mahoney and Sara Adams for their comments on earlier drafts of sections of the book. I am grateful to Lauren Osborne for helping me understand the mysteries of the book publishing process. Thank you to former and current series co-editors Rima Apple, Janet Golden, Susan L. Smith, and Nancy Tomes for taking on my book and carrying it to completion. Former and current Ohio State University Press editors Heather Lee Miller, Sandy Crooms, and Maggie Diehl have been wonderful people with whom to work.

I would like to thank the editors of *Nursing History Review; Women, Health, and Nation: Canada and the United States since 1945;* and *American National Biography* for permission to reprint previously published work. Portions of chapter 2 appeared in "Mary Breckinridge," *American National Biography,* Vol. 3, ed. John A. Garraty and Mark C. Carnes (New York: Oxford University Press, 1999): 462–63. Parts of chapters 2 and 3 appeared in an earlier form in "Nurse-Midwives, the Mass Media, and the Politics of Maternal Health Care in the United States, 1925–1955," *Nursing History Review* 7 (1999): 47–66. Sections of chapter 5 appeared in "Mission to Mothers: Nuns, Latino Families, and the Founding of Santa Fe's Catholic Maternity Institute," *Women, Health, and Nation: Canada and the United States Since 1945,* ed. Georgina Feldberg, Molly Ladd-Taylor, Alison Li, and Kathryn McPherson (Montreal: McGill-Queen's University Press, 2003): 144–60.

I am grateful to the staff at the following archives, libraries, and institutions for helping me find materials: National Library of Medicine, Maternity Center Association, Medical Mission Sisters Archives, University of Kentucky, University of New Mexico, Johns Hopkins University School of Medicine, University of Rochester, and Clarkson University. I especially thank Maureen Corry and Carol Sakala for allowing me access to the stored materials at Maternity Center Association, Stephanie Morris for helping me find materials on Catholic Maternity Institute at the Medical Mission Sisters Archives, and William Mitchell and the entire staff at Archives and Special Collections at the University of Kentucky for making my stays in Lexington such a pleasure. Preston Reynolds, a historian and physician, kindly pointed me to a wonderful series of photographs of African American nurse-midwives at the National Library of Medicine.

I would like to thank my colleagues at Clarkson University, who have been very supportive of my work and of me personally. In particular, I wish to thank Jerry Gravander, who, as dean of the School of Liberal Arts, was very generous in providing financial help for research trips and other expenses, as well as a one-semester teaching load reduction; Barbara Brady, who kindly helped to edit some of my work; and Rick Welsh, Mary Graham, Annegret Staiger, and Heidi Fritz, who are wonderful colleagues and friends.

Many nurse-midwives and nurse-midwife scholars generously shared their experiences, knowledge, and connections with me. In particular, I wish to thank Helen Varney Burst, Katy Dawley, Kitty Ernst, Ellen Craig, Sister Catherine Shean, Rita Kroska, Sister Paula D'Errico, Sister Anne Cauzillo, Sister Sheila McGinnis, Sister Mary Gavin, Sister Kathryn Gates, Julie Buenting, Susan McConaughy, Bunny Adler, Mary Rooks, and Kim Schoch. The last two women—Mary and Kim—helped bring my daughters into the world, and for that I will be forever grateful.

My friends have gone out of their way to offer support, encouragement, love, and importantly, grounding in reality. I could not have done this without them. Special thanks go to Nancy Bloomstein, Tracy Callahan, Maria Finch, Laurel Gabel, Gretchen Hollmer, Sarah Lieberman, Michelle McClellan, Pamela Schroeder, and Karen Tomann. Thank you also to Lyn Dominguez and Dave Obelkevich who gave me a fabulous place to stay in Manhattan while I was doing research. Other wonderful people have enriched my life during the years that I worked on this book.

One friend in particular deserves special mention. I could not have completed this book without the help of fellow historian and dear friend Alexandra Lord. Lexi not only reviewed my manuscript twice and listened for years to my stories and questions about nurse-midwives, but she also provided me with the moral support that I needed to know that I could do this.

Marge Howe has been a godsend. She came into my life when my older daughter, Alison, was an infant, and now she feels like part of our family. I am very grateful to her for her loving care of my daughters that enabled me to work on this book and teach at Clarkson. She also made possible a research trip to New York City with Alison.

My family has been incredible throughout this lengthy process. I thank my brother and his family, Dan, Catherine, Nick, and Steven Ettinger, and my sister-in-law and her family, Dara, Jason, Liam, Max, and Declan Lanier, for being there for me. My sister Kathryn Ettinger has made me laugh in a way that no one else can (and I needed that while I worked on this book!). My parents-in-law Judy DeLong and Gino Williams have been extraordinarily supportive and generous to me over the years; most recently, their babysitting services have been greatly appreciated.

I wish to dedicate this book to three important people in my life. My parents, Phyllis and David Ettinger, loved me unconditionally, taught me a love of learning, and told me I could do and be anything that I wanted. I could not have written this book or become who I am without their love and support. Their intellectual curiosity and commitment to their passions continue to inspire me. In addition, my mother's comments on the epilogue and my father's experiences as a physician have been very helpful to me.

My husband, Jondavid DeLong, has always believed in me, even when I have not believed in myself. For many years, he has been there for me, providing love, encouragement, a sense of humor, and a reminder to "stop obsessing about writing and just write!" The thanks that I owe him would require a separate book, but for now I dedicate this book to him with my love. I am blessed to share my life with him.

Our daughters Alison, born in 2001, and Caroline, born in 2005, have changed my life in too many ways to count. They keep me grounded, they remind me about what is important, and they make my world a better place. Their entrance into my life also has made me more sensitive to and even more invested in the subject matter of this book.

CHAPTER 1

# Conception

## Nurse-Midwives and the Professionalization of Childbirth

"IS nurse-midwifery the solution?" Sister M. Theophane Shoemaker, nurse-midwife and director of Santa Fe's Catholic Maternity Institute, asked in an article written in 1946. For Shoemaker, the answer was obvious: nurse-midwives, working in collaboration with physicians, could provide a permanent solution to the problem of poorly distributed and inadequate maternity care that had existed for decades in the United States.[1]

Born Agnes Shoemaker in 1913, Sister Theophane had become interested in nursing because she had wanted to help others and had admired an aunt who was a nurse.[2] After joining the Medical Mission Sisters and graduating from Catholic University with a bachelor's degree in nursing in 1941, she worked as a nursing supervisor in the maternity and newborn nursery units of a busy hospital. When the superior general of the Medical Mission Sisters asked her to study nurse-midwifery so Sister Theophane could establish a new nurse-midwifery service in Santa Fe, an area with high maternal and infant mortality rates and very few physicians, she eagerly accepted the challenge. As Sister Theophane explained, "I had been really quite unhappy with the way they [physicians] were treating maternity patients [in hospitals] at that time. They were giving them high doses of scopolamine [which causes amnesia], sometimes with morphine, and the women were really out of their minds . . . . They were really animalistic, and it was awful. . . . I'd never heard of nurse-midwives before, but I was willing to try it."[3] Different from many of her counterparts, Sister

Theophane's motivation for becoming a nurse-midwife had to do, at least in part, with her dislike of the way women acted—"animalistic" and not in control of their feelings—when they received the contemporary drugs of choice during labor.

After graduating from one of the only two nurse-midwifery schools then in existence in the U.S., Sister Theophane and another nurse-midwife founded Catholic Maternity Institute (CMI), a home delivery nurse-midwifery service, in 1944. She loved the change from her previous nursing job, as she perceived a huge difference between births attended by nurse-midwives and those attended by physicians. "We treated mothers as human beings—[seeing] mothers as part of families—and [making] maternity care a real physiological activity rather than a pathological activity. . . . It just was amazing . . . the difference . . . when a mother was conscious, knew what was going to happen to her, was able to control her feelings to some extent, was able to cooperate with you and was able to receive the baby with some kind of mental stimulation, some love. And to put the baby to breast right away after delivery, which we always did, . . . was a very physiologically healthy thing to do. And the simplicity of the whole operation—I don't want to call it an operation—of the whole procedure was just wonderful."[4]

In addition to providing a very different kind of maternity care from what physicians were providing at hospitals, Sister Theophane and her fellow CMI nurse-midwives also helped improve the health of women and children in the area they served. Her nurse-midwifery work, however, did not stop with this pioneering service and school in Santa Fe. In the 1950s, Sister Theophane fought to organize and unite nurse-midwives, playing a central role in the formation of a national nurse-midwifery organization and serving as its second president. She and her colleagues constantly faced opposition from a health-care establishment that sought to limit nurse-midwives' work. Physicians and nurses believed nurse-midwives were too independent and therefore threatened their positions. Physicians also charged that nurse-midwives were not sufficiently trained to practice obstetrics and that they used "bad," old-fashioned approaches to childbirth. Some physicians were even unaware nurse-midwives existed at all.

Sister Theophane was not alone. She was part of a group of pioneering nurse-midwives in the early and mid-twentieth century who successfully changed maternity care in select regions of the United States and constantly fought relentless prejudice against and ignorance about their profession. Today, American nurse-midwives attend a small but steadily growing percentage of births. In 2003, nurse-midwives attended 7.6 percent of American births, a rise from less than 1.0 percent in 1975.[5] Yet in an age when modern has been equated with scientific, nurse-midwives, primarily through association with traditional and "unscientific" midwives, have been perceived as a vestige of a distant, best-forgotten past.

Contrary to this view, nurse-midwives were and are licensed professionals, with formal education in both nursing and midwifery. But in the twentieth century, as modern births in America came to involve physicians, hospitals, technological interventions, and quick, routine procedures, nurse-midwives seemed increasingly anachronistic. They delivered babies at home, intervened less in the birth process, and took considerable time with their patients. Yet nurse-midwives, who worked, at least theoretically, under the supervision of physicians, also served as agents of the professionalization and medicalization of childbirth.

Despite most nurse-midwives' successful track records, the medical establishment, both directly and indirectly, discouraged the growth of their practice. Physicians actively sought to limit where nurse-midwives worked, whom they served, and the types of care they could provide. They also failed to promote nurse-midwives as modern health practitioners and to give them widespread support as birth attendants for the nation's women, or even just for the poor. Nurse-midwives provided quality health care to their female patients and offered women practitioners an unusual amount of independence. However, fears among medical professionals and cultural concerns about the place of the midwife in modern society resulted in a limitation of nurse-midwives' sphere, forcing these practitioners to make difficult choices about the directions their profession would take.

By exploring the birth of nurse-midwifery, my book analyzes the ways in which women professionals created a space of their own in the face of many obstacles. As the name "nurse-midwife" indicates, the profession was a hybrid. As nurses, nurse-midwives belonged to a profession whose members were not seen as autonomous professionals. Nurses were overwhelmingly women in a field dominated by male physicians. As historian Susan M. Reverby has shown, even nursing leaders were subordinate to physicians' and hospitals' needs, ordered to care in a society that did (and does) not value caring.[6] Yet nurse-midwives were also part of midwifery. While early nurse-midwives identified with their European counterparts, well-respected and well-educated women on whom they based their profession, the American public and health professionals identified them with traditional midwives, many of whom were immigrants or African Americans. Increasingly, these traditional midwives were viewed as dirty, backward, and ignorant. In the early to mid-twentieth century then, the nurse-midwife occupied a strange and ambivalent position.

She did have, however, some power, certainly more than many nurses or traditional midwives. Unlike many nurses, when nurse-midwives interacted with their patients, they made the important decisions, except in the relatively few cases where they needed to bring in physicians. Unlike traditional midwives, nurse-midwives had formal education and worked squarely within the mainstream health-care system. They supervised or replaced traditional midwives, and sometimes joined others in criticizing traditional midwives.

However, compared with physicians, nurse-midwives were much less powerful both because they were women in a male-dominated profession (obstetrics) and because they were not seen as fully credentialed. In many ways, they stood outside the health-care establishment, challenging the notion that childbirth required male physicians, hospitals, and interventions. They also challenged the health-care hierarchy: neither fish nor fowl, nurse-midwives could not be easily characterized. While individual physicians and nurses were supportive and active in the emergence of nurse-midwifery, the nursing and medical professions as a whole were not.[7] Troubled by nurse-midwives' unique place within the hierarchy, many physicians and nurses aggressively sought to stop or at least limit nurse-midwives' work. Nurse-midwives responded to the opposition by adopting a strategy of accommodation; they remained within nursing (unlike many European midwives), and they conceded a fair amount of authority to physicians.

This book also explores the changing practice of childbirth in America. In the United States, as in many other industrialized nations, childbirth gradually moved from home to hospital, birth attendants changed from female midwives to male physicians, and birthing practices replaced folk healing with scientific medicine. The history of nurse-midwifery provides an often-overlooked insight into these shifts. In a sense, nurse-midwives were and are an exception to the medicalization of childbirth during the twentieth century. They offered and continue to offer an important challenge to what scholars call the "male medical model" of childbirth. As Sister Theophane indicated, nurse-midwives offered their patients something radically different from what most physicians provided in hospital births. Nurse-midwives spent more time with their patients in labor and intervened less, and they saw birth as a normal, rather than pathological, process. Eventually, they also created collaborative, rather than hierarchical, relationships with their patients—an approach to patient care that ran (and runs) counter to modern notions of medical authority and treatment.

Finally, this book analyzes changing patterns of health care in the United States. The American health-care system was, and remains, chaotic. Unlike many economically developed countries, the United States has offered only private insurance (except for the very poor and the elderly, starting in 1965) rather than universal health insurance, demanding fee-for-service payments rather than providing universal care. Additionally, there has been no centralized planning for the distribution of health-care practitioners. Overall, this unique approach has not benefited Americans. Millions of Americans lacked and continue to lack access to professional health care because they are uninsured or underinsured, and Americans, on average, are less healthy and have a shorter life span than citizens of thirty industrialized nations.[8]

Nurse-midwifery was developed to target groups traditionally left out of the American health-care system. In a few select places starting in the 1920s, nurse-midwives dramatically improved the health of poor and minority women and families. However, they never got the opportunity to give large numbers of people better access to health care in any systematic way. Nurse-midwives' underutilization and marginalization indicates how unprepared Americans were to use innovative approaches to improve and more simply provide health care for *all* Americans.

## The Medicalization of Childbirth

In order to understand the birth of the American nurse-midwife, it is necessary to explore what writer and social critic Jessica Mitford called the "American way of birth."[9] Historians have explained that American childbirth went from a social event controlled by neighbor women to a medical event controlled by male physicians. This process, commonly called the "medicalization" of childbirth, involved two important transformations: a change in birth attendants from midwives to physicians, and a change in birth location from home to hospital.[10]

An understanding of changes in childbirth requires some background in American medicine. In the late eighteenth and nineteenth centuries, anyone could proclaim himself or herself to be a "doctor." In this democratic culture, no special license, certificate, or education was required. This meant that the care that women received varied widely from practitioner to practitioner. During this time, medical practitioners could be loosely divided into two groups: orthodox, or "regular," physicians and the others, including Thomsonian botanists, homeopaths, eclectics (who used a mixture of remedies from the Thomsonians, homeopaths, and others), "quacks," and midwives.[11] Orthodox physicians organized and tried to eliminate the competition by claiming that they were better educated (although many were not), that many of the "irregulars" relied on erroneous therapeutic concepts (although the "regulars" also tended to believe in theoretical medical systems), and that their remedies were more effective (although many of the treatments—such as massive bloodletting, purging, and heavy drugging—were not, and patients often disliked them). They tried to establish professional medical societies and licensing laws to advance their own interests and keep other practitioners out.[12]

Until the twentieth century, birth was a female activity that took place in the home. When a woman went into labor, she gathered her female relatives, friends, and neighbors around her. These women helped the laboring mother, sharing stories of their experiences, comforting the woman, walking around with her, and assisting her in delivering her baby. They also provided an important support system at a vulnerable time in a woman's life when she feared death during childbirth. Many of these women stayed for days or weeks after the birth to lend their continued support.

The midwife was just one of the many women in the "birthing room." Midwives usually had no formal training, but a lot of experience based on an informal apprenticeship with another midwife. No rules regulated these apprenticeships, and while some of these women were highly skilled, others were not. Nature and gravity were central to midwives' work. Indeed, midwives spent most of their time supporting the birthing woman and waiting.

In cases of difficult or long labors, midwives sometimes intervened by turning the fetus or by giving the mother liquor. While some used drugs and forceps, which urban male physicians by the mid-eighteenth century increasingly employed, most did not; they feared criticism for incorrect use of forceps (and most had not received training in their use). When faced with a very difficult birth, the best midwives often had little to offer a suffering or dying patient except comfort. After a birth, a midwife typically stayed for hours, making sure the new mother and baby were well, changing the bed linens, and spending time with the roomful of relatives and friends.[13]

Starting in the late 1700s, urban middle- and upper-class families began to employ male physicians, known as "man-midwives," to attend their babies' births. Man-midwives brought scientific medicine into the birthing room; this scientific medicine was male, white, and middle or upper class. Contrary to contemporary beliefs, however, the increased presence of these men and their so-called scientific methods in birthing rooms likely caused more problems for parturient women than did traditional, female midwives.

Just as female midwives' skills varied because of a lack of regulation, so too did those of man-midwives. Most had no formal training in anatomy and had never attended medical school. Yet male physicians had several attractions: 1) they used forceps and drugs that midwives generally did not use, 2) they were thought to have had formal education in anatomy, and 3) their sex conferred a certain amount of prestige.[14] More interventionist than midwives, male physicians felt that a doctor, as one explained, "must do something. He cannot remain a spectator merely, where there are many witnesses, and where interest in what is going on is too deep to allow of his inaction."[15] Physicians typically used bloodletting, chloroform (starting in the 1840s), and/or forceps. Bloodletting and chloroform accelerated the labor and relieved pain (among other things), while the forceps could deliver the baby in a prolonged, difficult labor, potentially saving two lives. Despite these tools, male physicians had serious limitations. Historians have shown that too often they were overeager to use forceps and caused disability and death for many mothers and babies.[16] In addition, the man-midwives, like female midwives, did not understand the cause and prevention of puerperal fever (bacterial infection of the genital tract shortly after birth)—the leading cause of maternal death in the nineteenth century. Doctors, like midwives, unknowingly spread the infection with their hands and their tools.[17]

Until the mid-nineteenth century, women who employed male physicians still maintained some control over the birthing process. They and their female support system (including the midwives) decided if and when to call on a physician, and together they decided what tools and techniques would be used during labor and delivery.[18] Many man-midwives, later called obstetricians, viewed midwives as competitors and sometimes attacked them. They denounced midwives in their writings, suggesting that women who practiced midwifery should have stayed at home in their proper sphere and that midwives were unsafe.[19] Over the second half of the 1800s, likely due in part to public, male-generated criticism of female midwives, a growing number of middle-class urban women chose physicians to deliver their babies, believing in the promise of science and medicine to make childbirth safer and associating a physician-attended birth with higher status. By 1900, 50 percent of American births were attended by midwives and 50 percent by physicians. At this point, midwives generally attended the births of rural, African American, or immigrant women, and shared the same background as the women they attended. Thus, among middle-class urban women giving birth, physicians were seen as status symbols, while midwives, commonly associated with the poor, were seen as déclassé.

The second transformation in the history of American childbirth occurred when birth moved into the hospital. In the nineteenth century, hospitals never attracted more than 5 percent of pregnant women, and even they did not come by choice. The women were usually poor or unmarried, and the maternity hospitals, called "lying-in hospitals" and established by private charities, were often dirty, dangerous places where patients frequently died from puerperal fever. These hospitals aimed more to provide moral uplift to the poor souls who ended up there than to guarantee safe labor and delivery to women (and their offspring) already perceived to be on the road to perdition.[20]

By the 1920s and 1930s, white middle- and upper-class women increasingly went to hospitals to deliver their babies. This change stemmed from several factors. By the 1920s, hospitals had transformed themselves into middle-class institutions by marketing modernity to paying patients; they advertised standardized medical procedures, notably surgeries and obstetrical deliveries, and a restful, modern environment—clean rooms, good food, radios, telephone, and call buttons for nurses.[21] Some obstetricians, armed with a basic understanding of the new science of bacteriology, also claimed that the hospital could be made into a more sterile environment for deliveries than the home.[22] In addition, obstetricians made increasingly systematic use of pain-relieving drugs, labor-inducing drugs, and technological interventions, such as forceps and episiotomy, in childbirth. They argued that these procedures, now seen as necessary, required access to nursing and anesthesiology staff that only hospitals could provide. Professional jockeying also motivated obstetricians, who tried a variety of ways to gain control of birth management from general practitioners who were attending the majority of physician-managed births.[23]

Women had their own reasons for choosing hospitals. First, they believed that the new science and medicine, and the institution that represented those things, would make birth less dangerous. Second, they liked the predictability of the new birthing procedures. A woman and her physician could decide in advance the day she would deliver her baby, and she could know that she would have medication to induce her labor, as well as medications to forget her pain. And finally, for urban women the traditional women's support network was often no longer available. With the increasing mobility of American society, many women did not have female relatives and friends living near them to assist once they went into labor, yet they still needed help. The hospital seemed like the perfect place to get such assistance.[24] In fact, as some women explained, a hospital birth provided new mothers welcome respite from busy home lives with older children and husbands demanding attention. Lillian Gilbreth, engineer, industrial psychologist, and mother of twelve, had her first eleven babies at home but chose to have number twelve in the hospital, which she found to be "marvelous": "'I would have to wait until my dozenth baby was born to find out how much better it is to have them in a hospital. The nurses here wait on me hand and foot. You don't know what a comfort it is to have your baby in the hospital.'"[25]

Yet, many women giving birth in hospitals felt isolated—"alone among strangers," as one patient explained.[26] Even more important, hospital births were actually, more often than not, *more* dangerous than home births because new mothers were exposed to other patients' germs, and because of the aggressively interventionist approach physicians practiced. In fact, maternal mortality rates actually *increased* from sixty-one deaths per 10,000 live births in 1915 to seventy in 1929, during the exact time that many women first chose to give birth in the hospital.[27] As historian of childbirth Judith Walzer Leavitt has argued, although a direct connection between the increases in hospital births and maternal mortality cannot be drawn statistically with available information, it is suggestive that both increases occurred simultaneously.[28] Indeed, three landmark studies of maternal mortality published in the early 1930s noted the connection as well.[29]

Joseph B. DeLee, a preeminent early-twentieth-century obstetrician, even concluded that "home delivery, even under the poorest conditions, is safer than hospital delivery."[30] At home, an expectant mother exposed herself and her fetus to germs every day, so her immune system built up natural defenses against the germs by the time she delivered her baby. However, new germs entered a hospital all the time, and there was no way to prevent completely the transmission of these germs, even under the best circumstances. Without natural defenses against the new germs, mother and baby were in danger of developing an infection.

Many obstetricians in the 1920s and 1930s agreed with DeLee that hospital births presented serious dangers to women's lives, often blaming their own profession for the deaths by citing excessive use of drugs and instruments in physician-managed hospital births.[31] These obstetricians—along with several important groups studying infant and maternal mortality—denounced the practice of "meddlesome obstetrics," whereby physicians too often used the invasive procedures of forceps, version (turning the fetus within the uterus to bring it into a favorable position for delivery), and Caesarean section, as well as drugs such as pituitrin, a uterine-stimulating drug that sometimes sent mothers into shock and/or ruptured their uteri, and the popular combination of scopolamine and morphine, which produced a semi-narcotic and amnesiac effect known as "twilight sleep" (described by Sister Theophane at the beginning of this chapter).[32] While these techniques did not cause a crisis in the majority of cases, such interventions sometimes led to disaster.

Despite these problems, over one-third of all American births took place in hospitals by 1935. The rate was 65 percent for white urban women, and 88 percent for white urban women with family incomes of $2,000 or more (in other words, middle-class families).[33] For those who could afford it, the ideal birth was one that was physician-directed and hospital-based.

## The "Midwife Problem": The Birth of the Nurse-Midwife and a Lost Opportunity

So where did the nurse-midwife fit into childbirth trends? To answer that question, it is necessary to understand how health and social-welfare professionals came to view the traditional midwife. At the same time that more births were attended by physicians and in hospitals, several groups, including social reformers, physicians, nurses, and public-health officials, claimed that the United States had a "midwife problem." Interest in the traditional midwife intensified around 1910 as mortality statistics showed American maternal and infant death rates to be substantially higher than those of most European countries.[34] Physicians and public-health officials tried to determine why these rates were so high, and what role the midwife might have played in creating them. They incorrectly argued that midwives were the cause of the problem.

The traditional midwife was an easy target. Typically, these women were African Americans or immigrants. During an era of anti-immigration sentiment and legalized racial segregation and discrimination, people who were not white and native-born were at the bottom of the social hierarchy. While midwives attracted birthing women because of their shared race, ethnicity, and language, those same qualities made white professionals deeply suspicious of them. Midwives' birthing practices and general lack of formal training also made them the targets of physicians and social reformers. Early twentieth-century health professionals commented frequently that midwives were ignorant and superstitious. Anna Rude, physician and director of the U.S. Children's Bureau's Division of Maternal and Infant Hygiene, reported that midwives "retain[ed] most of the practices, traditions and superstitions that have been transmitted for generations" among African Americans and the foreign-born. She condemned immigrant midwives for high rates of tetanus among newborns, "undoubtedly due to dirty cord dressings," and decried African-American midwives' use of raw pork pacifiers for newborns because of their supposed laxative effect, "supplemented at frequent intervals by curious and oft-times obnoxious concoctions known as 'teas.'"[35]

Concerns about medical professionalization played a role in debates over midwives. General practitioners cared for most American women not attended by midwives, while obstetricians attended the births of very few urban women. At this time, obstetrics, with weak training programs and low status, was not a popular specialty for physicians. Obstetricians worked to convince fellow physicians and the public that midwives had set back their field by decades. Noting that midwives were often foreign-born or African American, obstetricians described them as dirty, backward, unprofessional, and female. Many obstetricians conceded that the general practitioner often caused as much damage as the midwife, but they used the general practitioners' poor record to justify further why midwives should be eliminated. According to this line of thinking, midwives stood outside the legitimate medical hierarchy, degraded the profession of obstetrics, and discouraged potentially good practitioners from going into the field. General practitioners could be taught to refer complicated cases to obstetricians, and with the elimination of the financial and professional threat posed by midwives, obstetricians could increase their caseload and therefore the clinical material available to train better future physicians.

Obstetricians' discussion of the "midwife problem" coincided with demands by lay women for better obstetrics. A significant decrease in immigration occurred in the 1920s, which lowered the number of ethnic midwives attending births in immigrant communities. A decreasing birthrate, with an accompanying emphasis on the now fewer deliveries, further compounded the issue. As a result, the use of midwives rapidly declined in the 1910s and 1920s. In Washington, D.C., midwives attended 50 percent of births in 1903, but only 15 percent in 1912; in New York

City, midwives delivered 30 percent of the babies in 1919, but only 12 percent in 1929.[36] Decrease in midwife use was part of a social trend, begun in northeastern cities and eventually spreading to the rest of the United States.

Even popular literature eventually enshrined the idea that obstetricians were a better choice over midwives. In *A Tree Grows in Brooklyn,* a popular novel about immigrants in the early twentieth century, Sissy has ten stillborn babies, all delivered with midwives. In her eleventh pregnancy, when her husband "insisted on the doctor and the hospital," "her mother and sisters were stunned. No Rommely woman had had a doctor at childbirth, ever. It didn't seem right. You called in a midwife, a neighbor woman, or your mother, and you got through the business secretively and behind closed doors and kept the men out. Babies were women's business. As for hospitals, everyone knew you went there only to die." But Sissy stands her ground, insisting that her mother and sisters "were way behind the times; that midwives were things of the past." When Sissy pushes out her eleventh baby at the hospital, "she closed her eyes tightly [because] [s]he was afraid to look at it." Once again, Sissy fears that her child has died because the baby is blue and does not move. In anger, she questions God: "'Oh, God, why couldn't You let me have one? Just one out of the eleven? . . . Oh, God, why have You put Your curse on me?'" But then she watched her obstetrician use his magic—the latest science—to make the baby come to life. He gave the baby oxygen, and Aunt Sissy "saw the dead blue change to living white. . . . For the first time she heard the cry of a child she had borne." She names her baby boy after the obstetrician who saved his life.[37]

Despite the fact that Betty Smith's fictional character Sissy reflected a growing trend among women to turn away from midwives, and despite obstetricians' prejudices, midwives were only a small part of the problem. Many factors contributed to high rates of morbidity and mortality for mothers and babies. First, midwives, general practitioners, and obstetricians all needed better training. As medical education reformer Abraham Flexner explained in his famous report (later known as the Flexner Report) for the Carnegie Foundation in 1910, most medical schools had extraordinarily low standards or even no standards at all. They did not require their students to have a college, or for that matter high school, education prior to admission, and they offered little in the way of laboratory or clinical instruction. Flexner also warned that training in obstetrics was particularly abysmal.[38] Second, as noted earlier, physicians intervened too quickly and too frequently in the birthing process—often with disastrous results. Third, hospitals contributed to rising rates of infection for new mothers.

Finally, lack of prenatal care contributed to poor outcomes.[39]

Although public-health officials, social workers, and some pediatricians agreed with obstetricians that midwives provided poor obstetrical care, many argued that eliminating midwifery would not solve the problem. These professionals claimed that general practitioners and obstetricians needed better training. But given that a cadre of adequately trained physicians would take years to produce, the complete abolition of midwifery would be impractical if not impossible. In addition, as director of the New York City Bureau of Child Hygiene S. Josephine Baker argued in the 1910s and 1920s, many immigrant and African-American women preferred traditional midwives and could not afford the care of a physician. The solution to the "midwife problem," then, was not to eliminate midwives but rather to train, license, and regulate them.[40]

Supporters of the regulated, trained midwife pointed to the successes of the few American cities and states with comprehensive training and regulatory programs for their midwives. New York City and New Jersey, for example, had sponsored lectures, conferences, and other educational programs for their midwives, and had experienced corresponding reductions in maternal and infant mortality rates. In 1911, for example, New York City opened the Bellevue Hospital School for Midwives, the first municipally sponsored American midwifery school, and one with much higher standards than nonacademic, for-profit proprietary schools. At first six months long, the course eventually expanded to eight months, with instruction by physicians and nurses in prenatal and postnatal care, procedures for normal labors and deliveries, feeding and care of infants, and the "housewifely duties" to be performed by the midwife. Mostly Italian, German, Polish, and Hungarian immigrants, students were required to witness or assist at least eighty deliveries, deliver at least twenty babies, and pass oral and written examinations, administered by a visiting obstetrician, at the end of the course. Maternal and infant mortality rates for births attended by Bellevue-trained midwives were dramatically lower than the rates for births in New York City as a whole.[41]

A few physicians, nurses, and public-health advocates believed that a special type of trained, regulated midwife could solve the "midwife problem." These participants in the midwife debate invented a new type of birth attendant, the nurse-midwife. The first call for American nurse-midwives came from two leading public-health nurses, Lillian Wald and Carolyn Conant van Blarcom, who issued a proposal for "the nursing profession to extend its usefulness by including training for practice in midwifery for normal cases" at the second annual meeting of the American

Association for the Study and Prevention of Infant Mortality in 1911. The proposal generated controversy and was tabled after three months of debate.[42] In her Russell Sage Foundation–funded study of midwives in the United States, fifteen European countries, and Australia, van Blarcom concluded that the United States was "the only civilized country" that did not train, license, and regulate its midwives sufficiently.[43] In particular, she compared the United States to Britain, finding that while most American states allowed midwives to practice without restriction or regulation, the British required midwifery education, registration, licensure, practice, and supervision—with excellent results.[44]

Around the same time Wald and van Blarcom made their proposal, Clara Noyes, another nursing leader and superintendent of the nursing school at Bellvue Hospital (the same hospital that had opened a school for midwives), argued publicly that public-health nurses should be educated as midwives because they would be better equipped to do their nursing jobs. Like van Blarcom, she looked to Britain, noting that the British nurse automatically received midwifery training as part of her general education, thus "enhanc[ing] her value to the community and increas[ing] her prestige." Noyes continued:

> Someone has suggested that she [the nurse trained as a midwife] will encroach upon the territory of the obstetrician. Not at all, her superior training will enable her to distinguish abnormalities and serious symptoms far more quickly than does the partially trained midwife. It has been proven in England that far more calls are made upon the physician and greater discrimination shown in the selection of physician since the nurses have practiced midwifery than ever before, while the number referred to maternity hospitals and wards has increased very markedly.[45]

Noyes argued that the nurse with "advanced obstetrical training" could solve the American "midwife problem." She explained, "If the midwife can gradually be replaced by the nurse who has, upon her general training super-imposed a course in practical midwifery, which has been clearly defined by obstetricians, it would seem a logical economic solution to the problem. . . . We should be able to provide better teaching, better nursing and eventually better medical assistance to the less highly favored classes."[46]

While public-health nurses like Noyes called for nurses trained in midwifery, the term "nurse-midwife" was first introduced into the American vocabulary in 1914 by a St. Louis physician, Frederick J. Taussig, in a paper presented to the National Organization for Public Health Nursing. He suggested that the nurse-midwife could be a qualified nurse with obstetrical training who would attend normal births. Taussig argued that "the nurse-midwife will . . . prove to be the most sympathetic, the most economical, and the most efficient agent in the case of normal confinements."[47] According to these proponents of the trained, regulated midwife, nurse-midwifery would resolve the problem of ignorant, unsupervised, unlicensed, and untrained midwives.

Although American public-health nurses and physicians introduced the idea of the nurse-midwife in the 1910s, no attempts to put nurse-midwifery into practice were made until 1923. During that year, obstetrician Ralph Lobenstine at the Maternity Center Association (MCA) in New York City made one attempt, but it was derailed after the city's Commissioner of Welfare, along with many leading obstetricians and nurses, refused to lend their support.[48] Two years later, a New York City hospital specializing in maternity care, the Manhattan Maternity and Dispensary, managed to open successfully the Manhattan Midwifery School, the nation's first school to educate graduate nurses in midwifery. This school existed for six years and graduated at least eighteen students before closing due to a lack of patients to accommodate the training of both nurse-midwifery and medical students. Very little is known about this pioneering school.[49]

In 1931, the year the Manhattan Midwifery School closed and nine years after MCA's first attempt to establish a school, MCA finally began its program—the nation's second—to educate nurse-midwives. Students came to the school as registered nurses and graduated as nurse-midwives ten months later, after receiving instruction and clinical experience in midwifery. Public-health nurse Mary Breckinridge made a third attempt to begin the practice of nurse-midwifery in the United States, modeling her proposal on midwifery in Britain, where she had received training in both nursing and midwifery. With support from obstetricians, nurses, and social reformers, Breckinridge opened the first American nurse-midwifery service, Frontier Nursing Service (FNS), in the Appalachian mountains of eastern Kentucky in 1925.

In many ways, FNS and MCA faced different challenges. FNS was located in an isolated, rural area where few physicians wanted to practice, and served white, native-born, Appalachian patients, while MCA was located in the largest urban center in America and therefore had the advantages and disadvantages of proximity to physicians. While FNS cared for native-born women, MCA served African-American and Puerto Rican immigrant patients—patients on the margins of American society. (Actually, both sets of patients were on the margins of society, but Breckinridge claimed that unlike people from racial and ethnic minorities, FNS patients were the "worthy poor" who deserved help.) However, leaders at both FNS and MCA faced one similar roadblock: antagonism, and their anticipation of antagonism, by the medical establishment. Thus, both institutions conceived of the profession as one in which nurse-midwives would attend only women who were not otherwise served by physicians. The role of nurse-midwives was, in other words, limited from the very beginning.

## Lessons from Western Europe

The nurse-midwife's role did not have to be so limited. In Western Europe, well-educated midwives, including nurse-midwives, played greater roles and produced excellent results. Today, the international comparison is useful for American historians, health professionals, and public-policy makers trying to understand how and why American nurse-midwifery developed in such a circumscribed role.

In the early twentieth century, all Western nations saw childbirth, maternal and infant mortality, and midwives as key issues of concern. The general trend in Western childbirth was medicalization, but the move from home to hospital, and from midwives and general practitioners to obstetricians, occurred at different rates in different places.[50] In the United States in the 1930s, the debate over the midwife's place in childbirth seemed to be over. The American medical establishment had severely curtailed the midwife's role; middle-class women increasingly sought out physicians and especially obstetricians—and where middle-class women went, lower-class women followed; and the new nurse-midwife only practiced in a few areas. However, in this same decade, most other Western nations assumed that midwives would continue to have an important place in childbirth. These nations focused on expanding the midwife's education and redefining her responsibilities.[51] Thus, while Europeans regulated midwives, Americans tried to eliminate them. European physicians were less defensive about their professional status than American doctors and therefore had less need to push other health practitioners to the margins. European governments had long regulated physicians' education, and this education was generally superior to that of American physicians.[52] European physicians did not need to try to eliminate midwives, pharmacists, and other perceived competition to strengthen their position. In addition, almost all of the European nations were far more successful than the United States in decreasing maternal mortality. While the United States had high rates of maternal mortality, the Netherlands and the Scandinavian countries, for example, had low rates, with the much-praised Britain in the middle.[53]

In terms of midwifery, the Netherlands was, and still is, at the opposite end of the spectrum from the United States; the Dutch have held trained midwives in high esteem for a long time. The Dutch government began regulating midwives in the early nineteenth century, although training for midwives dated back to the late seventeenth century. Since the Medical Act of 1865, Dutch midwives have been able to practice independently with normal cases of pregnancy and childbirth. Early twentieth-century Dutch midwifery schools were very competitive, offering a three-year course, in which students witnessed on average 1800 deliveries and attended home deliveries under supervision during their third year. After deliveries, Dutch midwives turned postpartum nursing duties over to trained nursing assistants. These midwives enjoyed a status somewhere in-between nurses and physicians. Today, the Netherlands is known for the independence of its midwives (who attended 33.9 percent of all births in 2000, and approximately half of all births when counting those completed in cooperation with a gynecologist) and its high percentage of home births (30.3 percent of all births in 2000). These midwives operate within a health-care system that guarantees health insurance to all of its citizens.[54]

Scandinavian countries provide more examples of well-trained, well-regarded midwives in the early twentieth century—and today.[55] Renowned New York obstetrician and advocate of nurse-midwifery George W. Kosmak argued in 1927 that Americans could learn from the good work of Scandinavian midwives, after meeting some on a trip with the American Gynecological Club. "In the[ir] training schools for midwives," he found "bright, healthy looking, intelligent young women of the type from whom our best class of trained nurses would be recruited in this country, . . . whose profession is recognized by medical men as an important factor in the art of obstetrics, with which they have no quarrel."[56] Scandinavian midwifery schools provided their students with extensive, thorough training, and the results, Kosmak said, "are evidently excellent because the mortality rates of these countries are remarkably low and likewise the morbidity following childbirth."[57] Scandinavian countries' strong public-health systems also contributed and continue to contribute to their low maternal and infant mortality rates—and to their long history of a desire to create an excellent cadre of midwives to serve all classes of women.

The Danish model provides an interesting example of this phenomenon. In Denmark, trained midwives had existed since the early 1700s, when the government passed a law decreeing that midwives receive instruction from a physician, do an apprenticeship with an experienced midwife, and pass an examination from a Board of Midwifery. Despite the legislation, midwives, who attended most Danish births, did not enjoy high status. In the late nineteenth and early twentieth centuries, Danish physicians and midwives initiated a campaign to modernize the midwife—in other words, to make her use antiseptic procedures to prevent puerperal fever. They raised the status of the midwife by improving wages, encouraging a better class of women to apply to midwifery schools, extending the length of study, creating a more challenging curriculum, and pushing midwives to trade folk healing for science. By the early 1900s, the Danish midwife was well educated and highly regarded. By 1914, in a midwifery act, the medical establishment went on record saying that physicians did not want to attend normal births. Through the 1920s, midwives attended the births of women from all classes. In the 1930s, when women's demand for analgesics increased physician attendance at normal births, midwives and physicians jointly attended many births. For decades thereafter, the two types of health-care practitioners came together into the laboring woman's home, where the midwife generally guided the birth while the physician sat off to the side and intervened only if necessary.[58] Today Danish midwives attend nearly all normal births.[59]

In Sweden, the government and medical profession had controlled the training and regulation of midwives since the seventeenth century. By the early twentieth century, Swedish midwives received two years of instruction, delivered 100 to 125 babies under supervision, and worked for a month on probation before receiving final approval to become midwives. Once trained, they had a great deal of autonomy, as well as the ability to use instruments if physicians were not available.[60] Swedish midwives today provide 80 percent of prenatal care, attend all normal births in public hospitals, and manage labors but not deliveries in private hospitals.[61]

While the efficacy of Scandinavian models was widely admired, early-twentieth-century American public-health leaders frequently cited and praised British midwifery. American nurses van Blarcom, Noyes, and Breckinridge, as well as Mary Beard, another public-health nursing leader, all looked to Britain for a model. In Britain, unlike in the previously mentioned countries, midwifery became a part of nursing. In 1924, the Rockefeller

Foundation invited Beard to study "maternity care in England, with special reference to the relations of midwifery to nursing."[62] Based on this study, Beard promoted the nurse-midwife as the answer to the nation's "midwife problem," and eventually convinced the Rockefeller Foundation to provide money for tuition and living expenses for twelve of the first twenty-five nurse-midwifery students at the MCA Lobenstine Midwifery School.[63]

In fact, although early-twentieth-century British midwives held higher status and encountered less opposition from physicians than their American counterparts, Britain lagged behind continental Europe in the training, regulation, and, therefore, status of its midwives. Unlike its continental neighbors, the British government was less involved in public health care. Additionally, because the British were more devoted to the principle of laissez faire, they were less likely to support professional regulation. As a result, British obstetrics was less prestigious, and general practitioners and obstetricians feared competition from midwives.

The Midwives Act of 1902 changed the situation of the British midwife. That act created the Central Midwives Board, which examined and supervised midwives and established a roll of midwives. While the act prohibited practice by uncertified midwives, it continued, for practical reasons, to certify untrained midwives (called "bona fides" because they were certified "by virtue of bona fide practice"), although their numbers declined steeply after the passage of the act. For the new kind of midwives who took and passed an examination from the Central Midwives Board, the act required three months of training; later this was lengthened to two years, and, eventually, as developers of the act had hoped, most certified midwives were also trained nurses. The board required midwives to call physicians in difficult, dangerous cases.

In another important piece of legislation, the Midwives Act of 1936, British midwives received more status and recognition. This new act required local health authorities to provide a salaried midwife service to meet the needs of local communities, mandated that certified midwives be provided free or at reduced cost, and said that certified midwives would be employed as maternity nurses in situations when general practitioners directed deliveries. Developers of the act specifically wanted to raise midwifery's status, and many would say they succeeded. By the 1930s, British midwives attended approximately 60 percent of births, compared with 50 percent in 1909.[64] In Britain today, midwives attend 70 to 80 percent of normal births.[65]

Just as Americans created a circumscribed role for their nurse-midwives, Europeans encouraged the creation of a large group of well-trained, well-regulated midwives, offered—and in some cases guaranteed—maternal health care to their citizens, and had relatively low maternal mortality rates. The United States had none of this. Instead it had a weak, fragmented public-health system, a lack of commitment to providing health care for all of its citizens, physicians engaged in turf wars, traditional midwives dying out, and a small group of nurse-midwives providing care for a few poor women outside the purview of most Americans.

## Independent Women

Although American nurse-midwives were intended to serve as a stopgap only until physicians could attend the births of all women, the women who became nurse-midwives saw an opportunity in this new occupational sector. Nurse-midwifery gave its practitioners a power that many of their contemporaries did not have. These women controlled only a small space—and even then they never had full control over it—but still the women who became nurse-midwives enjoyed a kind of independence and power unusual for their era.

This new occupation came at an opportune moment; increasing numbers of women from educated backgrounds were choosing to enter the workforce in the 1920s. This era saw the full-blown emergence of what came to be known as the "New Woman." No longer content to be bound to the home, the "New Woman" spoke her mind, joined organizations, and worked in the public eye as a secretary, salesclerk, teacher, librarian, social worker, or nurse. Many of these women became involved in government programs and social reform efforts directed toward women and children (such as the U.S. Children's Bureau and the Sheppard-Towner Act).

Even when they remained within the home, so-called modern women professionalized homemaking and motherhood. This period also witnessed the development of both "scientific motherhood," the belief that women needed expert advice to raise their children in a healthy way, and maternalism, the argument that women's unique capacity for motherhood united all women, regardless of race, religion, or class. Under this model, all women were responsible for caring for all children, and since mothers produced the state's citizens, they deserved the government's help.[66]

Nurse-midwifery was part of the larger trend of expanding job options for women and of increasing numbers of women working with needy women and children. But because of the isolated, marginalized nature of the profession, nurse-midwives had more autonomy than the salesclerk, secretary, teacher, or social worker. In addition, although nurse-midwifery was a female occupation like the others, it remained an odd choice for a woman to make in the 1920s or 1930s, and even later. In those early years, becoming a nurse-midwife generally meant leaving one's family for one's job. Nurse-midwifery then was akin to joining the Peace Corps today, offering excitement, adventure, and independence to the idealistic and dedicated.

It is unlikely that the women who chose nurse-midwifery in the 1920s and 1930s would have opted for medicine instead. The medical profession at that time was changing and contracting, and women physicians, in particular, declined in numbers. Several factors discouraged women from applying to medical school. In the wake of the Flexner Report, many medical schools, including nearly all women's medical schools, closed, and the remaining schools required more time and money of their students than they had previously. This era also saw the decline of the general practitioner and the ascent of the hospital-based specialist who spent less time on direct patient care. While some women physicians pursued careers as specialists, many remained committed to more traditional ideals of what historian Ellen S. More calls "medical benevolence." Further compounding this was the fact that women in hospital medicine often faced discrimination.[67] While medicine offered fewer opportunities for women, nurse-midwifery gave women a chance to pursue a relatively autonomous profession with the safety of a more traditionally female role involving nurturing and direct patient care.

Given the nature of the job, it is not surprising that many women who became nurse-midwives, both leaders and rank-and-file, were single and devoted their lives to the fields of maternal and child health.[68] Early leaders of Frontier Nursing Service and Maternity Center Association embodied these trends. FNS founder Mary Breckinridge dedicated her life to improving the health of women and children after the deaths of her own two young children and divorce from her husband.[69] MCA general director from 1923 to 1965, Hazel Corbin planned to become an Army nurse during World War I, and instead became involved with the precursor to MCA, beginning her lifelong commitment to maternal and infant care, public health, and nurse-midwifery.[70] Rose McNaught, who worked at FNS in the 1920s and then at MCA starting in 1931 as supervisor of the new Lobenstine Nurse-Midwifery Clinic and teacher at the new Lobenstine School, remembered making a conscious decision not to marry: "'I had no wonderful chances, but I could have married. . . .Yeah, I had a couple of chances, but I couldn't see it myself. I wanted to go around and see the world. . . . I saw a pretty good part of the world in my day and that's what I enjoyed. I couldn't be bothered to get married and [rear] children.'"[71]

Nurse-midwifery presented special potential conflicts for married women. Because so few nurse-midwifery schools existed, student nurse-midwives usually had to attend school far from home. Following graduation, many nurse-midwives moved to isolated regions, such as Indian reservations in the West or rural areas in the South, where they supervised traditional midwives or public-health nurses. These jobs were impossible for most married women.

Women who chose nurse-midwifery were able to make this choice for other reasons. Most were white and native-born (like most other kinds of nurses), many were from the middle and upper classes, and many were well educated, often receiving college degrees (usually in nursing) prior to entering nurse-midwifery school.[72] These women generally had familial and financial backing that allowed them to pursue their passion.

In the interwar years and even much later, many of these women took a missionary approach to their jobs. Although, as chapter 5 explains, missionary nuns founded one important nurse-midwifery service and school during World War II, most nurse-midwives were not necessarily missionaries per se.[73] They wanted to serve those in need, and devoted their lives, or a portion of their lives, to the cause of maternal and infant health. For these women, nurse-midwifery was not just a job; it was their mission. MCA reported that its graduates traversed the globe preaching the MCA way of maternal and infant health. In Iran, one MCA alumna worked to change beliefs that nurses and midwives did not need education. In Korea, another MCA graduate on a Presbyterian mission reported setting up a midwifery course for graduate nurses, and trying to raise obstetric nursing education to a higher level. In Mexico, an MCA-trained nurse-midwife tried to teach new mothers to abandon harmful superstitions, such as waiting forty days after the birth before washing their hands. These nurse-midwives believed in the "universal applicability of the [MCA] philosophy, methods, and attitudes."[74] Many FNS nurse-midwives also had a missionary zeal.[75] A former FNS nurse-midwife recalled that before the existence of such organizations as Peace Corps or VISTA, "FNS was one of the few places adventuresome young women could find creative, idealistic jobs other than with missionaries."[76]

Many women liked the challenge and adventure involved in nurse-midwifery. While the traditional image of the nurse centered on the white, starched uniform and an unwillingness to improvise, the public-health nurse and nurse-midwife was "rough and ready," making do whenever necessary. Helen Browne explained that the "challenge of the rural area" brought many women to FNS, located in the Appalachian Mountains. When FNS nurse-midwives switched from riding horseback to driving jeeps in the 1940s, Browne and other FNS staff feared the work might lose "its glamour," but found "it was still rural enough that it made a challenge."[77]

By the late 1930s and early 1940s, many of the women who attended nurse-midwifery school sought something beyond what their regular nursing education provided them. They had experience in maternity nursing, but wanted a different and fuller knowledge of the maternity cycle, as well as more autonomy and responsibility in caring for their patients. Although it is sometimes difficult to determine whether nurse-midwifery attracted women for these reasons or whether they liked these aspects of nurse-midwifery in hindsight, at least some women clearly went to nurse-midwifery school because of the possibilities for greater knowledge, responsibility, and independence. These women enjoyed taking responsibility for every aspect of pregnancy, labor and delivery, and postpartum care. They also wanted to be able to handle deliveries by themselves when necessary. According to a group of six MCA alumnae, nurse-midwifery school filled gaps in their maternity nursing education; these gaps had left them feeling unprepared to attend births without a physician, something they had all faced.[78]

The quality of independence, fostered by their nurse-midwifery education, was both an advantage and disadvantage for nurse-midwives struggling to gain recognition for their new profession. On the plus side, their independence helped them succeed in challenging jobs in places off the beaten path, geographically and/or medically. Also, the profession's independence provided them with something they wanted—authority over their daily work lives. But as independent nurses, midwives, and women, they ruffled the feathers of both physicians and nurses, who sought to keep them in their place. They upset the status quo of the American medical establishment—and of the larger culture. That is why, despite the great potential of nurse-midwives to transform American maternity care, they were forced into a limited role.

*Nurse-Midwifery* is the first book-length study to document the emergence of nurse-midwifery in the United States. By documenting the education, training, practice, and professional development of nurse-midwives, this book shows the professional tightrope that they and their nursing and medical allies walked because of the opposition of the medical and nursing establishments. It reveals the limitations that nurses, physicians, and nurse-midwives placed on the profession of nurse-midwifery at the outset because of the professional interests of nursing and medicine. My book argues that nurse-midwives challenged the "male medical model" of childbirth, but the cost of the compromises they made to survive was that nurse-midwifery did not become the kind of independent, autonomous profession it might have been.[79]

Several works on midwifery and women's health explore the creation of the nurse-midwife, but few sources have placed nurse-midwifery in a larger social and historical context and only Frontier Nursing Service has been analyzed in any detail.[80] In an excellent article on FNS, Nancy Schrom Dye analyzed the struggles Mary Breckinridge faced as she tried to establish her pioneering organization, and Dye argued that despite the service's successes, nurse-midwifery was seen as irrelevant as "operative intervention, hospitalization, and universal medical management became the hallmarks of American birth management during the 1920s and 1930s."[81] My work on FNS builds upon Dye's by explaining in greater depth the nurse-midwives' approach to birth and health, the reactions of the local people, and the romantic imagery Breckinridge and her friends used to gain support for FNS. In addition, I contribute an original interpretation of FNS through a focus on eugenics, race, and nativism and by placing FNS in the broader context of other nurse-midwifery organizations.

This book also adds to a growing literature on the development of nursing and the complex roles women have played in the medical profession. Analyzing the history of women in medicine, Regina Morantz-Sanchez and Ellen S. More have shown that women physicians experienced many conflicts: between their commitment to "sympathy" and "science," between their interests in home, work, and community, and between their desires to advance their careers and the barriers they faced in educational and professional settings.[82] Unlike women physicians, nurse-midwives were in a female profession, and did not experience the same conflict between their professional values and their lives as women. However, like women physicians, they encountered barriers to advancement from a medical profession that simultaneously looked down on and was threatened by them. Morantz-Sanchez and More also explain that women physicians tried to resolve their multiple, and seemingly competing, interests by using holistic methods of care despite contemporary medical trends, and by entering specialties seen as feminine, such as obstetrics, gynecology, and pediatrics, as well as public health. Nurse-midwives, already in a feminine specialty, bucked nursing trends and emphasized the importance of looking at all aspects of their patients' lives—social, psychological, and physiological. Along with these other historians, my book argues that many women in the health professions have focused on looking at a patient as a whole person, rather than simply an individual diseased part.[83]

Susan M. Reverby and Barbara Melosh have shown that nurses historically have disagreed about what constituted "good" nursing, the education necessary to become a "good" nurse, and reasonable work conditions, arguing with one another as they faced "patriarchal constraints imposed from above by hospitals, physicians, and the broader culture."[84] I found that nurse-midwives, like nurses in general, faced both internal and external conflicts, even as they had more in common than nurses as a whole did. Other historians, like Darlene Clark Hine and Karen Buhler-Wilkerson, have examined specific groups of nurses.[85] Hine explored the issue of race and American nursing, showing how black nurses, denied access to all-white training schools, hospitals, and nursing organizations, fought to become trained nurses, even though their numbers were limited. In chapter 5, I augment Hine's work by analyzing the development of two schools of nurse-midwifery for African American women. While the number of African American nurse-midwives was very small (and thus my discussion of them short), their story is important and complicates our understanding of nurse-midwifery. Race and ethnicity are important themes in this book. Mary Breckinridge, founder of the Frontier Nursing Service, used her racism, and that of her potential supporters, to raise money for FNS, which served mostly white women and families. The other four early schools of nurse-midwifery (not counting the Manhattan Midwifery School about which little is known) trained nurses to supervise and ultimately replace traditional African American and Latina midwives; these nurse-midwives had varying degrees of sensitivity to the women with whom they worked and their traditions.

Buhler-Wilkerson demonstrates that public-health nurses had a central place in the American health-care system at the turn of the twentieth century, but that this role diminished in the 1920s as infectious disease declined and as more patients sought hospital, rather than home-based care. My book expands our understanding of public-health nursing by studying one group of public-health nurses (since nurse-midwifery began within the context of public-health nursing). And a major goal of this book, like Buhler-Wilkerson's, is to analyze "why a movement that might have become a significant vehicle for delivering comprehensive health care [or in nurse-midwives' case, maternal health care] to the American public failed to reach its potential."[86] As I indicated earlier, the United States was unique; while professional midwives in many other countries played a central role in twentieth-century maternal health care, they did not do so in the United States. This book examines and explains how that happened.

This book is organized both chronologically and topically. Part I, "Early Labor Pains, 1925–1940," explores the creation and development of America's first long-standing nurse-midwifery services and schools, Frontier Nursing Service in eastern Kentucky and Maternity Center Association in Harlem, as well as the compromises these organizations had to make to avoid criticism and craft a place for nurse-midwives. Chapter 2 focuses on FNS, where Mary Breckinridge carefully constructed her nurse-midwives as exotic frontierswomen, riding horses to save native-born white babies in the Appalachian Mountains. She used the then-popular language of eugenics to gain acceptance and funding for her radical-seeming nurse-midwifery service. Chapter 3 focuses on MCA, whose leaders slowly convinced New York City's physicians that nurse-midwives were not their competitors. MCA nurse-midwives received more supervision from physicians than their FNS counterparts did, and they worked with a minority clientele whom physicians had no interest in serving. Chapters 2 and 3 also analyze FNS and MCA nurse-midwives' approach to birth, and conclude that they offered their patients something different from many obstetricians, general practitioners, and traditional midwives. They attended their patients at home, providing frequent prenatal care, good care in labor and delivery, with few unnecessary interventions, and close contact with mothers and newborns after birth. In spite of serving low-income people, many of whom had poor nutrition and housing, early nurse-midwives lost astoundingly few mothers at a time when maternal mortality was high.

Part II, "Active Labor, 1940–1960," analyzes nurse-midwifery as it expanded in new directions and faced new challenges as the fledgling profession sought to become more mainstream. Chapter 4 explains that many nurse-midwives began working in hospitals because that was where the majority of births were taking place. Some established nurse-midwifery services at major medical centers like Columbia, Johns Hopkins, Yale, and Downstate Medical Center, State University of New York; nurse-midwives at these elite institutions provided prenatal and postnatal care, managed labor and delivery, and took part in demonstrations of the new "natural childbirth" method. Most nurse-midwives, however, were unable to find work in their profession, so they served as more subordinate maternity nurses and maternity nursing supervisors in hospitals. When compared with counterparts who attended home births, hospital nurse-midwives were not on the margins. But they lost autonomy as they became part of the male-dominated, physician-dominated hospital hierarchy. Chapter 5 follows the nurse-midwives who continued to attend home births in the World War II and post-war era, with a focus on Santa Fe's Catholic Maternity Institute. In an age of increasing hospitalization and medical technology, these nurse-midwives bucked the national birthing trends more than ever. They show that medicalization of childbirth did not go unchallenged. Chapter 6 discusses nurse-midwives' arguments among themselves over how to deal with misunderstandings about and intense opposition to their work. Ultimately, they chose to accommodate physicians. This strategic choice made sense given the way nurse-midwifery developed and the opposition that its practitioners faced. Nonetheless, accommodation created limitations on individual careers as well as setting up unintended roadblocks for the future of nurse-midwifery as a profession.

The epilogue brings nurse-midwifery up to the present. Since the 1970s, the profession has grown significantly under the influence of the women's health and consumer movements and sky-rocketing health-care costs. But today the profession still is both misunderstood and ignored; nurse-midwives continue to face opposition from some physicians and hospital administrators, and they continue to be underutilized. The book ends by explaining the strengths that nurse-midwives have as they labor to improve the health care of American women and babies, and the barriers they face as they try to do so.

# PART I

# Early Labor Pains, 1925–1940

# CHAPTER 2

# Eastern Kentucky's Frontier Nursing Service

## Mary Breckinridge's Mission, Survival Strategies, and Race

### Introduction

Born in 1899 in Oxfordshire, England, Betty Lester worked as a nurse and then completed her midwifery training at the York Road General Lying-In Hospital in London.[1] One of her classmates at York Road was Alice Logan, an American nurse who told stories about an idyllic place back in the United States where she planned to return to practice midwifery. According to Logan, this place offered midwives a wonderful life, with horses, dogs, beautiful mountains, and frontier living. Lured by her classmate's tales, Lester applied to work at Frontier Nursing Service (FNS). Her parents were dead, she was single, she had no particular ties to England, and she loved the idea of riding a horse through the mountains to attend births (especially as she had ridden horses throughout her girlhood). "I want[ed] to go so badly," she remembered thinking. "All I thought about was having a horse and a dog."

But her British instructors told her that she could not go unless she did a six-month postgraduate course in midwifery so that she could be of more use to her new employer. Finally, after completing her postgraduate work, Lester made the eight-day voyage to America, arriving on the Fourth of July, 1928. She landed in New York City, took an overnight train to Lexington, Kentucky, and then another overnight train to Krypton in the Appalachian Mountains. Next, she rode a horse for seventeen miles to the tiny town of

Hyden, home to FNS. Shortly after her exhausting trip, Lester was given midwifery license number thirteen, becoming the thirteenth nurse-midwife in the United States. Except for a brief return to Britain to serve her country as a nurse during World War II, she lived the rest of her life in Hyden. She served FNS in many capacities: as a district nurse-midwife, field supervisor, superintendent of the hospital, director of social services, and even as the star of the 1927 silent film about FNS, *The Forgotten Frontier*. Lester officially retired from FNS in 1971 at age seventy. However, she continued to work for the service as a speaker, tour guide, and member of the Mary Breckinridge Hospital Auxiliary until her death in 1988.

Betty Lester and her FNS colleagues were the first practitioners of nurse-midwifery at the first nurse-midwifery service in the United States. Mary Breckinridge (1881–1965), an American public-health nurse with British training in midwifery, established FNS in 1925 in the Appalachian Mountains of eastern Kentucky, a region with one of the highest maternal and infant mortality rates in the nation. The stated purpose of FNS was to protect the lives and health of mothers and children by providing trained nurse-midwives in a geographically isolated area without access to health professionals.[2] FNS nurse-midwives denounced the work of the local "granny" midwives as a way to promote their own professional status. They then gradually replaced "grannies" as the region's birth attendants. Breckinridge and her staff offered their Kentucky patients midwifery service, general medical care of families, and preventive medicine at low cost, and dramatically improved their health. Although some local people initially resisted the service's efforts, most eventually took advantage of at least some of its services. In 1939, FNS also opened the Frontier Graduate School of Midwifery to train registered nurses to work as nurse-midwives in remote rural regions. FNS still exists today, and its school, renamed the Frontier School of Midwifery and Family Nursing, continues to have a significant impact, training almost one-quarter of the nurse-midwives in the United States through a special community-based distance-education program.[3]

Breckinridge faced financial, professional, and image problems as she created and built up FNS. Her Appalachian patients could not afford to pay for health care, and her attempts to secure government funding failed. Because nurse-midwifery was new and different, it was believed to represent a potential threat to the medical establishment's ideas about birth and to their incomes. Finally, health professionals and the lay public often associated nurse-midwives with "granny" midwives, whom they saw as dirty, ignorant, and unprofessional. The names were similar, and many feared their approaches to maternity care might be similar too.

In response to both the constraints Breckinridge faced and her own biases, she carefully constructed FNS nurse-midwifery. She limited her work to rural Appalachia, a region off the beaten path of other health professionals. She raised money for FNS by tapping into contemporary racist views, claiming that her patients were the "finest old American stock"—that is, white, Anglo-Saxon Protestants—people with the "right" genes who needed some help in order to thrive. She also portrayed her horseback-riding, mountain-mother-serving nurse-midwives as mythical figures, rather than serious professionals who might threaten physicians or the American health-care status quo.

Given Breckinridge's tactics, myths about FNS were and remain persuasive. While FNS, unlike the other aspects of this book, has received some attention from historians, it has been the subject of even more attention in the popular and nursing press both because of the extensive public relations efforts by Breckinridge and her friends and because of its appeal from the beginning as an organization functioning in a place that seemed to be from another era. Building on the scholarship of Nancy Schrom Dye, Carol Crowe-Carraco, and others, my work analyzes in depth the service's unique approach to birth and health, offers a new focus on the reactions of eastern Kentuckians to the service that received so much attention from outsiders, and, most important, contributes a new interpretation of Breckinridge's cleverly crafted use of eugenics, nativist beliefs, and racism to gain support for FNS.[4]

## Mary Breckinridge's Mission

Mary Breckinridge was FNS. Although FNS could not have succeeded without the support of physicians, nurses, and donors, Breckinridge was both its sole creator and guiding light until her death in 1965. Thus, it is impossible to separate FNS ideology and history from Breckinridge. In many ways a typical Progressive (a supporter of a variety of reforms popular after the turn of the twentieth century), Breckinridge believed that the terrible health problems of rural mothers and babies could be solved. Using the latest social scientific techniques, she studied these problems (with the help of others), publicized them, and came up with a solution: use professionally trained nurse-midwives to provide health care and education for rural families. Tough, energetic, and single-minded in her focus, Breckinridge devoted half of her long life to FNS, inspiring others, especially

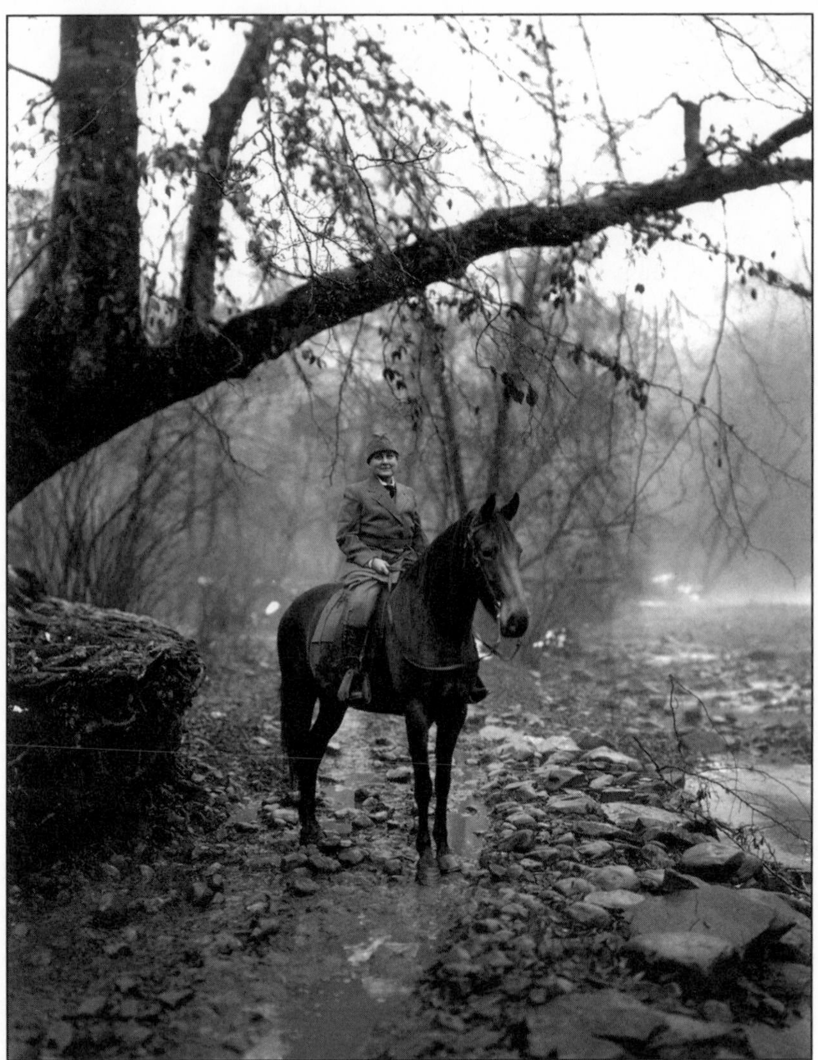

FIGURE 1. Frontier Nursing Service founder Mary Breckinridge on horseback. Courtesy of the Audio-Visual Archives, Special Collections and Archives, University of Kentucky Libraries.

women, to join her crusade against maternal and infant mortality and morbidity. Although part of a generation of single Progressive women who focused their energies on social reform causes, Breckinridge was also a nonconformist.

Despite her blue blood, she disdained many of the trappings of her class. Ignoring the fashions of the day, she always kept her straight hair short and plain, and she defied social convention by refusing to wear a hat. A short woman who was somewhat hunch-backed as a result of a horseback riding accident at age fifty, Breckinridge undoubtedly raised more than a few well-shaped eyebrows when she gave talks to the upper crust in New York, Cincinnati, and Detroit to raise support for her beloved FNS.[5] But if the upper crust found Breckinridge unconventional at fifty, they would have been shocked to have met her earlier in her career. When Breckinridge first came to eastern Kentucky, she openly and frequently swore, but she changed after her father repeatedly told her in his summer visits to Hyden that ladies did not use that kind of language.[6]

According to her staff, Breckinridge was a force to be reckoned with. Betty Lester described her as "commander-in-chief" and said that when Breckinridge came into the room, you felt like you had to stand. She was the "five-star" general of FNS.[7]

Breckinridge's background gave her the financial backing, connections, and motivation to head FNS. Born in 1881, she came from a distinguished southern family.[8] Her father was a congressman and ambassador to Russia, and her grandfather was vice president of the United States under James Buchanan.[9] Breckinridge married twice. Her first husband died young and her second marriage ended in divorce. She had two children with her second husband; her son "Breckie" died at age four and her daughter Polly died just six hours after birth. According to Breckinridge, the deaths of her children and her experiences in World War I prompted her lifelong commitment to improving the health of mothers and babies.[10]

Prior to developing FNS, Breckinridge, a registered nurse, worked for the U.S. Children's Bureau and in a post–World War I massive relief program for France. As director of Child Hygiene and District Nursing for the American Committee for Devastated France from 1919 to 1921, she coordinated food and medical relief for approximately seventy villages, and organized a visiting nursing service to provide general and maternity nursing. Her experiences first in France and then in London with British nurse-midwives prompted her to write in her autobiography: "After I had met British nurse-midwives . . . , it grew upon me that nurse-midwifery was the logical response to the needs of the young child in rural America."[11]

Breckinridge's experience in World War I also influenced her to compare motherhood with war, arguing that "maternity is the young woman's battlefield. It is more dangerous, more painful, more mutilating than war, and as inexorable as all the laws of God. . . . But for her there will be no drums beating or trumpets blaring."[12] In fact, she argued: "We have lost more women in childbirth in our history as a nation than men in battle."[13]

Breckinridge used the military comparison to justify her nurse-midwifery service to potential donors. Americans' lack of concern for maternal mortality as compared with wartime deaths also troubled Breckinridge on a personal level. In her private correspondence during World War II, she suggested that Americans seem to pay more attention to the suffering of war than the suffering of peace, including death in childbirth.[14]

On returning to the United States, Breckinridge took refresher courses in public-health nursing at Teachers College, Columbia University, from 1922 to 1923. She then began to make plans for a demonstration site in nurse-midwifery in eastern Kentucky. She chose this region because of her family connections in the area, her belief that rural mothers and children were in greater danger than those in urban areas, and her conviction that success in a region so remote and poor would prove nurse-midwifery could succeed anywhere. Her first step was to ride through the eastern Kentucky mountains to survey local midwives. She found these midwives providing inadequate care to their rural patients; most had no formal training and did not offer prenatal or postnatal care. A minority of midwives received instruction from nurses working under the State Board of Child Hygiene in conjunction with county health officers. Yet, even these midwives continued "unhygienic practices" unless they received instruction from physicians who made extra efforts to teach them.[15] Despite Breckinridge's perception of them, the midwives Breckinridge interviewed often proudly proclaimed they "never had to call a doctor yit," citing their own abilities and geographic distance as the main reasons for not involving physicians.

For Breckinridge, the local midwives served as both an inspiration and a marketing tool. Her 1923 survey, "Midwifery in the Kentucky Mountains: An Investigation," supported her argument that Leslie County desperately needed modern medical care. Breckinridge eventually used the survey to denounce the midwives in her publications and speeches, and to show outsiders why they should support nurse-midwives in eastern Kentucky. She always contrasted the old, "bad" ways of the "granny" midwives with the modern, "good" ways of trained nurse-midwives.

Breckinridge visited fifty-three local midwives from three counties in the Appalachian Mountains of Kentucky in summer 1923. She visited the midwives in their homes, and typed up notes after each interview. Her reports on Susan Stiddum and Nancy Brock were typical. Born in Leslie County, forty-five-year-old Susan Stiddum had practiced midwifery for sixteen years. Breckinridge found numerous problems with her. Stiddum's home and husband were not up to standard: "Dirty untidy rough plank house, with [her] children working, bringing up wood, and mother not at home. Found her several miles off, working in the field for Uncle Clavis Lewis, while her preacher husband sat in the shade nearby." According to Breckinridge, Stiddum had used bad judgment in raising her own children: "Raised 5 [and gave birth to eight] but oldest is now only 15 and has stopped school when only in 2d reader, to work, although mother says she has 'fainting fits' since her 'health come on her.'" Stiddum could not read or write, and she had become a midwife for "economic reasons." To Breckinridge, her obstetrical practices were abysmal: she "rubs her hands with castor oil or other grease for examination, and makes no other preparation [such as cleaning her hands]. In answer to all questions as to what she would do if the baby did not breathe, if mother had convulsions, etc., she made the one reply, 'aint never had none yit.' And she had not thought what she would do should any of these complications arise." Breckinridge concluded that Stiddum was a "dirty, untidy, poor drudge of a woman"—and obviously not fit to deliver babies.[16]

Breckinridge thought much more highly of another local midwife, Nancy Brock. Also born in Leslie County, fifty-year-old Brock had practiced midwifery for eight years because she was "called on by neighbors." According to Breckinridge, Brock had a "clean, neat" appearance, as well as a "clean and tidy," "extraordinarily picturesque old double log house, with big white oak tree behind it, and apple trees in front." With her farmer husband, she had had nine children, eight of whom lived. Breckinridge approved of Brock's connections to the formal health-care system in Leslie County. She had registered as a midwife six years prior to the interview on the advice of the registrar, and she carried a clean washable bag with birth records and drops of silver nitrate for her babies' eyes to prevent blindness in case the mothers had gonorrhea. Brock called a doctor when a mother in labor went into convulsions, showing her willingness to get help at least in some situations. She also "attended state conference at Beach Fork [instruction for midwives given by nurses from the State Bureau of Child Hygiene in conjunction with the county health officers] last year and appears to have profited by it to some extent." However, even this midwife had her problems. Despite Brock's contact with the health-care system, she admitted using some folk remedies, such as "pepper tea for chilling" the mother. Although she scrubbed her hands, Brock used no disinfectant on them. She also admitted that she had had some infant deaths due to prematurity, and her neighbors noted that she had had three stillbirths recently.[17]

After gathering information on Brock, Stiddum, and fifty-one other midwives, Breckinridge wrote her report. She found that the midwives did have a few good qualities; some had "native intelligence," even if they could not read or write. At least fifteen midwives and their homes were "exceptionally neat and clean," according to Breckinridge, although she described ten midwives and their homes as "filthy," with the rest in-between. As expected, Breckinridge found more bad than good. None had formal midwifery training; the little instruction they received had come from watching other midwives. Their obstetrical practices were poor. For example, very few carried equipment bags, and none provided postnatal care. When a mother started to hemorrhage, the midwives used "superstitious practices," such as giving teas or spices, "cording the leg," putting an ax under the bed, or reading a passage from the Bible. Worse, most midwives failed to recognize when they needed to call for medical assistance, and if they did, they called "pseudo-doctors," rather than licensed physicians. They also were generally unprepared for and unconcerned about complications. Breckinridge cited one example after another to show the disastrous results of their approach to birth. Although she claimed that she did not want to "'point the moral' of the data collected," ultimately she insisted that the story of these fifty-three midwives would continue to be a "problem" until a solution had been found and applied.[18]

While conducting her 1923 survey of local Kentucky midwives, Breckinridge asked her friend Dr. Ella Woodyard, from the Institute of Educational Research of Teachers College, Columbia University, to perform random intelligence testing of Appalachian children. Woodyard found the median intelligence quotient to be 99.5, somewhat higher than the national median. She concluded that while most Appalachian children possessed good native intelligence, very few lived in an environment conducive to stimulating these abilities.[19] Breckinridge would later use this data to show potential donors and supporters of FNS that eastern Kentuckians were worth helping, and would improve in the right atmosphere.[20]

## Roadblocks, Racial Myths, and Romantic Imagery

Despite Breckinridge's efforts to establish her potential patients' native abilities and their great need for improved maternal and infant care, her initial attempts to set up a nurse-midwifery demonstration site failed. The major roadblock she faced came in the form of the director of Kentucky's Bureau of Maternal and Child Health, Dr. Annie S. Veech, whom Breckenridge derisively called "Mr. Ready-to-Halt" in her private correspondence.[21] Veech refused to support Breckinridge's proposal for a nurse-midwifery service, thus preventing her from getting funds from the American Child Health Association (ACHA), which required state support, or from state agencies. In fall 1923, just after completing her midwifery survey, Breckinridge applied for money from the ACHA for what she titled the Children's Public Health Service, a five-year demonstration site in nurse-midwifery in eastern Kentucky. Her plan was to create a free health-care program, offered by public-health nurses with advanced education in midwifery, for children from the prenatal period through school age. In her proposal, Breckinridge promised the support of the few physicians from this remote region. She also argued that because the people of eastern Kentucky could not afford to pay for the majority of the program, it needed to be funded by government money, specifically through the recently passed Sheppard-Towner Act, which had allocated funding to improve maternal and child health. Although members of the ACHA liked Breckinridge's project, the organization, which was funded by the Commonwealth Fund (a private philanthropic organization dedicated to improving health care) needed state approval for the project before granting its support.[22]

But approval was not forthcoming from the project's state evaluator, Veech, who rejected the plan on several counts. First, she felt that Breckinridge was too independent, unwilling to take the advice that Veech and her staff offered. As Veech chided Breckinridge in personal correspondence regarding the matter, others were "willing to take absolutely our outlined policy for [child health] work in the state" whereas Breckinridge was not. Similarly, while others "have not come to us suggesting how we should do things, but knowing our experience here have come asking how they could help to do the things as we thought best," Breckinridge thought that she knew best.[23] Second, Veech believed the plan for a nurse-midwifery demonstration site was impractical.[24] She disagreed with the idea of nurse-midwives: "After all, a nurse-midwife is only a midwife. There appears to be a tendency among certain groups of nurses towards practicing medicine for which they are in no way prepared without graduating in medicine." Furthermore, Veech argued, a less costly solution to maternal and child health-care problems was to train "granny" midwives, rather than hiring nurse-midwives. Her comments suggested that she viewed "granny" midwives as more willing than nurse-midwives to submit to state control.[25] Finally, she found Breckinridge's report of her midwifery survey to be very disturbing. In fact, Veech refused to publish the report, telling Breckinridge that she was exploiting the people of Appalachia:

> Your suggestion that the report of your observations of the midwife condition in our mountains be published by us was very unexpected. I told you I would have it printed before I realized it was your intention to broadcast this report. It seems to me our distressing midwife problem is our own, and does not concern the great public. Our mountain people are hypersensitive—already they have been greatly exploited. . . . Broadcasting such a report as yours is like making public family skeletons or shouting one's sorrows on the housetops. I fear in your enthusiasm to be of service, you failed to get this viewpoint.[26]

Stopped in her tracks by Veech, Breckinridge was unable to pursue further the possibility of financial support from the ACHA or the state of Kentucky. A few years later, looking back at her run-in with Veech, Breckinridge maintained she was glad that FNS did not get Sheppard-Towner money:

> we would have been hampered with red tape at every turn, with no compensating financial assistance, and a position less strong as regards the nursing association, and the bureau of nursing. . . , and the medical profession, than we have at present with our direct contact with [Dr. Arthur] MacCormack [State health officer] independently of any bureau. . . . I am thoroughly in favor of Sheppard-Towner as a principle; but in our American tradition nothing ever yet *began* in a governmental way in new movements in health and education. Private initiative and voluntary aid is our tradition for the *creation* of all such work.[27]

In part, Breckinridge likely was rationalizing her rejection by Veech, but she also genuinely believed she was better off not having to deal with the bureaucratic roadblocks associated with government funding.[28]

Despite Veech's rejection of her plan, Breckinridge remained convinced that she should establish her program in eastern Kentucky. Before doing so, she went to Britain to learn more about its system of nurse-midwifery. She attended the British Hospital for Mothers and Babies in the Woolwich section of London from 1923 to 1924 to become a midwife, and was certified by the Central Midwives Board, a regulatory body established by parliament in 1902. Breckinridge took a four-month midwifery course, typical for British trained nurses who wanted certification. She and her fellow students served rotations at prenatal clinics, labor wards, mothers' wards, nurseries, and in the districts, and delivered, with supervision, a minimum of twenty normal childbirths. Breckinridge also benefited from delivery room and bedside teaching by physicians and nurses, as well as classroom lectures.[29] She then spent several months in Scotland studying the Highlands and Islands Medical and Nursing Service, an organization staffed by nurse-midwives to provide skilled health care to a poor rural population. As Breckinridge stated, "the system used by the Frontier Nursing Service is an adaptation of the methods used in the Highlands and Islands work." Located in an area similar geographically to eastern Kentucky, the Scottish service was decentralized, administered by local volunteer committees, and financed by private donations with the help of government grants.[30] Nearly prepared to begin her Kentucky project, Breckinridge returned to England, where she enrolled in postgraduate courses in midwifery at the Post Certificate School of the York Road General Lying-In Hospital in London in 1924.

Back from Britain, Breckinridge applied what she learned from her experiences there. Given her failed attempts to secure public funding, she created a private philanthropic organization, the Kentucky Committee for Mothers and Babies (renamed Frontier Nursing Service in 1928), to serve mothers and families in a 700-mile area extending into four southeastern Kentucky counties. Modeled after Highlands and Islands, FNS had three parts: 1) the hospital and nursing center in Hyden; 2) the administrative headquarters, nursing center, and Breckinridge's home five miles away in Wendover; and 3) by 1930, six outpost centers. Breckinridge believed strongly in a decentralized organization because of the difficulties of traveling through the rough Appalachian terrain. Additional benefits accrued to local families who were able to develop relationships with their district nurse-midwives and comment on center operations through a center citizens' committee. Local citizens also donated labor and money to help build the centers. Each outpost center, the gift of a wealthy benefactor from outside the mountains, housed two nurses responsible for the general health of all the families within their district. Districts covered an approximately five-mile radius around the outpost, meaning that nurse-midwives would never be farther than an hour's horseback ride to families in the area. First by horseback and later by jeep, FNS nurse-midwives traveled through the mountains offering prenatal, labor-and-delivery, and postnatal services for women, as well as general nursing care and public-health programs for men, women, and children.

Financing this new organization proved very difficult. Fees for FNS services were low compared with typical health-care providers. Until the late 1940s, FNS charged five dollars for complete midwifery care, including prenatal care, care during childbirth, and nursing visits for ten days

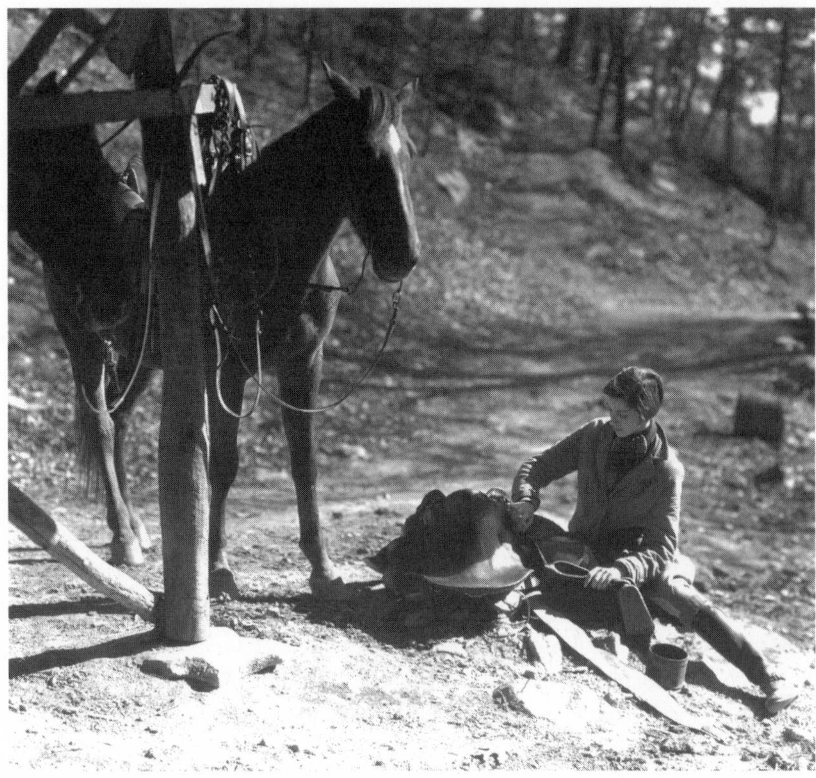

FIGURE 2. Betsy Parsons from Hartford, Connecticut, "Courier at Work," pictured on the cover of the Winter 1934 issue of *The Quarterly Bulletin of the Frontier Nursing Service, Inc.* Courtesy of the Audio-Visual Archives, Special Collections and Archives, University of Kentucky Libraries.

after the baby was born. The service charged each family one dollar a year for general nursing care, and never denied care based on lack of ability to pay.[31] Because patients often lacked cash, they sometimes paid with animal fodder, eggs, butter, corn, potatoes, chestnuts, apples, rhubarb, or honey. Sometimes, women paid by making quilts, and men by making chairs. At other times, fathers or sons worked at FNS, mending fences, chopping wood, and whitewashing barns to pay their families' bills.[32] These payments, whether in cash, work, or produce, covered only a fraction of the cost of the services. Yet the poverty of the patients meant they could not possibly meet these costs. In 1932, the average family income for residents of Leslie County, where FNS was located, was $416.50 per year, with only $183.53 of that in cash, or $36.70 in cash annually for each person in an average family of five.[33] In 2006 dollars, that translates into an average family income of $5,947.86 per year, with only $2,620.92 of that in cash.[34]

Because FNS lacked money from both patients' fees and government funding, it needed private contributions and marketing. To provide FNS with both, Breckinridge, who was extraordinarily savvy in marketing and public relations, created a system of mixed-gender volunteer committees in the Northeast and Midwest to form the backbone of FNS financial support.[35] FNS committee members were among the most prominent and wealthy in their cities (in other words, the opposite of FNS patients), and they came from a wide range of political and social perspectives. At various times, the committees included Eleanor Roosevelt; Sophonisba P. Breckinridge, Mary's cousin and professor and founder of the University of Chicago's School of Social Service Administration; Joseph B. DeLee, a leading obstetrician; and Clara Ford, wife of conservative automobile magnate Henry Ford. Committee members donated money to open FNS outpost centers, and, in return, FNS named the centers after benefactors' relatives. Committee funds also financed FNS operations. In addition, Breckinridge set up a program for "couriers," young horse-riding debutantes who came to the Kentucky mountains for several months, or sometimes several years, to care for the nurse-midwives' horses and otherwise assist them. She used these couriers to advertise FNS to the blue bloods back home, whom she hoped would donate money to the service.[36] Many, if not most, couriers became members of FNS committees after their service in Appalachia, and maintained lifelong connections to FNS.

Anticipating criticism about nurse-midwives and knowing from experience that physicians such as Veech could injure her nurse-midwifery service, Breckinridge carefully designed both her service and its publicity. FNS deviated from increasingly popular views of childbirth as a medical process, yet these deviations did not turn away potential donors or alarm physicians, mostly because of the patients FNS served. Media materials created by FNS staff and volunteers helped the public see nurse-midwifery as anomalous—employed only by people on the margins. They emphasized not the unusual approach FNS took to birth and health, but the needs of its poor, white, Appalachian patients, thus shielding FNS from potential opposition and hostility from the medical establishment. However, the media coverage also prevented the public from taking the FNS approach or nurse-midwives seriously as potential birth attendants for the middle class or even for other poor people with some access to physicians. Although this careful crafting worked at the outset to garner support for and deflect negative reactions to the service, it would ultimately circumscribe the authority given to the nurse-midwives who worked for FNS.

From the beginning, Breckinridge and her staff, as well as FNS volunteers and friends, published articles touting their experiences with FNS, took hundreds of photographs, and produced several films of nurse-midwives in homes, on horseback, and in jeeps in Appalachian Kentucky.[37] Breckinridge spent at least twelve to fifteen weeks a year outside the mountains, speaking to FNS committees and using films, books, and magazine articles created by her staff, couriers, and friends to add to the FNS coffers.[38]

The words and images FNS supplied to journalists emphasized the class, culture, and race of FNS patients and the difficult circumstances in which nurse-midwives worked. These portraits perpetuated and extended myths about Appalachia in an attempt to prompt potential donors to give money, and to encourage volunteers, students, and nurse-midwives to join the FNS. Starting after the Civil War, novelists, missionaries, and journalists created a series of positive and negative images of Appalachian people and Appalachia, the place. They described the region as natural, undeveloped, and beautiful, separate from civilization and industrialization. They described the mountaineers as hillbillies, moonshiners, feuders, bushwhackers, and inbreeders—as quaint, primitive, and, yet of pure stock, as descendants of Anglo-Saxons. As William Goodell Frost, long-time president of eastern Kentucky's Berea College at the turn of the twentieth century, explained, Appalachia was a remnant of eighteenth-century civilization, "a contemporary survival of that pioneer life which has been such a striking feature of American history," while the mountaineers were "our contemporary ancestors," descended from Revolutionary War heroes.[39]

Two forces in the 1920s made Americans receptive to the romanticization of Appalachia. First, the 1920s saw a resurgence of nativism and racism, resulting in large part from the influx of a "new" kind of immigrant between 1880 and 1920 (many of whom were Southern and Eastern European), as well as from the nationalism accompanying the United States' entry into World War I and the Red Scare following the Bolshevik Revolution. Nativism and xenophobia helped create the severe immigration restrictions of the early to mid-1920s, Americanization campaigns, the founding of numerous nativist organizations, such as the National Patriotic Council, and the revival of the Ku Klux Klan.[40] For the upper-class women and men Breckinridge tried to reach, Appalachians were true Americans; saving Appalachians provided an opportunity to save the "old stock," even if they came from the wrong class (and even as that stock was under threat). Second, in the 1920s, timber buyers and coal speculators continued a tradition from the late nineteenth century of depleting Appalachia's natural resources, using mountaineers to do the logging and mining and then leaving Appalachian people with ruined land susceptible to the ravages of floods.[41] As upper-class outsiders exploited Appalachian land and people, they glorified the culture they were also helping displace. Like many other Appalachian social-service programs, schools, and institutes, FNS reflected its founder's upper- and middle-class "outsider" values, as well as a desire to preserve Appalachian culture.[42]

Articles and films produced by FNS romanticized its patients as mountaineers of this so-called true American heritage. In a typical article, a student of the Frontier Graduate School of Midwifery argued that her patients reminded her of a glorious past: "There was something excitingly different about these mountain people who seemed to have resisted the standardizing influence of modern communications systems, and clung to the customs and habits which were brought over and handed down to them by their British ancestors. One senses a curiously whole-hearted friendliness in their attitudes. Their mountain twang sounded delightfully strange to the ear of an 'outsider.'"[43] According to a former courier, Breckinridge did "a lot of research" to trace the Anglo-Saxon roots of eastern Kentuckians.[44] She, her staff, and friends sought to convince their audience that eastern Kentucky patients were the "worthy poor"—people whose lives could be improved, and who deserved the improvements.[45] In a 1928 article penned by Breckinridge, the caption under a photograph of an elderly woman with a child read: "A fine old grandmother. The people of this lonely mountain region are pure English stock."[46] FNS committee pamphlets explained that Appalachians were "people of old American stock," and that "nowhere is the stock truer to type."[47]

In fact, FNS public-relations materials made a point of explaining that unlike the immigrants and African Americans who seemed to be taking over urban areas, its clients were "just like you and me," only poor. Elizabeth Perkins made this point clearly when explaining the purpose of *The Trail of the Pioneer,* a film on FNS she codirected and which Breckinridge used in her lectures around the country:

> The one great thing for us all to remember is that we pure blooded Americans must stand solidly together, whether we come from the South or the North, for we Americans are the inheritors of this wonderful country, and we are very distinct from the foreign born element which is overpowering us in the great cities.

> It is with every desire to preserve the coming generation of Americans that we want to acquaint all America through the medium of pictures—with the knowledge of the uncontaminated race to be found in our mountain regions. It is with the hope that those whose lives lie in the maelstrom of cities may appreciate the quietness of the mountains, and send their own people such assistance as may help to continue for generations the best examples of sturdy, upright, God fearing Anglo Saxon race.[48]

Nativism prompted Perkins to make her film, and she hoped that "pure blooded Americans" would respond to her nativist appeal by giving money to FNS. FNS simultaneously portrayed the mountaineers as backward and excellent raw material; as different, but in a good way; and as "good old American stock handicapped only by geographical conditions."[49]

Even as they tried to appeal to eugenic beliefs, Breckinridge, Perkins, and other supporters of FNS were wrong about the heritage of FNS patients. Appalachian people predominantly were not Anglo-Saxon, but "Scotch-Irish," people whose ancestors originally came from Northern Ireland, the lowlands of Scotland, and northern England. In other words, the ancestors of FNS patients had lived in the British borderlands, just as they did in Appalachia. As residents of these marginalized regions, the "Scotch-Irish" had been considered suspect by the "true" English; this view persisted in America where English Americans regarded them as barbarian and non-English. Tellingly, at the time of the Revolutionary War, this "heroic stock" was viewed as marginal, and certainly not of "good" stock, as FNS claimed fewer than two hundred years later.[50]

FNS media materials also played on existing gender roles to romanticize Appalachians. Breckinridge and other writers on FNS viewed Appalachia as a remnant of a better past, when men were men and women were women. As Breckinridge explained, eastern Kentucky men feuded to keep their honor—just as "men of the intellectual ability of Hamilton, Jackson, and Clay" had done in a previous century—and practiced "the utmost chivalry for women."[51] In another article, Breckinridge argued that "in the country, the mother is the heart of the household in a way that has come to be old-fashioned in city life." While the man handled the timbering, plowing, and raising of crops, the woman tended the garden, dried the beans, turned raw produce into food, milked cows, fed chickens, and quilted covers for beds in an eighteenth-century–style household economy. Breckinridge claimed: "In all of this, she has the help of her children whose lives revolve around hers. In a country home, the mother is irreplaceable."[52]

The media produced by FNS seemed to long for a past when men and women held roles different from the ones found in the early to mid-twentieth century—a past they claimed to find in eastern Kentucky. However, other sources show Appalachian gender roles to be less distinct than FNS portrayed.[53] According to recent scholars, both contemporaries and academics have portrayed Appalachian women in simplistic, romantic ways, ignoring the nuanced realities of women's lives and relations between men and women.[54]

To gain support for the FNS cause, Breckinridge, her staff, and her friends emphasized the high birthrate of Appalachian women. They used racial stereotyping to perpetuate myths about eastern Kentucky in an era of great concern about high fertility rates among immigrants and African Americans and low fertility among native-born whites.[55] One of the more exaggerated examples of this emphasis on eastern Kentuckians' fertility can be found in a letter from actor, author, and humorist Will Rogers. Breckinridge encouraged Rogers to write to several New England newspapers supporting an FNS cruise to the West Indies. This was just one of many newspaper advertisements for local and national fundraisers and benefits for FNS. Rogers began his letter with the salutation, "Well if it aint Mary Breckinridge." He explained that as an actor he did not have the time to take a cruise. He continued: "The trip I want to make is right out in that virgin baby country of yours. I can talk to those people that are breeding these babies, but I never could understand a black Negro in Jamaica that spoke English better than Lady Astor [one of the cruise stops was Jamaica]. . . . So when I get some time off I am heading for this incubator country of yours. You can't beat old Kentucky for a breeding ground. It's the limestone in the soil, and the corn in the jug that does it."[56] Rogers clearly intended the letter to be funny, but his humor shows how Breckinridge and her supporters used racial arguments to solicit money for FNS.

Breckinridge and FNS used the mass media to romanticize not only the Kentucky mountaineers but also the mountains themselves and rural life in general. The media images FNS generated and supplied to the press had a sort of tension; on one hand, the place and people were wild and different; on the other hand, they were simple and reminiscent of a better time. By the 1920s, the majority of Americans lived in urban areas. Yet, Ernest Poole, an author who worked closely with Mary Breckinridge for an article about FNS in *Good Housekeeping,* quoted Breckinridge as saying, "fully eighty percent, I am told, of the men who direct our great corporations came from rural regions." She argued that "the vigor and youth of a nation are born again in its children, and most of all in the country districts," and therefore we must "help mothers to have their children well born."[57] Poole himself suggested that "nobody hurries in the hills. Life is quiet down there. You hear only soft halloos."[58] FNS created articles and supplied information to journalists portraying eastern Kentucky as a simple place that deserved attention because it produced so many fine citizens—and as a kind of exotic, foreign-seeming region, a place with "Swollen Rivers and Rocky Mountain Trails"—"The Last Frontier."[59] FNS writers figured the more exotic FNS seemed, the more likely it would attract potential donors.[60] They also appealed to a long-standing and persistent American myth—that the "real" America was in small towns and rural areas, where people continued to have good values.

Media shaped by FNS also glorified nurse-midwives as "Heroines on Horseback," emphasizing their role in saving mothers and babies in a region with few resources.[61] Just as the Model T was becoming more widely available in the United States, Breckinridge emphasized the horses nurse-midwives rode.[62] As she explained, Appalachia had "no railway, no highway, no automobiles, no physicians":

> All of our work is carried forward on horseback. . . . Each nurse saddles and feeds and grooms her own animal. . . . The riding is always difficult and dangerous. During the winter, when the cold spells come and the streams freeze over, the horses, shod with ice nails, slip and stumble and often crash through with bleeding hocks. Sometimes a way must be made for them out to the rapids, where one commonly finds the fords, by a chivalrous mountaineer with his axe. When the "tides" come the fords of the unbridged river are unpassable.[63]

Breckinridge praised the nurse-midwives—and the horses—who worked against the odds for "all-American" mothers and children. Her cousin, Mary Marvin Breckinridge (known as "Marvin"), who came to FNS as a courier in summer 1927 after graduating from Vassar College, made a silent film, *The Forgotten Frontier,* portraying the difficulties nurse-midwives and their patients faced. She opened with the question: "Do you know that America is still a frontier country for about fifteen million people with almost no medical, nursing, or dental care?" The film, with local actors portraying real events connected with FNS, showed nurse-midwives crossing swollen rivers, a woman giving birth with the assistance of an FNS nurse-midwife, one man shooting another and nurse-midwives dealing with the aftermath, and nurse-midwives inoculating a group of children.[64]

In addition to the lack of motorized transportation, the difficult topography, and a dearth of professional medical care, ignorant "granny" midwives were another difficulty that eastern Kentuckians faced, according to Breckinridge, her staff, and friends. Repeatedly, Breckinridge told potential donors that FNS brought modern health care to poor, deprived Appalachians, who suffered at the hands of these backward women. She used the information from her 1923 midwifery survey to gain support for FNS. Breckinridge's condemnation of local midwives was part of a strategy to contrast traditional midwives and the new nurse-midwives to foster the perception of nurse-midwives as modern professionals. This tactic helped Breckinridge to establish her service but created some problems for nurse-midwifery in the long term. No matter how hard nurse-midwives tried to portray themselves as modern, many people—both potential patients and health professionals—associated them with the traditional midwives whom Breckinridge and other nurse-midwives criticized.[65]

Breckinridge, her staff, couriers, and friends then used a variety of strategies to help FNS get off the ground and survive. They glorified and romanticized the people of eastern Kentucky, rural life, and nurse-midwives while condemning "grannies." They argued that FNS could uplift Appalachians, who deserved such efforts because of their presumed Anglo-Saxon heritage. But in the process, they indicated that the nurse-midwife only served people on the margins, and that the nurse-midwife did not engage in a modern profession, but in an exotic, romantic pastime. FNS certainly promoted the good works its own nurse-midwives performed, but did not attempt to encourage the general expansion of nurse-midwifery around the nation.

Despite the myths, FNS was a perfect solution to the health problems of Appalachians, providing excellent care and avoiding condemnation from physicians. Certainly, FNS could not have succeeded without medical support, both backing up the nurse-midwives and lending authority to the organization. Breckinridge formed a national medical advisory board, composed of some of the country's leading obstetricians, including George Kosmak, editor of the *American Journal of Obstetrics and Gynecology,* but the board did not have a regular influence on FNS work. Physicians who supported FNS realized that very few doctors worked in Leslie County, and no hospitals existed there until FNS opened one in 1928. As physicians knew from both a study by Johns Hopkins statistician Raymond Pearl and their own experiences, poor, rural areas lacked good medical care for two reasons: physicians could not make money in such places and they disliked being isolated from modern, technological medicine.[66] Thus, FNS medical advisors saw nurse-midwives as the best alternative to physician or hospital care and even suggested that nurse-midwives' presence encouraged a few qualified physicians to locate in Leslie County.[67] Some physicians may have lent support to the "nurses on horseback" because they believed nurse-midwives received proper obstetrical training and up-to-date medical supervision, while local general practitioners and midwives had little to no training in obstetrics.[68] Supporting FNS may have assuaged the guilt of some physicians, who were dedicated to improving maternal and infant care yet unwilling themselves to practice in poor, rural areas—or to encourage their students to do so. Finally, they also may have promoted the program because they endorsed the racial myths and romantic imagery surrounding FNS and its patients.

## The Local Perspective

What did eastern Kentuckians think of the way that Breckinridge and her colleagues portrayed them—and their land—in the media? The available evidence suggests that some people did not like it. Interestingly, these people were middle or upper class, and not FNS patients. They understood that Breckinridge and FNS staff needed to appeal to rich outsiders to raise money, but believed that the appeal could be made in a different way—one that depicted Appalachians more accurately. Mary Brewer, who came to Leslie County in 1939 as a social worker with the Works Progress Administration, wrote a book to correct erroneous images of her adopted home and its people:

> Mary Breckinridge . . . was the first one, I guess, that put the people in this area on the map by going out and soliciting aid, and naturally most of their material was slanted toward the poorer class of people. They didn't tell anything about the fine homes that were here. It was always the little shacks on the hillsides and people going without clothing and half-starved and barefoot. So that most people . . . outside of Kentucky, they got the wrong idea, and I . . . thought that ought to be corrected.[69]

An erudite Leslie County resident, M. C. Roark, wrote an angry letter to the editor of the county's newspaper in 1927 after it reprinted a *New York*

*Times* article about the Sophie Smith and Elizabeth Perkins film *The Trail of the Pioneer* about FNS discussed early in this chapter. Roark praised FNS, but indicated his frustration with its method of fundraising:

> We welcome, and will be glad to support any organized work in Leslie county, and hope to say nothing to lower their efforts and goal, and especially honor Mrs. Breckinridge for her work in our behalf.
>
> But we feel that we pay in the sacrifice of our honor when the support is agitated and purchased by the Miss Smith and Perkins plan. We don't like to see the worst possible conditions that can be described and exaggerated peddled upon as the fruits and products of Leslie county. It seems to me that any organization would find a higher plane upon which to raise funds than to come down to the wornout plan of exaggerating conditions.[70]

Clearly, some local people resented the picture FNS painted of them, but what did they think of FNS itself? Their feelings were mixed and varied. Some actively welcomed FNS, others actively disliked and rejected FNS, while many responses were in-between those two extremes. However, after some initial resistance and even hostility toward the service, most people came over time to like or at least accept FNS.

Breckinridge and her staff members' official writings proclaimed widespread acceptance of and cooperation with FNS. In her autobiography, Breckinridge wrote that as she rode through Leslie County trying to gain support for the new FNS, she found a crowd of mothers "begging for a nurse for their part of the county."[71] Nurse-midwife Betty Lester explained how wonderfully the local people came together to make "the clinic the neighbors built." All of the local men with whom she met agreed to donate timber to build a new outpost center. In fact, most donated more than the 200 feet for which she asked. Once the men built the clinic, local women cleaned the building, wallpapered the walls, and decorated two rooms for the grand opening.[72]

The statements of some Leslie County residents who were interviewed in the 1970s and 1980s support the notion that local people liked FNS. These interview subjects pointed to local respect and admiration for Breckinridge and her desire to improve area health care. Born in 1901, Frank Bowling was working for the Fordson Coal Company (a subsidiary of the Ford Motor Company) at the time he met Breckinridge in 1928. But he had heard wonderful things about her long before that meeting:

> Well, everything that I'd heard about her was . . . good. . . . Miss Breckinridge was well respected in this section of country. Everybody looked up to her. She come in here . . . and helped people when they couldn't help theirselves back yonder. . . . Everybody owed an awful lot to Miss Breckinridge.[73]

Hallie Maggard, a Hyden native who was interviewed in 1978 at age ninety, retained a clear picture of Breckinridge from when the FNS founder first arrived in the area. Maggard said that the local people "honored her. I mean they helped in every way they could. People was glad to have her. And they tried to help her in what she'd come here . . . to do. . . . She took care of mothers and babies. That was a great relief to people."[74]

However, there clearly was some resistance to FNS, at least during its first few years. Rumors of terrible things FNS nurse-midwives did to mothers and babies were common. FNS nurse-midwife Grace Reeder mentioned that early on the locals believed that nurse-midwives took their female patients' rectal temperatures because "they were fixing the little girls so that they could never have babies."[75] Other local people refused to use the service, or to help FNS in any way. Lester said that "at first people didn't want their children to have . . . these needles shoved into them. They thought it was cruel. They didn't see any sense in having a needle shoved into a child."[76] Some locals wondered about FNS motives. Ruth Huston, who first visited Hyden in 1924, stayed to work with a Presbyterian school, and became a member of the first local FNS committee, explained that the local people "weren't sure what she [Breckinridge] was there for. They got the idea that they were missionaries at first. They didn't understand what she was doing, although she had a meeting in the courthouse trying to explain it."[77]

Resistance seems to have been strongest during the earliest years of the service. Several oral histories indicated that once FNS had established itself and people learned to trust the nurse-midwives, even those who initially resisted FNS accepted at least some of the services it offered. For example, Lester explained that "after a time" the same people who resisted vaccinations "began to tell us when their typhoid shots, and this, that, and the next thing, were due."[78] And, according to Huston, eventually Leslie County residents understood Breckinridge's motives and accepted her: "They finally got onto the fact that it [FNS] was medical and that she wasn't a missionary."[79] Breckinridge and her staff ultimately gained the trust and support of many local people.

## The Depression and World War II: Financial Troubles and the Opening of a School

The Depression severely damaged FNS work. Cancellations of FNS subscriptions and a decline in donations caused staff reductions and nonpayment of staff for several years; as late as 1947, FNS owed back payments to its employees. During the early 1930s, the FNS Executive Committee debated closing some outpost centers, but decided to maintain them with reduced services.[80]

Financial decline during the Depression also hampered Breckinridge's goal to extend nurse-midwifery to other isolated areas of the United States. In 1930, the FNS St. Louis Committee, one of many volunteer committees designed to provide funding for FNS, requested that FNS survey certain Ozark Mountain counties to determine whether it should bring its services to these remote rural regions. In fall and winter that year, two FNS nurse-midwives and one FNS secretary spent two-and-one-half months surveying seven counties in northern Arkansas and southern Missouri. Despite an interest in expanding their services, FNS officers and trustees decided against going into the Ozarks because of a lack of funding.[81] Eastern Kentucky turned out to be the only place where Breckinridge established a demonstration site in nurse-midwifery.

World War II forced FNS to make changes as well. The first occurred when FNS began receiving some government money. After Breckinridge's 1923 attempt to gain government funding failed, Breckinridge did not try again until World War II, when FNS participated in the Emergency Maternal and Infant Care Program, whereby the government reimbursed FNS for its care of servicemen's wives. The second change entailed the creation of a nurse-midwifery school. Since nurse-midwives did not exist in the United States prior to FNS, the service had originally employed mostly British public-health nurses, like Betty Lester, who had also trained as midwives. Sometimes FNS sent American nurses to England and Scotland on scholarships to receive midwifery training. However, World War II terminated these options. Once again, Breckinridge created another survival strategy for FNS: the development of an educational program to maintain its staff. FNS probably would have closed if Breckinridge had not opened a new school for nurse-midwives, the Frontier Graduate School of Midwifery, in 1939.

FNS staff had made some earlier attempts at nurse-midwifery training. In 1932, FNS nurse-midwife Mary B. Willeford outlined a plan for a nurse-midwifery school in her dissertation, "Income and Health in Remote Rural Areas," at Teachers College, Columbia University. Willeford proposed a school that would train graduate nurses to meet the health-care needs of the rural poor.[82] In 1935, FNS provided midwifery training, as well as instruction in "our frontier technique in bedside nursing and public health," to two Native American nurses, at the request of the National Society of Colonial Dames of America in Pennsylvania; Colonial Dames in other parts of the country provided financial support for the nurses' year at FNS. (Colonial Dames were women of Breckinridge's class and ethnic background who could trace their ancestors back to the colonial era.) Upon completion of their training, the two nurses worked for the Bureau of Indian Affairs on reservations in Wyoming and Nevada.

In the mid-1930s, Breckinridge had wanted to open a nurse-midwifery school affiliated with the University of Kentucky, with the nurses completing most of their fieldwork at FNS. Although the president of the university supported the idea, Breckinridge's repeated attempts to find financing failed, thwarting the school's creation.[83] Originally, Breckinridge had thought FNS could obtain money under a clause in the new Social Security Act which sought to appropriate one million dollars for research into and care of maternity cases in rural areas. However, Congress struck out this clause when it passed the legislation, thus eliminating the possibility of federal funds for an FNS school. In addition, the Carnegie Foundation rejected the service's request for money to conduct studies of schools for midwives in northern Europe, which FNS had hoped would help in the development of plans for its own school.

In 1939, FNS opened the Frontier Graduate School of Midwifery, since by then Breckinridge felt she had no choice but to open her own school.[84] That year, many British nurse-midwives employed by FNS returned home to help Britain fight the war. The war also cut FNS off from British educational opportunities for American nurses who wanted training in midwifery. The Frontier Graduate School of Midwifery offered midwifery training to registered nurses, with the goal of meeting the service's personnel emergency and then supplying nurse-midwives to other agencies working in "frontier outpost areas." The school started by training two nurses at a time in a four month course, with each student receiving scholarship money. In 1940, the school expanded to training three students at a time, and extended the course to six months.[85] Early classes were small because FNS lacked the facilities and staff to teach more students. To meet its staffing crisis, FNS sent two graduate nurses to Maternity Center Association's Lobenstine School in New York City.[86]

Once the Frontier Graduate School met the service's staffing needs, FNS hoped to expand its mission to train nurse-midwives for work in other isolated rural areas, and "at last to respond to the calls so frequently made upon us to provide frontier nurses for American outposts from the Caribbean to Alaska and including the Indian reservations."[87] In 1941, the U.S. Children's Bureau asked FNS to expand its school to train more nurse-midwives, who would then return to their home states to work in maternal and infant health care. FNS complied, and later that year beginning with its fourth class in 1941, the school expanded to four students, funded by scholarships from the U.S. Children's Bureau, private donations, and churches, which helped sponsor missionary nurses.[88] Each student promised to work for FNS for two years after her training, receiving the regular salary paid to first- and second-year nurse-midwives.[89]

Modeled after British midwifery schools, the Frontier Graduate School of Midwifery offered something unique in the United States—instruction in theory combined with practical experience in rural midwifery. Students learned "to work with what they have," and to develop their judgment in observing problems affecting their patients' pregnancies and/or births, recognizing the abnormal, and applying necessary emergency measures until a physician arrived. Student nurse-midwives heard thirty lectures in midwifery from the medical director and took thirty classes with the instructor, a nurse-midwife with a master's degree in public health. Classes involved frequent discussions and tests. The medical director and instructor used a life-size mannequin in demonstrations and for practice as well as forty-seven preserved specimens to demonstrate fetal development and abnormalities. Students had access to a reference library with British and American midwifery textbooks.

Under supervision, FNS students provided prenatal, labor-and-delivery, and postnatal care in a variety of settings. They gave prenatal and postpartum care in patients' homes, in outpost nursing centers, at clinics held at the FNS hospital in Hyden, and to a lesser extent, at the hospital itself. They learned to conduct detailed prenatal examinations, including abdominal examinations, a test for albuminuria, blood pressure, vaginal smears and blood for the Kahn test to diagnose syphilis, measures for hemoglobin, and measures for blood coagulation time. Carrying out part of Willeford's original plan of teaching students broad issues in public health, the school instructed student nurse-midwives "how to supervise the diet of the low income rural group," including methods for eradicating intestinal parasites. Students handled both home and hospital deliveries, attending at least twenty women under the supervision of an instructor. In addition to their regular twenty deliveries, they had the option of assisting the medical director in abnormal deliveries. During the postpartum period, students provided bedside care to mothers and babies. Upon completing the course and fieldwork, FNS students took a final examination, with written, oral, and practical components, given by the Kentucky State Board of Health. When students passed the examination, they received diplomas from the Frontier Graduate School of Midwifery and certificates to practice midwifery in Kentucky, as well as the right, granted by the Kentucky State Board of Health, to use the letters C.M. (Certified Midwife) after their names.[90]

Grace Reeder was a member of one of the Frontier Graduate School's first classes and a typical student in those early years. Originally from Ohio, Reeder had graduated from the Columbia University School of Nursing, and then worked as a private duty nurse. After hearing Breckinridge speak about FNS in Cincinnati, she became "very intrigued," so she went first to FNS as a non-midwife nurse volunteer in the hospital, and then two years later worked as a paid staff member, chief of the hospital outpatient department. Approximately six months later, she entered the Frontier Graduate School of Midwifery. While a student, Reeder had the "responsibility of total care for . . . patients," and remembered getting to know them very well. She had no difficulty logging her twenty required deliveries, all but four of which took place in patients' homes. At the end of her course, Reeder remained at FNS as a district nurse-midwife for three years, after which she left for New York City to pursue her bachelor's degree and eventually her master's degree. Reeder repeatedly returned to FNS to relieve nurses in need of vacation, and she later returned to eastern Kentucky on a full-time basis to take over the outpatient department of the United Mine Workers Hospital in Harlan. Late in her life, she worked as a nurse in hospitals in central Kentucky and Appalachian Virginia. Reeder was so attached to FNS that she returned once again to the area when she retired.[91]

## Frontier Nursing Service's Approach to Birth and Health

### *Prenatal Care*

Grace Reeder, Betty Lester, and the many other women who dedicated themselves to FNS provided unusually comprehensive care to their low-

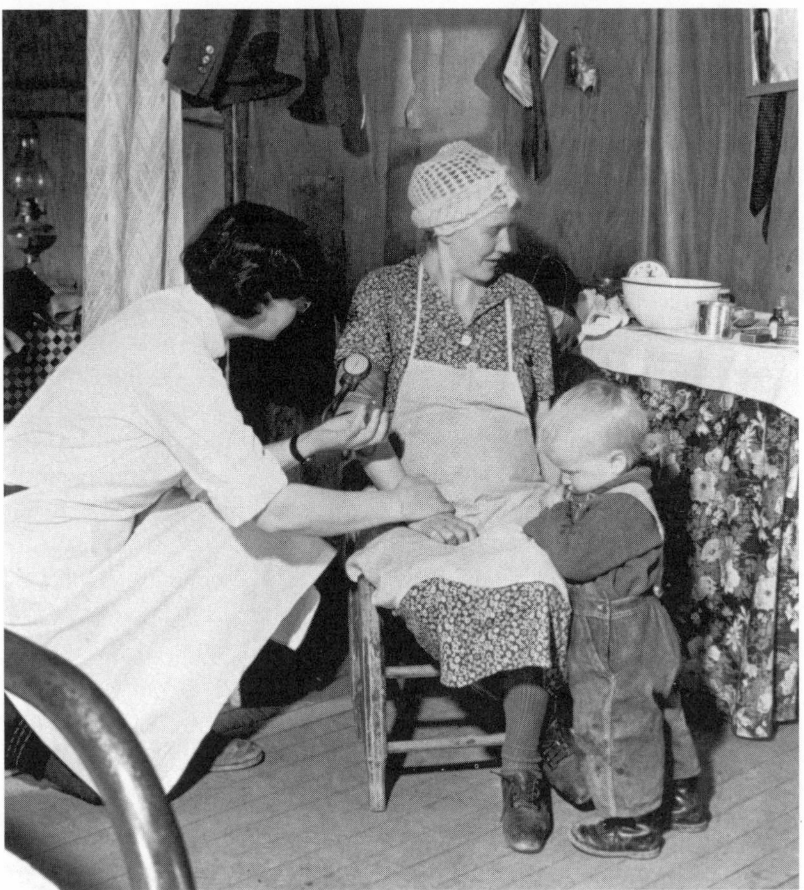

FIGURE 3. Shown in a 1937 article in *Life,* the caption above this photo read: "Prenatal visits during which the blood pressure is taken are part of the routine for the busy Kentucky Frontier Nurses. Note the primitive plainness of this Kentucky mountaineer's well-scrubbed home, the sturdy well-bred features of its hard-working mistress." ("Frontier Nursing Service Brings Health to Kentucky Mountaineers," *Life* 2, no. 24 (14 June 1937): 35.) Courtesy of the Audio-Visual Archives, Special Collections and Archives, University of Kentucky Libraries.

income patients. From their first year of practice in 1925, FNS nurse-midwives advised their patients to seek prenatal care early and often. They urged prenatal care for all expectant mothers, even those planning to deliver with a "granny" midwife. As founder and director Mary Breckinridge said, "'You've got to take care of the baby before it's born,'" and frequent antepartal visits allowed nurse-midwives to detect abnormalities immediately.[92]

Lester explained, "That's what we midwives are for, to take care of the normal and recognize the abnormal."[93] In the 1920s, Lester and her fellow FNS nurse-midwives went directly to their patients for the most part, often traveling two or more hours by horse to reach the cabin where a patient lived; by the mid-1930s, many prenatal patients visited weekly clinics at one of several FNS nursing centers.[94] Ideally, FNS nurse-midwives saw their prenatal cases every two weeks until the seventh month, and then every week until delivery. In reality, most cases delivered by nurse-midwives had at least one month's prenatal care; by 1930, only 21.4 percent of the service's pregnant patients saw a nurse-midwife before the sixth month of gestation.[95] By 1937, FNS saw a rise in its prenatal care record, with 32 percent of patients registering before the sixth month.[96]

On each prenatal visit, Lester took blood pressure, inspected breasts, performed an abdominal examination, checked for edema, examined urine for albumen and sugar, and took external measurements to see that the fetus was properly positioned. She discussed preparation for delivery, baby clothes, rest, and diet.[97] Malnutrition was a serious problem for expectant mothers in eastern Kentucky.[98] FNS staff taught prenatal patients how to use a limited diet to serve their needs, especially since rural mothers generally received the least food in their families.[99] As the delivery date neared, an FNS nurse-midwife gave instructions on what to do once labor began: "have a big fire burning, a kettle or lard bucket full of boiling water, clean gown or dress, clean sheet, newspaper pads, plenty of coal oil in the lamp, and [do] not to wait too long before sending for the nurse."[100]

FNS nurse-midwives believed that familiarity with the patients and their families allowed them to provide good care. Each FNS nurse-midwife had a district, usually limited to a three- to five-mile radius from the nursing center where she worked.[101] As former FNS district nurse-midwife Reeder explained, "as a practicing nurse-midwife on the district . . . you were so familiar with your patient that if . . . there was any abnormality, you were well aware that there was a problem before it came time for the actual delivery. You really knew your patients very, very well."[102] FNS nurse-midwives were not the only ones with this familiarity. Despite the service's criticism of "granny" midwives, they were the neighbors, friends, or relatives of the birthing women and likely knew much more about their patients' daily lives, needs, and concerns than did the nurse-midwives, who were outsiders to Appalachia and often foreigners. However, in the 1920s and 1930s, FNS nurse-midwives' provision of prenatal care was unique. At that time, only obstetricians offered prenatal care to their elite clientele, while traditional midwives and general practitioners, who attended the majority of births before World War II, for the most part did not.[103]

Nurse-midwives' prenatal patients usually saw physicians for an initial exam, and after that only if they had abnormalities. FNS nurse-midwives first tried themselves to deal with the abnormalities, such as a fetus in a breech position, following the medical routines authorized by the service's Medical Advisory Committee. If unable to deal with the situation or uncertain of what they found, FNS nurse-midwives sought help, first from the midwifery supervisor and then, if necessary, from the service's medical director.[104] Alternatively, nurse-midwives convinced pregnant patients, such as one "expectant mother who seemed to be having more than the customary discomforts," to attend a physician's clinic.[105] Sometimes the nurse-midwives had difficulty getting prenatal patients who were in need of medical assistance to see a physician. Poor roads and rivers that could not be forded often prevented patients from coming to the hospital; in those situations, the medical director made home visits with a nurse-midwife, and outlined a course of home treatment.[106]

When providing prenatal care, Lester and her colleagues looked not only at the expectant mothers' bodies but also at their life circumstances. This approach differed significantly from most physicians (at least those untrained in public health), who tended to be narrower in focus. FNS began providing formal assistance to patients through its social-services program during the Depression. In 1931, the Alpha Omicron Pi national sorority voted to create and support a social service department at FNS as its national philanthropic project. This sorority wanted to help handicapped children; in choosing to assist FNS, one member argued, "Is there anywhere a more environmentally handicapped child than the mountain child?" The social-service director, supported by the Alpha Omicron Pi fund, distributed food, clothing, and books; placed dependent children in homes; provided family casework; and arranged for patients to pay what they could afford for hospital stays outside the mountains and return train rides.[107]

During the Depression, FNS provided material aid to the people of Leslie County in other ways. The Depression brought many unemployed people who had worked in railroad and coal-mining towns back to Appalachia, just as a terrible drought in 1930 created near-famine conditions.[108] Many people survived the drought only because of a $2.50 per person monthly allowance they received from the American Red Cross. FNS pushed the Red Cross to help, by hiring a Leslie County man to survey families in the 700-mile area covered by FNS to determine how much (or in this case how little) corn each family had for the months ahead. FNS also assisted local people by employing male heads of households, and by giving away milk and cod liver oil to pregnant women and children, as well as clothing and shoes to those in need.[109] FNS staff saw the direct benefits of this kind of assistance. For example, several FNS nurse-midwives, with some assistance from the service's volunteer chairman and social-service department, and free labor from neighbors, helped one young couple create a home with a cooking stove, utensils, food, and a mattress. The service's help meant that the woman did not have to work in the fields for several months; after two previous stillbirths, likely caused by overwork, this woman bore a healthy child.[110]

In addition to extensive prenatal care and aid, FNS nurse-midwives also offered education for mothers and pregnant women. They traveled to local county fairs equipped with model baby beds and cribs; model sanitary toilets to be placed away from water sources (as opposed to the more typical privy where human waste was dumped into the same streams from which people got their drinking water); life-sized demonstration dolls; and posters on infant care.[111] At weekly clinics held in the nursing centers, nurse-midwives advised mothers about child hygiene and urged fathers to build sanitary toilets and baby cribs and to screen their houses to keep out disease-carrying mosquitoes.[112] The nursing centers also sponsored mothers' clubs, where FNS staff gave speeches. At one club meeting, Mary Breckinridge spoke about "the development of the mind of the little child up to school age, using the simplest language and illustrations."[113] Thus, while general practitioners and traditional midwives, who attended most births in the 1920s and 1930s, provided little, if any, prenatal care, FNS nurse-midwives pioneered some of the most thorough and accessible prenatal and postpartum care and education in the United States.

## *Labor and Delivery*

Betty Lester told her maternity patients to send a man to get her as soon as they felt their first labor pains. Once the man arrived, Lester dressed in her special blue-grey uniform and gave her bags to the man, who saddled her horse. Then the two rode out to the patient, day or night. Sometimes a patient was in false labor, but that did not bother Lester. She maintained that she always stayed long enough to ensure that her patient was doing well.[114] If her patient was indeed in labor, she watched and waited, and then delivered the baby on her own. If the birth became complicated, Lester left the home and called the FNS medical director, who then helped her with the delivery. Lester's approach to labor and delivery was typical of American nurse-midwives in the 1920s through 1940s. This approach, combined with nurse-midwives' emphasis on prenatal and postpartum care, was very successful in reversing high rates of maternal and infant mortality and morbidity.

Lester and her fellow FNS nurse-midwives, in comparison with many traditional midwives, were well trained in the latest obstetrical and aseptic procedures and knew when to hand over their patients to obstetricians with whom they had established relationships (although the obstetricians could not always get there in time). The nurse-midwives delivered women at home, with less chance of infection than in the hospital where infection spread from patient to patient. While they used anesthesia and forceps in delivery, they did so less frequently than their physician counterparts. The reasons for this varied and included a lack of qualifications to use the necessary equipment and techniques and lack of access to the equipment. Unlike obstetricians, who typically spent little time with their laboring patients, nurse-midwives used a time-intensive approach, which discouraged the automatic use of anesthesia and forceps and focused on the women's needs.

However, the FNS approach to childbirth had its limitations. For example, the nurse-midwives used enemas to promote cleanliness in the name of germ theory, but such a procedure produced new problems for and opposition from birthing women. FNS nurse-midwives were simply following nursing protocol of the day. Up until the 1980s and even in some cases today, medical personnel believed enemas would reduce infection rates by decreasing the chance of the expulsion of feces during labor. However, recent evidence has shown that enemas do not accomplish this goal; rather, they cause significant pain and distress for women, who often dread receiving them.[115]

FNS nurse-midwives handled the overwhelming majority of deliveries without physicians. Between 1925 and 1937, FNS nurse-midwives obtained physicians' services during one or more stages of labor only 166 times out of 3000 deliveries, or around five-and-one-half percent of the time.[116] Although the nurse-midwives were supposed to attend normal deliveries only and to use physicians as backup, the difficulties of traveling long distances over rough terrain meant that physicians were often unavailable, even in emergencies.

From the beginning, FNS had a medical advisory committee of Lexington physicians, which included several of Breckinridge's cousins.[117] This committee wrote the *Medical Routines* manuals for nurse-midwives to follow, as they realized physicians might not be available when nurse-midwives needed them.[118] Committee members also served as consultants for more complicated cases and held special health clinics for FNS patients. Visiting medical specialists from Lexington and Louisville also volunteered to provide clinics in obstetrics, trachoma, hookworm, orthopedics, pediatrics, dentistry, nose and throat, and ear and eye at FNS. In addition, FNS benefited from the services of a visiting surgeon in a mining town twenty-four miles from Hyden. Unlike most surgeons, this one charged his patients based on ability to pay, and performed many free operations.[119] FNS also used the services of other local physicians whenever possible, but often faced problems, especially in the early years, getting these physicians to the patients when nurse-midwives called. An FNS annual report explained:

> Medical care was obtained with great difficulty during the winter, owing to the illness or absence of the two nearest physicians. For one abnormal obstetrical case we were over thirty hours in getting assistance and twenty-one hours for another. The doctors were, as always, splendidly cooperative when they came, and answered the call at the earliest moment possible. One physician, from Bell County, who came in from an emergency eclamptic (the one who was twenty-one hours getting to us), had not been in his bed for two nights in succession. His territory covers a thousand square miles.[120]

In 1928, FNS finally established a twelve-bed facility, Hyden Hospital, and hired a resident medical director both to lead it and to attend to emergencies in the districts.[121] Adding a hospital and a medical director meant that FNS could provide more consistent medical care. The hospital treated patients with appendicitis, burns, dysentery, and gunshot wounds, as well as women in childbirth with complications.[122] Even after the founding of Hyden Hospital, outside specialists continued to hold health clinics at FNS, and when the service's hospital in Hyden did not meet patients' needs, they were sent to hospitals in Louisville, Lexington, Cincinnati, or Richmond, all of which had ties to FNS. Still, because of the mountain topography and long distances between the hospital and patients' homes, nurse-midwives continued to handle most home deliveries without additional medical assistance. In an era when increasing numbers of births took place in the hospital with physicians, FNS nurse-midwives successfully attended the majority of births at home without physicians.

Given their isolation, FNS nurse-midwives obviously had to be prepared for whatever occurred during labor and delivery. The contents of their midwifery bags combined with their delivery routines showed a keen concern with cleanliness. Delivery bags held a rubber apron, an operating gown, a cap to cover their hair completely, gloves, soap, and a scrub brush. They also brought a thermometer, an enema tube and funnel, artery clamps, a hypodermic set, scissors, umbilical cord ties, several basins, rubber sheeting, dry sterile gauze and cotton, perineal pads, and towels. In advance, they made sure that the home had pads made of clean rags and newspaper for the delivery bed, as well as baby clothes. Nurse-midwives also carried several drugs and medical supplies, including Lysol as a disinfectant; silver nitrate for babies' eyes to prevent blindness; ergot, a fungus-derived medication causing the contraction of muscle fibers, to prevent and check postpartum hemorrhage; pituitrin, a hormone causing uterine contractions, which was also used to stop postpartum hemorrhage; and sedatives for the first stage of labor.

FNS nurse-midwives tried to reach their laboring patients as soon as possible. According to Breckinridge, "the support and help given through the long hours of the first stage has a bearing on the outcome."[123] *Medical Routines* instructed FNS nurse-midwives to greet the patient upon arrival and ask about when labor had begun, the strength and time between contractions, and the woman's overall health. She was also to make sure there was a fire, hot, sterile water, and if possible, cold, sterile water. In the first stage of labor, the nurse-midwife was to wash her hands well with soap in the patient's basin, and then boil the necessary articles she carried in her midwifery bag, including a pair of gloves and a hypodermic syringe and needles. She was then to conduct an abdominal examination; take the patient's temperature, pulse, and respiration; and perform a vaginal examination, if necessary, after scrubbing for five minutes with soap and warm water and soaking in a Lysol solution for three minutes. If there was time, the nurse-midwife could give her patient an enema. Except in cases of breech presentation or fatigue, both first-time mothers and others were to be up and walking in the first stage, and taking hot drinks and food, predominantly carbohydrates, at regular intervals. However, the nurse-midwife was to encourage the patient, especially a first-time mother, to rest with sedatives, as circumstances required. If she arrived in time, she was also to give the patient, again especially a first-time mother, an ounce of castor oil, which acted as a laxative, at the beginning of the first stage.[124] Breckinridge explained, "our aim is to get a quiet first stage."[125]

The nurse-midwife's goal in the second stage was to protect the perineum and avoid tears "by delivering between pains when the head is fully crowned, and with a minimum of bleeding. We usually deliver on the left side, as we were taught, keeping careful pressure on the fundus [top of the uterus] and following down with the left hand."[126] While physicians commonly used forceps, such deliveries at FNS were rare. FNS staff used forceps in only nine out of the first 1000 midwifery cases, four out of the second 1000, and one out of the third 1000 performed through the service—and most likely physicians, not nurse-midwives, actually delivered the babies in these instances.[127] The FNS medical director, upon being called by a nurse-midwife, apparently used forceps only if the patient had been in labor for an unusually long time.[128] Other interventions were also uncommon at FNS. Only four of the first 3000 midwifery cases (1925–1937) required Caesarean sections; just two needed episiotomies; one required a Duhrssen's incision (an incision of the cervix to facilitate delivery) with low forceps; and four needed internal versions with ether.[129]

As Breckinridge explained, "the third stage [of labor] causes us the deepest anxiety, because upon our judgment alone hangs the life of the patient should the third stage not be normally complete, as medical aid could not possibly reach us until too late."[130] At that stage, the nurse-midwife was directed to "hold [the] fundus firmly without stimulating for twenty minutes after the birth of the baby. If, at the end of that time, the midwife knows by the usual symptoms that the placenta has separated and is in the vagina, and the patient does not expel it, the midwife may express it through the abdominal wall, as she has been taught." After delivery and examination of the placenta, the nurse-midwife was to give the patient ergot to prevent hemorrhage, leaving the family to give more ergot to the patient in three to four hours. Then, the nurse-midwife was to give the patient perineal care, and again take the temperature, pulse, respiration, and fundus height. She was also to destroy the placenta after examining it, preferably by burning, while remaining at least one hour after the placenta was delivered. As soon as the baby's head emerged, the nurse-midwife cleansed the eyes with dry, sterile cotton. Once the baby was born, the nurse-midwife clamped and cut the cord, and placed him or her in a blanket in a safe, warm place. After the mother's needs were met, the nurse-midwife scrubbed up for the baby, dropped silver nitrate in each eye, tied the umbilical cord twice and applied a dry dressing, oiled, weighed, and dressed the baby, and placed the baby at the mother's breast for five minutes. Finally, the nurse-midwife was to clean both patients and the room before leaving.[131]

The stories FNS nurse-midwives told about births show that they spent extensive time, and often went to great lengths to be with their patients during labor and delivery. In February 1930, two nurse-midwives at an FNS nursing center reported a mini baby boom, with six deliveries in one four-day period, and one labor lasting thirty-one hours with "slow but steady progress." Usually the two nurse-midwives saw each other frequently, but the large number of deliveries prevented them from working together. The sixth birth occurred a little later than the rest, and thus the nurse-midwives were able to attend the event together, arriving at the home at 7:00 P.M., nine-and-one-half hours before the birth.[132] It was not unusual for FNS nurse-midwives to spend hours with a laboring woman in addition to occasionally spending hours *getting* to her house. One Saturday night in winter 1932, an FNS office secretary accompanied a nurse-midwife on a call from the husband of a pregnant woman who lived outside the FNS districts. The two FNS staff members rode horseback for two hours, arriving to find the expectant mother frightened about having as long a labor as with her first child. According to the secretary, the nurse-midwife "reassured her, and it almost seemed miraculous to me the way she succeeded in transferring her calmness to the mountain woman." The patient gave birth to a daughter four hours later, and the nurse-midwife stayed another two hours to make the mother feel comfortable and to clean and dress the infant.[133] Both the service's prescriptive literature, such as *Medical Routines,* and reports of actual deliveries reveal that nurse-midwives typically stayed with their patients through the entire labor and delivery.[134]

## *Postpartum Care and General Nursing Care*

The nurse-midwife/patient relationship did not end with the delivery. Betty Lester stayed with a mother and her newborn for at least one-and-one-half hours after the delivery. She took care of each to ensure that both were healthy, clean, and comfortable. Plus, "you had to stay . . . to make sure that everything was all right because you might be five miles away from home. . . . A woman could hemorrhage, she could do anything. A baby could get asphyxiated, anything can happen."[135]

Postpartum care did not end there. Once a woman gave birth with Lester's help, she and her baby both received regular care and assistance. This regular at-home nursing care, along with an emphasis on breastfeeding, which provided many health benefits to baby and mother, made

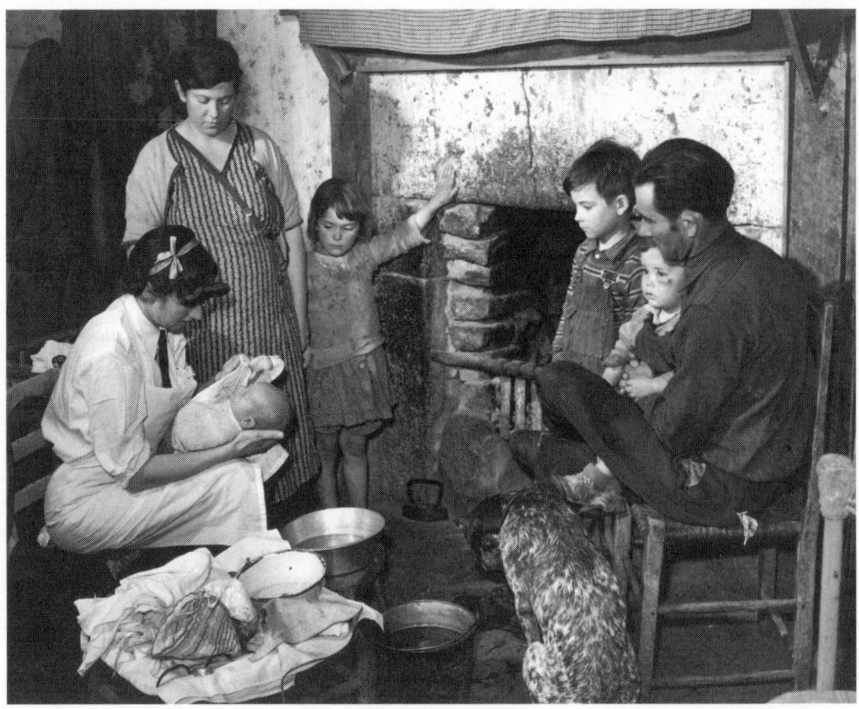

FIGURE 4. A Frontier Nursing Service nurse-midwife makes a postpartum home visit to a mother and her family, c. 1930s. Courtesy of the Audio-Visual Archives, Special Collections and Archives, University of Kentucky Libraries.

nurse-midwives' postpartum care different from that provided by other birth attendants. Traditional midwives also emphasized breastfeeding, but focused more on housekeeping and care of older children than on the mother's health. During this period, physicians of all types did not especially encourage breastfeeding, and by the mid-twentieth century, artificial infant feeding had become the norm.[136] General practitioners provided little postpartum care. Obstetricians kept their patients in the hospital for ten to twelve days after delivery; in the hospital, new mothers received attention to their health along with relief from household chores and older children, but they also dealt with alienating, impersonal hospital routines and what they sometimes saw as insensitive obstetric nurses.[137]

FNS nurse-midwives had close contact with patients after delivery. *Medical Routines* instructed FNS nurse-midwives to visit each mother and new baby for the first ten days, on a daily basis if the patients lived within a three-mile radius of the nursing center, and every other day if they lived within three to five miles of the center. Nurse-midwives' work with the mother included bathing, checking temperature, pulse, and respiration, dressing the perineum, helping the family with the mother's diet, asking about urination and bowel function, and "giv[ing] very careful attention to breasts, especially as the milk comes in, as the baby's food supply for the year depends largely upon getting lactation well established in the beginning." The nurse-midwife gave a laxative to the woman on the second day after delivery; had her sit up in bed after the first nursing visit; and had her out of bed on the tenth day. During those first ten days, nurse-midwives also paid careful attention to the newborn, giving sponge baths, dressing the umbilical cord, retracting and cleaning the foreskin if necessary, weighing at birth, the fourth day, and the tenth day, asking about urination and bowels, and assuring that the baby was getting enough milk through nursing. After the first ten days, nurse-midwives visited the mother and baby every week until one month after delivery. The manual also gave instructions on what to do in case of abnormalities.[138]

Although it is hard to determine to what extent nurse-midwives followed the manual's instructions, statistical and anecdotal evidence shows they spent a significant percentage of their time on postpartum care. Tabulating the service's first 1000 midwifery cases (1925–1930), statistician Louis I. Dublin explained that FNS nurse-midwives followed up with all new mothers for one month after delivery, and reported that ninety-six percent of these women were in satisfactory condition.[139] FNS monthly reports show that in the 1920s and 1930s, postpartum visits for mothers and babies made up a significant percentage of nurse-midwives' visits. For example, in May 1929, FNS had sixty midwifery cases, with twelve deliveries, 118 visits with prenatal patients, 115 visits with postpartum mothers, and 109 visits to newborn babies. Assuming that visits to postpartum mothers and babies generally occurred simultaneously, postnatal care comprised 39 percent of nurse-midwives' midwifery work, in terms of number of visits to patients, that month; and took up 103.2 hours, or 38 percent of the time nurse-midwives spent on midwifery care.[140] In November 1930, FNS had 111 midwifery cases, with twenty-four deliveries, 204 visits with prenatal patients, 241 visits with postpartum mothers, and 341 visits to newborn babies. Postnatal care comprised 60 percent of all midwifery visits, and 189.05 hours, or 42 percent of the time nurse-midwives spent on midwifery care.[141] The other monthly reports indicate that nurse-midwives spent many hours providing postnatal care.

Stories of nurse-midwives' work also illustrate the extent to which nurse-midwives attended to the needs of their postpartum patients. On one Saturday morning in 1931, an FNS nurse-midwife made her regular visits to her patients: "In the next home there is a brand-new baby. The mother too is new, being only seventeen and this her first child. . . . The lusty-lunged infant is bathed, instructions as to regularity of feedings are given. The nurse will return the day after next."[142] In another case in that same year, a family called in a nurse-midwife after trying a patent medicine to cure their very ill thirteen-month-old, and after failing to understand a doctor's directions on how to make a special formula. The nurse-midwife demonstrated to the mother how to make the formula and give it to the baby; she then returned the next day to ensure that the mother understood the procedure and that the baby was improving.[143]

Fannie Huff, a patient whose five children were delivered by FNS nurse-midwives, explained that the nurse-midwives "come ten days after the baby was borned, and dress you, and get you cleaned up and . . . take care of your beds. And you didn't have the things to take care of 'em with, why they'd bring their own things, you know, their sheets and everything they needed." Huff also said she could buy a layette, including baby clothes, blankets, towels, and soap, from the nurse-midwives for just one dollar.[144]

Betty Lester said that not only did she see her patients every day for the first ten days after delivery, and every week for the first month, but also every month for the first year. In fact, Lester and her colleagues took care of women, children, and even men long after the babies they delivered passed out of the newborn stage. They saw children twice a year while they were in school, and saw adults on an as-needed basis.[145]

Stories from the nurse-midwives confirm not only the amount of time FNS staff spent on postpartum care but also their emphasis on breastfeeding. Lester noted that in the service's early years all of its mothers breastfed their babies. As Lester explained, breastfeeding was both what she and her fellow nurse-midwives advocated and what mothers wanted. She claimed "all our babies stayed on the breast for nine months to a year."[146]

FNS nurse-midwives provided more than comprehensive maternity care. They also offered general nursing care, and preventive actions and public-health education for families. They provided patients with this wide range of services in a period when American public-health nurses focused more narrowly on instruction and prevention. Breckinridge explained her rationale for this broader approach:

> The nurse who tends the sick only, and teaches nothing and prevents nothing, is abortive in her work. On the other hand the nurse who

> attempts instruction and prevention without combining with them an appreciation for the sickbed, and without meeting its appeal, has failed in the one element which differentiates her profession from all others and out of which it was created.[147]

FNS district nurse-midwives held weekly clinics not only for prenatal examinations but also for vaccinations and advice on child hygiene and sanitation, and they sometimes held special clinics on the outer bounds of the districts, since the mountainous terrain and lack of roads and transportation often made travel difficult even to the outpost centers.[148] In the first month of its service, FNS staff bandaged the wounds of fifty adults and forty-one children, treated several hundred nonmaternity patients, vaccinated thirty adults and 114 children for typhoid at the request of the Kentucky Board of Health, and worked on persuading people of the need to maintain stores of smallpox vaccine and toxin-antitoxin to prevent diphtheria.[149] By 1932, FNS had given more than 46,000 inoculations and vaccines against such diseases as typhoid, diphtheria, and smallpox.[150] From its earliest days, FNS believed that in areas with few or no physicians, "prevention is more than ever the life-saver."[151] FNS nurse-midwives also held numerous classes for children, especially girls, in general health and hygiene, on topics such as "Germs and How They Are Spread," and home hygiene and care of the sick.[152] They hoped to prevent disease and ensure that eastern Kentuckians knew how to provide basic care for themselves, especially given the long distances they needed to travel to receive medical or nursing care.

## *Statistics*

An examination of maternal mortality statistics for FNS during the interwar period shows that the service's emphasis on early and frequent prenatal care, on home deliveries with few interventions, and on close contact with patients and their families in the postpartum period appeared to pay off. As seen in table 2.1, FNS had an astoundingly low maternal mortality rate. This is especially remarkable given that one would expect exactly the opposite simply because the service's patients were low income and often had poor nutrition and housing—factors that typically contribute to higher rates of maternal mortality.

It was no accident that FNS compiled statistics on its rate of maternity mortality. FNS anticipated criticism, or at least skepticism, about its work,

**Table 2.1** Frontier Nursing Service and Comparison Groups: Maternal Mortality Rate (per 10,000 births), 1925–1937[153]

| | |
|---|---|
| Frontier Nursing Service (3000 deliveries, 2 maternal deaths) | 6.6 |
| Kentucky (white population only) | 44–53 |
| White women delivered in hospitals by physicians in Lexington, Kentucky | 80–90 |
| United States: | |
| Total population | 48.9–69.5 |
| White population | 43.6–63.1 |
| Non-white population | 85.8–121 |

and knew that it needed to prove that it provided patients with good outcomes. FNS hired Louis I. Dublin, statistician and a vice president at Metropolitan Life Insurance Company, to help gather the data. A well-known, well-respected statistician with a PhD in mathematics from Columbia University, Dublin believed that statistics as applied to public health could benefit humankind. Employed at Met Life from 1909 to 1952, Dublin was president or director of many public-health institutions, including the American Public Health Association, and he had expertise as well as an interest in maternal and child health.[154] Hired by FNS in the late 1920s, Dublin issued his first report on the organization in 1932, after he analyzed data from the first 1,000 deliveries. He continued to compile and analyze the statistics for FNS through its first 10,000 deliveries in 1954.[155] FNS broadcast the statistics in its literature, hoping to promote its good work and to combat assumptions that nurse-midwifery would not improve maternal health.

There were potential shortcomings with this collection and analysis: Dublin was sympathetic to nurse-midwifery and FNS hoped to prove itself to health professionals and the public, in part by using these statistics.[156] However, Dublin was a highly esteemed statistician whose reputation would have been damaged had he lied about the statistics. In addition, he worked for a life insurance company; the job of a life insurer is to assess risk, and thus he or she would tend to err on the side of an increased possibility of morbidity and mortality. Furthermore, to this day, no one has been able to counter or disprove Dublin's statistics for FNS.

## Conclusion

FNS provided much-needed, comprehensive maternity and general health care to people in a large area of eastern Kentucky, as well as a school to train nurse-midwives in service to the rural poor. However, the ways in which Breckinridge, her staff, and friends promoted the new service limited the development of nurse-midwifery as a profession. The service's media messages focused on the exotic and romantic sides of nurse-midwifery in Appalachia and on the "backward" patients of supposed "fine old American stock" rather than on the nurse-midwife as a legitimate professional type. Readers and viewers were left with the notion that nurse-midwives were mainly good for ignorant mountaineers living in rough and rugged Appalachia. No matter how much Breckinridge believed in the ability of nurse-midwives to make a difference in Americans' health, she had to compromise in order to launch and sustain FNS. Additionally, she had to find ways to appeal to local people, who were not used to seeking out health care from professionals and outsiders. But Breckinridge encountered challenges much greater than recruiting patients. Because the nurse-midwife was new, because outsiders confused her with the much-maligned traditional midwife, and because she represented a potential threat to obstetricians and what was becoming the American way of birth, Breckinridge faced a host of problems. How would she win approval from physicians—necessary for FNS to function (since nurse-midwives required physician backup) and garner cooperation from outsiders? How would she get support from nurses, members of her own profession who sometimes felt threatened by the independence of the new nurse-midwife? How would she raise money? Finally, how would she get support for FNS when the American health-care system generally disregarded poor patients?

To answer these questions and overcome the service's potential problems, Breckinridge appealed to racist beliefs. She used her passion to help women and children, her incredible network of family and friends, and her excellent public relations skills to paint a picture of the FNS nurse-midwife and her poor, white, and worthy charges that both health professionals and the lay public could support. She simultaneously ensured that FNS would flourish and that nurse-midwifery would be seen as a noble and romantic calling rather than a real profession.

CHAPTER 3

# New York City's Maternity Center Association

## Educational Opportunities and Urban Constraints

### Introduction

Born in 1893 in Holyoke, Massachusetts, Rose McNaught, known as "Rosie," came from a family that immigrated to the United States just after the Revolutionary War.[1] Her father was superintendent in a paper mill, and her mother stayed at home to raise McNaught and her four siblings. McNaught actively chose not to marry and have children because she wanted to travel and be a professional woman. When picking a career, she, like other girls of her race and class, had few real options. She attended normal school and prepared for teaching, and even taught primary grades for a few years due to family pressure, but ultimately she realized she did not want to teach. So, during World War I when recruiters came to her hometown from the Army School of Nursing in Washington, D.C., McNaught jumped at the chance to change her life. She began her nursing training at Camp Devens in Massachusetts and finished it at the Army School of Nursing at Walter Reed Hospital in Washington, D.C. After completing her nursing degree, she returned to Holyoke to work as head nurse at the obstetrics department in the local hospital. In 1922, McNaught pursued her interest in public-health nursing, finding employment as a nurse and supervisor at the Henry Street Settlement House in New York City. While at Henry Street, she learned about nurse-midwifery—through both a lecture by Maternity Center Association's Hazel Corbin and exposure to two Frontier Nursing Service (FNS) nurse-

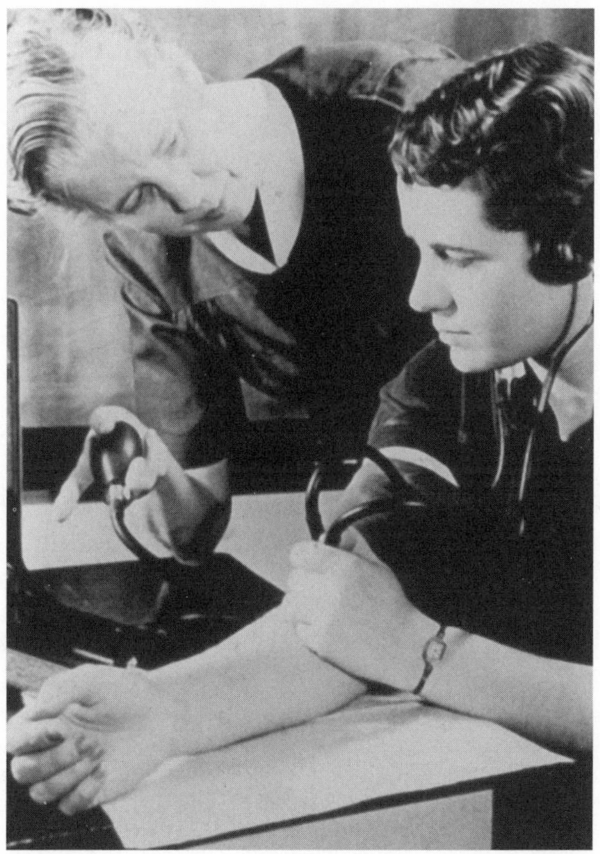

FIGURE 5. Maternity Center Association's Lobenstine School of Midwifery instructor Rose McNaught teaches student nurse-midwife Margaret Thomas how to take a patient's blood pressure, late 1930s. From the personal collection of Helen Varney Burst, CNM; originally from the Maternity Center Association.

midwives who had done field work at Henry Street while getting master's degrees at Columbia University. Further shaping her decision had been the frustration she experienced as a Henry Street nurse while attending births—a field in which she had no training.

These experiences led McNaught to FNS and Kentucky. She worked there for a year as a staff nurse, and then, in September 1928, FNS sent her on scholarship to the midwifery program at York Road General Lying-In Hospital shortly after Betty Lester had finished her midwifery training there.[2] After passing the British midwifery examinations, McNaught returned to Kentucky, working as a nurse-midwife until fall 1931, when FNS founder and head Mary Breckinridge sent her to New York City to help set up the new nurse-midwifery service and school at Maternity Center Association (MCA). Although at first hesitant to leave her mountain life, McNaught devoted the rest of her career to MCA. The first nurse-midwife to practice at MCA's Lobenstine Clinic and therefore in New York City, McNaught was nurse-midwifery supervisor at the clinic and instructor at the school until 1958.[3] She was a strict teacher who both gave and expected much from her students. As one former student explained, sometimes she was "a very hard task-master. If you did something she did not like she would yell at you!" When physicians asked her why she chose nurse-midwifery, she said that women had always attended childbirth, but "then the men took over and some are very, very good but a lot of them are very, very . . . nothing." Students and colleagues, while intimidated at times by her tell-it-like-it-is approach, deeply admired McNaught, felt her influence for years to come, and loved her great sense of humor. Before her death in 1978, McNaught received several honors from the American College of Nurse-Midwives in recognition of her accomplishments.

While the Appalachian Mountains offered the first location for nurse-midwives to practice, New York City provided the first American site for them to get an education. Actually, it provided the first *two* nurse-midwifery educational sites. The first, Manhattan Midwifery School (MMS), opened from 1925 until 1931 and affiliated with Manhattan Maternity and Dispensary, appears to have been invisible both to historians and contemporary public-health officials and to maternal and child health advocates in New York City. Proposed by Emily Porter, superintendent of nurses at Manhattan Maternity and Dispensary, the school admitted graduate nurses and trained them in midwifery, first for four months and later for six months. The school combined clinical work, during which students assisted in hospital deliveries and managed home deliveries, with classes, which were taught by obstetricians and nurses. Approved by the New York State Board of Health, the MMS graduated at least eighteen students, most of whom worked as missionaries in foreign countries or in American public-health settings. Two went on to work at FNS, and some taught obstetric nursing or worked as obstetric nursing supervisors in hospitals. The school closed because the maternity hospital lacked enough patients to train both medical and nurse-midwifery students. Although MMS played a pioneering role in American nurse-midwifery education, it was not well known either by contemporaries or by later nurse-midwives looking back at their history.[4]

New York City's—and the nation's—*second* nurse-midwifery school, the one Rose McNaught helped establish, is this chapter's focus. The school and accompanying clinic had a long-lasting impact on American nurse-midwifery. Opened by MCA in 1932, the Lobenstine School of Midwifery was named after Ralph W. Lobenstine, a prominent New York obstetrician and one of the school's founders. The school taught public-health nurses to supervise traditional midwives practicing in rural areas and to provide skilled care to some rural populations, under the guidance of obstetricians. At the same time, MCA established a nurse-midwifery clinic—the second in the United States after FNS—to give students the opportunity to apply what they learned in the classroom. The clinic served poor women in Harlem, offering complete maternity care to women who wanted home delivery and for whom a normal pregnancy and childbirth were expected.

Compared with FNS, MCA had a radically different location and clientele, a different purpose, and different challenges. Leading male obstetricians helped create and shape MCA, and years before the association advocated nurse-midwifery, it performed pioneering work in maternity-care education. In the 1920s and early 1930s, MCA's physician and nurse pioneers struggled to establish a nurse-midwifery school and practice clinic. They experienced difficulty persuading already-established health professionals that the nurse-midwife would not "follow in the trail made already by the granny midwife."[5] After several aborted attempts, MCA finally opened a nurse-midwifery school and clinic in the early 1930s, but faced several obstacles. While most early graduates of MCA's nurse-midwifery school went on to supervise traditional rural midwives or nurses, performing important work to change the state of maternal health care, they remained few in number and isolated. MCA's clinic, a professional home-delivery service in Manhattan, was radical, opening just as middle- and upper-class city dwellers were establishing hospital deliveries as the standard. The clinic served mostly African Americans and Puerto Ricans, a clientele that white America scorned. Compared with FNS practitioners, MCA's urban nurse-midwives posed a greater threat to physicians, and thus local practitioners kept a more watchful eye on their activities. In response to this suspicious environment, MCA educated its student nurse-midwives with the assumption that upon graduation they would work in rural areas rather than stay in New York City. MCA administrators also downplayed the role of the new kind of birth attendant their school was training; instead, they emphasized less threatening messages aimed at educating the general public about the need for early prenatal care and early registration with physicians.

## Early Pioneer in Maternity Care Education

Long before opening its nurse-midwifery school, MCA led New York City and the nation in attempting to reduce high infant and maternal mortality rates. Obstetricians, social reformers, and public-health nurses had established MCA in New York City in 1918, with well-known Progressive Era reformer Frances Perkins (who later became the first female cabinet member in the United States as Secretary of Labor under President Franklin Roosevelt) as its executive secretary. Unlike FNS, which specifically aimed to create a nurse-midwifery service, MCA was founded to provide maternity care education. In 1919, MCA public-health nurses began holding mothers' classes, attended mostly by recent immigrants living in tenements.[6] At these weekly classes, MCA nurses offered games, refreshments, and simple instructions on how to prepare for a new baby. They taught the prospective mothers how to keep cow's milk fresh and unadulterated, how to streamline household duties, and the importance of prenatal care and seeing a physician early in pregnancy.[7] By 1920, MCA had opened thirty maternity centers, three of which they operated in conjunction with the New York Milk Committee and the Women's City Club. Located in churches and storefronts all over Manhattan, these centers offered prenatal care and instruction by nurses, social workers, and laypeople.[8] Infant and maternal mortality dropped significantly for families who utilized the center's services. MCA centers' infant mortality was 25.1 per one thousand babies, compared with 36.6 per one thousand in New York City as a whole; MCA maternal mortality was 40 per ten thousand, compared with 50.9 per ten thousand in New York City.[9] By 1921, MCA changed its emphasis from prenatal care to complete, intensive care through all phases of the maternity cycle at one center.

MCA quickly became a model for community maternity care for other communities that wished to establish similar programs. In 1922, MCA began a demonstration project of its maternity work within a square-mile district in Manhattan, providing prenatal and postnatal clinics staffed by public-health nurses, nursing assistance during delivery, and instruction in all aspects of maternity care. Again, MCA staff encouraged patients to make physician or hospital arrangements early in their pregnancies, and even when patients preferred traditional midwives, the staff prompted them to stay in close contact with clinic physicians. Analysis of the demonstration project's records from 1922 to 1929 reveals a maternal mortality rate of 2.4 for the 4,726 patients who received maternity care at MCA, compared with a rate of 6.2 for patients living in the same district but not under MCA's care.[10] This project also provided public-health nurses with field experience. Between 1921 and 1928, 2,500 nurses came to MCA, staying anywhere from one day to six months, to work and observe its approach to maternity; 240 stayed at least three months with the service. These nurses then returned to their own communities, where they often organized and conducted services similar to MCA's.[11]

From the early 1920s on, MCA focused more on education than practice. An MCA report from 1921 concluded:

> It is clearly the function of the Association to be a great educational agency; first, in arousing the public to the importance of the problem with which it is concerned, and, second, in stimulating public health agencies to a desire to participate in the solution of the problem. . . .The little work that it can do in the direct handling of patients in its clinics and centers can, at best, reach only a small proportion of the city's total pregnant women. Our main conclusion is that the Maternity Center Association must more and more become an educational and experimental agency rather than a large local public health or nursing society.[12]

By 1925, MCA had distributed 14,000 copies of its book, *Routines for Maternity Nursing and Briefs for Mothers' Club Talks*, a handbook of instructions to public-health nurses on informing pregnant patients about maternity care, as well as outlines for a series of classes for mothers. *Routines for Maternity Nursing* included a series of short talks on prenatal care, nutrition for pregnant and nursing women, maternity clothes, baby clothes and other items, how to give baby a bath, preparation for delivery, and aftercare.[13] Also by 1925, MCA had sent out 500,000 copies of *Twelve Helpful Talks*, a series of pamphlets addressed to prospective mothers and fathers explaining the value and content of maternity care; 20,000 maternity care record forms; and 150 educational exhibits to public agencies, private services, and individuals throughout the world.[14] Starting in 1929, MCA taught public-health nurses about all aspects of prenatal and postnatal care in maternity institutes conducted throughout the country.[15] By the time MCA opened its nurse-midwifery clinic in 1931 and school in 1932, it had become the leading advocate for prenatal and adequate maternity care in the United States and excelled in training public-health nurses in prenatal, labor and delivery, and postnatal care.

## Aborted Attempts to Establish a School and Practice Clinic

Despite MCA's resounding successes by the early 1930s, the road to establishing a nurse-midwifery school and clinic at MCA had been long and difficult. Several of New York City's leading obstetricians on MCA's Medical Advisory Board led the campaign to create a school and clinic to improve maternity care for the poor. These men believed that nurse-midwives could retrain traditional midwives and handle normal labors and deliveries. Noting that traditional midwives attended over 8 percent of the deliveries in New York City in the early 1930s, George W. Kosmak, founding editor of the *American Journal of Obstetrics and Gynecology*, suggested midwives could not be eliminated immediately, "even if their final elimination might prove desirable," because they worked with a needy population that valued their services. Kosmak argued the "only solution" to the problem of poorly trained midwives was to create "a body of more highly trained midwives from the registered nurse group, who shall act as teachers and supervisors" to traditional midwives.[16] Lobenstine, one of the founders of MCA, agreed, explaining that nurse-midwives should focus on training the large numbers of midwives in rural areas because "there are not now in the United States enough doctors in rural or small communities to attend women at the time of delivery or during pregnancy."[17] Lobenstine added that some nurses already supervised midwives but that they lacked training in attending childbirth, making their supervisory role "both difficult and ineffective."[18]

According to MCA's medical advisors, in addition to training midwives, nurse-midwives could also learn to attend births when normal labor and delivery were expected. Frederick W. Rice, professor of obstetrics and gynecology at New York University's medical school and obstetrician at Bellevue Hospital, argued that nurse-midwives should attend births in rural areas where there were few physicians because he wanted poor women to have access to "modern" medical care (as opposed to care by "granny" midwives).[19] Lobenstine suggested that mortality and morbidity would decline if all rural physicians had nurse-midwives working with them.[20] He also thought that nurse-midwives should handle normal cases "in large foreign communities" if authorities restricted the practices of traditional midwives through strict supervision and gradual elimination.[21] Making an even more radical argument than either of his colleagues, Benjamin P. Watson, professor of obstetrics and gynecology at Columbia University's medical school and chair of the department from 1926 to 1946, stated that *all* physicians who delivered babies should have one or more nurse-midwives conduct deliveries in normal cases. He noted that although his proposal might seem unorthodox in the American context, a similar plan had worked well in Europe.[22]

MCA's forward-thinking medical men believed that educating nurses in midwifery would call attention to the problems poor people faced. They believed that not only inadequately trained birth attendants but also "deplorable" economic conditions caused high infant and maternal mortality rates.[23] They hoped, as Lobenstine explained, that nurse-midwives' "presence in the different states, particularly where they will act as supervisors of midwives, will at once stimulate interest and improve the standards and the care given to the very poor."[24]

According to MCA obstetricians, the nurse-midwife would stir public concern not only about the plight of the poor but also about the sad state of American obstetric care. MCA medical advisors, along with leading obstetricians in other cities, argued that general practitioners deserved a good part of the blame for high rates of maternal and infant mortality. Lobenstine was one of many obstetricians who noted that most medical students received little hands-on experience in obstetrics, and that general practitioners often interfered unnecessarily during childbirth. As Lobenstine explained, "meddlesome midwifery accounts for many deaths, many needless complications and much invalidism."[25] Rice agreed with Lobenstine, arguing that "meddlesome midwifery" occurred precisely because physicians lacked knowledge about normal labor and delivery.[26] Rather than waiting for a normal childbirth, they insisted on interfering. Rice, Lobenstine, and their colleagues believed that with appropriate training, nurse-midwives would be better birth attendants than general practitioners. Even more than that, they hoped that the presence of well-trained nurse-midwives would push the American public to demand better maternity care from physicians. As Rice said, "When this demand becomes overwhelming and not until then, are we going to have the medical profession interest themselves in obtaining better obstetrical training."[27]

Finally, some MCA obstetricians noted that nurse-midwives would actually *improve* their professional and personal lives. John Osborn Polak, professor of obstetrics and gynecology at Long Island College Hospital from 1911 to 1931, said the nurse-midwife would "relieve [the physician] of much of the wear and tear of his work."[28] Watson believed that if nurse-midwives performed normal deliveries, obstetricians would deal with fewer complications during and after childbirth, perform fewer Caesarian sections, have more time to read medical journals and attend medical meetings, and become richer.[29]

Prominent MCA nurses also strongly advocated nurse-midwifery. Hazel Corbin, Louise Zabriskie, and Nancy E. Cadmus all were involved in conferences designed to investigate and promote an MCA affiliation with Manhattan's Bellevue Hospital School for Midwives (the first city-sponsored school to train American traditional midwives) for the purpose of training nurse-midwives.[30] Corbin (general director of MCA from 1923 to 1965) drew up a plan for training nurses in midwifery in her 1929 "Suggestions for Improving Existing Maternity Service in New York City."[31] In 1930, she urged Lobenstine to write to the Commonwealth Fund, a private philanthropic organization to which FNS founder Mary Breckinridge also appealed, to explain why he thought the nurse-midwife was so important.[32] Compared with the obstetricians, MCA nurses said less—at least in the available documents—to promote nurse-midwifery before the Lobenstine School and Clinic opened. As women and as nurses, they believed (and likely were told) that their voices carried less weight than that of the obstetricians. Still, their support prior to the establishment of the school and clinic, along with their life-long commitments to nurse-midwifery afterward, indicate that MCA nurses played an important role in establishing nurse-midwifery education in the United States.

Despite the many justifications for a nurse-midwifery school and clinic, these programs faced numerous barriers from both physicians and nurses. To address these hurdles, MCA organized a conference in 1921 of physicians and nurses to discuss training and using nurse-midwives.[33] Although many opposed the idea, several leading obstetricians associated with MCA, as discussed earlier, supported it. In the mid-1920s, the National Organization for Public Health Nursing organized a committee, which included MCA nursing leaders, to investigate the possibility of starting a nurse-midwifery school, and the nurses talked about how much opposition they anticipated facing. Throughout the 1920s, MCA made several failed attempts to establish an affiliation with Manhattan's Bellevue Hospital School for Midwives. In the early 1930s, MCA tried to work with New York Nursery and Child's Hospital to establish a field service for nurse-midwives; again, they failed. MCA leaders finally gave up trying to work with established institutions and decided to found their own nurse-midwifery school and clinic.

One cause of MCA's difficulties in establishing a nurse-midwifery school and clinic was the attitude of nursing leaders, which letters and minutes from meetings about the attempted Bellevue-MCA partnership reveal. The partnership was designed to give public-health nurses a course in midwifery, "known as an advanced course in obstetrics," for a total of six months—two months at MCA, one at Bellevue Hospital to observe clinic work, and three at Bellevue School for Midwives to gain delivery experience.[34] The goal was to train public-health nurses "1. to practice as midwives in rural communities; 2. to supervise the work of the now existent midwives; 3. to supervise the work of obstetrical nurses; 4. to do obstetrical nursing in the public health field, taking care of midwifery where the need arises."[35] MCA administrators planned for nurse-midwives' rural patients to be "under medical control," and they hoped to work out an arrangement with physicians from local bureaus of child hygiene to have them determine which of the cases were routine enough for MCA students to care for.[36] In 1923, after internal discussions between Bellevue and MCA about their plan, MCA gathered together public-health nursing leaders from New York City and around the country, and sent out questionnaires to divisions of maternity and child welfare in every state, to explain and solicit opinions about the plan. Although many nurses supported the plan, noting the "disgraceful record of large numbers of the mothers still not receiving proper care" and benefits to both nurses and mothers if nurses were prepared to deliver babies in emergencies, nurses' voices were some of the loudest in opposition to training nurses in midwifery. Their words help clarify MCA's long struggle to create a nurse-midwifery education program.[37]

One reason given for opposing the Bellevue-MCA plan was that nurses would not want to assume midwives' responsibilities. Two nursing leaders—one with extensive experience with urban public-health nurses and the other with rural public-health nurses—argued that few nurses would be interested in midwifery because they already felt prepared enough to handle occasional emergency deliveries and would not want to extend their duties beyond that. Edna L. Foley, superintendent of the Visiting Nurse Association of Chicago, noted that she knew British nurses who also had certificates in midwifery. These women "did not like the midwife part of their work at all, [because] . . . too much responsibility was placed on them and . . . it was not as easy to secure physicians for complicated cases as it sounded."[38] Elizabeth G. Fox, from the National Organization for Public Health Nursing (NOPHN), indicated that many rural nurses had expressed that they were far too busy to add midwifery to their duties.[39]

Some nurses opposed the Bellevue-MCA plan, arguing that nurses *should* not assume responsibility for deliveries because they would upset the "medical fraternity."[40] Fox argued:

> I think it is the definite duty of the medical profession [to assume responsibility for the delivery of patients]. Whether they fall down or not is not for me to say. . . . I cannot quite see that the way to influence the medical group is through our undertaking to deliver patients ourselves. I am inclined to think that the way to influence them is through our doing better pre-natal and post-natal work, and better service as nurses; that doctors should do the actual delivery, rather than by our taking upon ourselves the practice of midwifery, whereby to show the medical profession how it ought to be done. I think our influence will be much more acceptable, much more likely to reach the goal [of improving maternity care] which [MCA's] Dr. Rice wants us to reach, if we approach it through those avenues which are *properly ours*, rather than through a field which the medical profession itself essays.[41]

Fox wanted to avoid stepping on physicians' toes, or appearing to take over their territory, for fear of hurting public-health nursing. Although her comments seem obsequious, she was, in some ways, right; throughout their history, nurse-midwives have faced physicians who saw (and continue to see) nurse-midwives as competition and who have worked to limit them.

Even prominent nurses who supported nurse-midwifery expressed deep concern about physicians' responses. In 1927, Elizabeth F. Miller, nursing consultant for Pennsylvania's Department of Welfare and chair of NOPHN's Committee to Study the Need of Midwifery for Nurses, and Isabel M. Stewart, director of nursing education at Teachers College, Columbia University in New York City and a member of Miller's committee, corresponded about the need for caution when presenting nurse-midwifery to physicians. They strategized about who would approach certain physicians with proposals and talked about "the delicacy of the problem and the need for much preliminary inquiry and the need for stimulating thought," as well as the fact that they were "confronting some very definite handicaps."[42] Nurses like Fox, who opposed the Bellevue-MCA partnership, felt that such a delicate problem was worth avoiding.

Finally, nurses opposed the Bellevue-MCA plan to train nurses in midwifery because it would potentially hurt public-health nurses' status within the medical profession by more directly associating them with much-maligned traditional midwives. As Fox said, "there is a tremendous controversy within the medical profession as to the place of the midwife, and as to its obligation or duty to that group of workers, the importance of having such a group, which also influences me in feeling that it would be rather unfortunate to interject the public health nurse question into that controversy when it is so far from being settled in the minds of the medical profession itself."[43]

Prominent nurses who opposed the Bellevue-MCA plan sought to tread lightly and not anger physicians. Recognizing that their status depended on association with physicians, they insisted that nurses should not assume full responsibility for patients. They also were aware that the profession of nurse-midwifery might ultimately hurt nursing because physicians saw midwives as unprofessional and dangerous.

Of course, nursing leaders were not the only ones with concerns about training nurses in midwifery. New York City Commissioner of Welfare Bird Coler was the man who actually ended any dreams of a Bellevue-MCA plan just as it appeared to be coming to fruition. Coler argued: "I see midwives only as poor women trained to take care of poor women. If graduate nurses are trained to be midwives they will charge such prices that women in the lower income level will not be able to afford them." An MCA report explained that the commissioner "didn't see the nurse-midwife as a paid public servant or as part of a public health organization."[44] Few known surviving documents specifically reveal which physicians opposed MCA's nurse-midwifery plans before 1931. However, judging from nurses' concerns and from documents dating to the early years of the MCA nurse-midwifery school that mention physician resistance, resounding physician opposition to MCA's plans clearly existed.

When the Bellevue-MCA plan failed, MCA leaders tried to collaborate with New York Nursery and Child's Hospital to create a nurse-midwifery school. Lobenstine, chair of MCA's Medical Advisory Board and a tireless advocate of a school and clinic, received an appointment at the hospital, "with the understanding that as soon as funds could be raised, the long awaited school for nurse-midwives would be opened under his direction." Although Lobenstine became gravely ill, MCA's Board of Directors continued to work with the hospital under the assumption that the partnership could still work. After Lobenstine's death, however, "his medical associates in the Nursery and Child's Hospital, who had helped in planning for the opening of the new school, immediately vetoed it and refused to cooperate."[45] MCA's leading obstetricians and nurses were foiled again.

## Educating Agents of Change

After a decade of efforts by MCA physicians and nurses to convince their colleagues of the value of establishing a nurse-midwifery school and two failed attempts—one at Bellevue Hospital and one at New York Nursery and Child's Hospital—to establish a practice clinic for nurse-midwifery students, MCA leaders decided to forge ahead on their own.[46] In early 1931, they established the Association for the Promotion and Standardization of Midwifery, Inc. The new association's certificate of incorporation included three men and one woman: Ralph Lobenstine, George Kosmak, and Benjamin Watson, who were members of MCA's Medical Advisory Board, and Hazel Corbin, a nurse who was MCA's general director. The Board of Trustees consisted of these four people, as well as other leading obstetricians and nurses, including FNS's Mary Breckinridge.[47] When Lobenstine died in March 1931, Evelyn Field, ex-wife of Chicago department store heir and banker Marshall Field, led approximately sixty women, friends and patients of the deceased obstetrician, to pledge enough money to maintain a clinic and school for three years. The Lobenstine Midwifery Clinic was established in November 1931 and the Lobenstine Midwifery School in February 1932. Both organizations were licensed by the New York City Board of Health and supervised by the Health Department's Bureau of Maternal and Child Hygiene; the clinic also received licensure and supervision from the New York State Department of Social Welfare.[48] The Lobenstine Clinic provided students with field experience, and gave prenatal, labor-and-delivery, and postpartum care to women expecting a normal pregnancy and delivery who wanted home delivery.[49] The Lobenstine School taught midwifery to public-health nurses to enable them to 1) supervise and teach untrained midwives and 2) bring skilled maternity care, under the direction of obstetricians, to women in remote rural areas.[50]

It may come as a surprise that MCA was so concerned with educating nurse-midwives to serve in *rural* areas given that it served a poor African American and Puerto Rican population in the middle of the largest American city. Several factors seem to explain this irony. First, a number of leading physicians on MCA's Medical Advisory Board argued that rural communities had the highest need for professional maternal care because they lacked access to physicians and continued to employ local midwives in large numbers.[51] Second, the percentage of midwife-attended births in the urban northeast continued to decline dramatically over the 1920s and 1930s, as the Lobenstine School was being conceived and developed, and therefore, residents of northeastern cities would theoretically have less of a need for nurse-midwives.[52] Third, and most important, the physicians and nurses who invented the Lobenstine School were being realistic. In the early years, some of the members of MCA's Medical Advisory Board had suggested that professionally trained nurse-midwives could serve women in urban areas.[53] But most recognized that even in poor urban areas where few physicians wanted to work, physician resistance to nurse-midwives would be very high. Thus, the physicians and nurses affiliated with MCA crafted a plan with the greatest chance for success: the creation of a school to train nurse-midwives primarily to supervise traditional midwives (and to a lesser extent provide professional maternity care) in remote areas of the United States and in developing countries, where they would be invisible to most health professionals.

MCA spent the first eight months of 1932 developing a curriculum, selecting staff, formulating policies regarding student and patient admission, fostering relationships with cooperating hospitals and social welfare agencies, creating standing orders for the clinic, and trying to gain the acceptance of local welfare agencies, nurses, and physicians. The school and clinic opened with one resident physician and four attending obstetricians. Hattie Hemschemeyer, a public-health nursing educator and director of the school and clinic, who then completed her nurse-midwifery degree in the first class at Lobenstine, and Rose McNaught, the American nurse-midwife with British midwifery training who had worked for several years at FNS, were also on staff. The first nurse-midwifery class at the Lobenstine School graduated in 1933 with seven students.[54] The school required applicants to have four years of high school and be graduates of an accredited school of nursing; they also needed at least "two years of professional experience, one of which has been spent in public health nursing" and to be registered to practice nursing in at least one state.[55] As an MCA publication later explained, "exceptions were made for applicants whose professional accomplishments justified special consideration, or who were referred by organizations training local personnel to become midwife supervisors."[56]

With no American nurse-midwifery schools in existence, MCA looked to European, especially British, examples to develop its curriculum. British nurses took a six-month midwifery course, and non-nurses took a one-year course; in 1938, the program lengthened to one year for nurses and two for non-nurses. MCA modified the British experience to meet American needs; its students were nurses with three months of obstetric training as part of their nursing degree. Although the school's admission requirements included public-health nursing experience, most of the early students did not have formal coursework in the subject. Thus MCA established a ten-month program, with the first four in instruction, supervision, and practice in public-health nursing, through the Department of

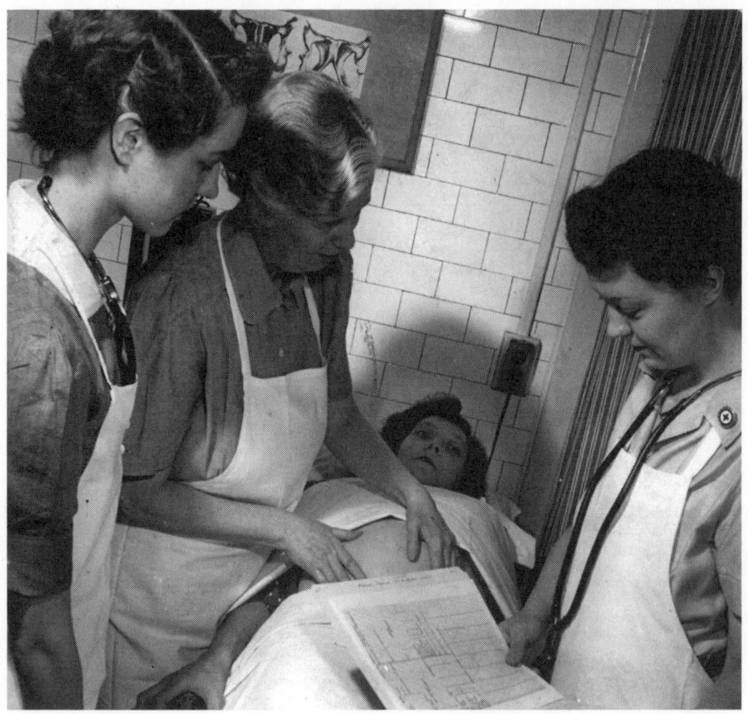

FIGURE 6. Rose McNaught teaches student nurse-midwives at Maternity Center Association's Lobenstine School of Midwifery, c. 1930s. Courtesy of the Maternity Center Association.

Nursing Education, Teachers College, Columbia University, and the last six months, spent at MCA, in instruction and practice in midwifery.[57] During the six months at Lobenstine, nurses attended lectures and watched demonstrations by obstetricians and supervising nurse-midwives. They gained practical experience by working with prenatal and postnatal mothers at the clinic, as well as teaching mothers' classes and working with social-welfare and health agencies to help their patients. An MCA student delivered twenty babies during her program, while many medical students observed only six deliveries during their training. In general, the Lobenstine School taught its students "how to provide good obstetric care under conditions which they may find in their own communities, and . . . how to improvise with small financial outlay a clinic which will provide safe care to mothers and babies."[58]

MCA gradually changed and adapted the curriculum to fit new needs. In 1935, at the Rockefeller Foundation's expense, Hazel Corbin and Hat-

**Table 3.1** Employment of the First Twenty Graduates of the Lobenstine School of Midwifery (Years of Graduation, 1933–1935)[62]

| Number of Graduates | Place of Employment |
|---|---|
| 4 | The State Departments of Health in New York, Kentucky, Florida, and Alabama |
| 1 | Frontier Nursing Service |
| 1 | Victorian Order of Nurses in Canada |
| 1 | Midwife instructor in Spain |
| 2 | Maternity instructors in schools of nursing |
| 1 | United States Children's Bureau; holds midwife institutes to teach traditional midwives |
| 1 | Director, Brooklyn Maternity Center |
| 1 | Director of rural public health nursing program in Ramsay, New Jersey |
| 1 | Nursing supervisor in tuberculosis maternity hospital |
| 1 | Attending college full-time to prepare herself to teach obstetric nursing in a nursing school |
| 1 | Ill |

tie Hemschemeyer studied midwifery schools and services in England, Scotland, France, Norway, Sweden, Denmark, and the Netherlands, countries with low rates of maternal morbidity and mortality. Eager for Lobenstine graduates to meet the educational standards of other nations so that their nurse-midwifery training would be recognized regardless of where they worked, Corbin and Hemschemeyer applied knowledge from their visits back home.[59] Later in the 1930s, MCA eliminated the four months of public-health nursing because most applicants had bachelor's degrees in public-health education, or had taken courses in public health and the social sciences. However, it maintained a connection with the Department of Nursing Education at Teachers College, albeit one which did not affect directly its own nurse-midwifery students. In later years, MCA provided field experience in obstetric nursing for interested public-health majors, and members of the MCA staff taught various courses at the college.[60]

Graduates of the Lobenstine School brought the philosophy and practices of nurse-midwifery to communities around the country.[61] Of the first twenty graduates, who received their degrees between 1933 and 1935, most worked in public health, supervising or teaching midwives; a few supervised or taught nurses. (See table 3.1 for specific places of employment.)

One example of early Lobenstine graduates' work can be seen in Maryland. In 1936, with money from the Social Security Act earmarked for maternal and child health, especially in rural areas hit hard by the Depression, J. H. Mason Knox, director of the Maryland State Department of Health's Bureau of Maternal and Child Hygiene, contacted the Lobenstine School with a request for help in educating Maryland midwives.[63] Just thirteen years before, Knox had indicated his disapproval of nurse-midwives, explaining that he "question[ed] [the] advisability of public-health nurses doing obstetrical work in Maryland" because it was the "medical profession's responsibility."[64] By the mid-1930s, however, his opinion of nurse-midwifery had improved enough that he hired Lobenstine graduates Elizabeth Ferguson and Martha Solotar to work for the Maryland State Department of Health, where they started "a demonstration in the supervision, teaching, and control of indigenous midwives" in a rural region of southern Maryland.[65] Each worked in a different rural county, mostly with African-American midwives. Both Ferguson and Solotar registered the midwives, taught them about obstetrics, cleanliness, postpartum care, and when to contact a physician, got to know the families the midwives served, observed their deliveries, kept records of their work, and, when necessary, reported problems to local authorities. The two nurse-midwives also conducted prenatal care clinics for local families. Ferguson, employed in a county with a part-time public-health officer, mostly worked on her own "with a minimum of medical help," while Solotar and her county's public-health officer worked together—although Solotar conducted many deliveries on her own.

Available accounts discuss the demonstration's success. Rates of maternal mortality and morbidity declined in the demonstration areas, and Johns Hopkins Medical School obstetricians were impressed by the results.[66] One argued that a good nurse-midwifery service improved rural obstetrics more than any other available method of maternity care. In particular, the Johns Hopkins obstetricians appreciated that Ferguson and Solotar instructed their charges to seek medical help if necessary. One frequently told story was that of Ferguson and a particular "mammy midwife" whom she had taught. This midwife "made a very clever diagnosis of the wrong position of a baby and got the patient into Johns Hopkins Hospital in time [although thirty miles away] for the doctor to deliver the patient of a live baby and secure health for the mother." After Ferguson told this story at a professional meeting, "the obstetricians at Hopkins arose and confirmed this statement and said that if American obstetrics were to be improved in Maryland, at least, we must have more midwives like Miss Ferguson."[67] While the "mammy midwife" was the one who made the diagnosis, Ferguson received the praise because the Hopkins obstetricians and MCA leaders assumed that the midwife would not have done this without Ferguson's influence and teaching. MCA leaders hoped that with more successes like Ferguson's and with more supporters like Hopkins obstetricians, nurse-midwifery would grow. Despite such success stories, the Lobenstine School failed to expand due to financial difficulties along with medical and lay ignorance about the nurse-midwife's efficacy.

## A Clinic with a Clientele No One Wanted

Ferguson, Solotar, and their fellow Lobenstine School alumnae gained nurse-midwifery experience at Lobenstine Midwifery Clinic. Nurse-midwifery was so controversial that MCA had established a separate organization to create the clinic in 1931; Lobenstine Clinic was not officially affiliated with MCA, even though most of the clinic's officers were members of MCA's Medical Advisory Board or staff.[68] Later events proved the wisdom of MCA's strategy. In 1934, MCA consolidated the clinic under its own organization after some felt that the clinic had proven itself. H. J. Stander, H. C. Williamson, and James A. Harrar, all prominent obstetricians at New York Hospital and members of MCA's Medical Advisory Board, resigned in protest.[69] Harrar explained that he regretted his resignation, "as I have always been a great admirer of the work the Maternity Center Association has accomplished; but I am not in sympathy with plans to educate any more midwives, whether as nurse-midwives or as midwives educated to be supervisors of midwives."[70] Now that MCA's Medical Advisory Board had "the medical responsibility for the Lobenstine Midwifery Clinic," these men wanted no part of MCA, or of this new kind of birth attendant, the nurse-midwife.[71]

The MCA Medical Advisory Board, Board of Directors, and staff always considered physicians' response to nurse-midwifery when making decisions about Lobenstine Clinic. In order to diminish physician opposition, the clinic specifically targeted patients who could not afford to pay the fees of private physicians.[72] As chair of the Medical Advisory Board George Kosmak explained in a letter to 200 physicians in the clinic district, "It is our aim to interfere in no way with the private obstetric practices in the district."[73] MCA had to prove to local physicians, who were skeptical about Lobenstine Clinic and the new nurse-midwives, that it was not in competition with them. As Rose McNaught said, it "took years" for the obstetricians and other physicians to get used to the nurse-midwives.[74] Despite the ambitions of Benjamin Watson, the member of MCA's Medical Advisory Board who thought nurse-midwives should conduct all normal deliveries, Lobenstine Clinic claimed (at least publicly) its only aim was to serve people who would have never been seen by physicians in the first place.

Lobenstine Clinic patients, like those at FNS, were generally poor. Through the 1940s, the clinic asked patients with the ability to pay to contribute five dollars (the same amount FNS asked of its patients); if the patient was unable to contribute that sum, the clinic asked for two or three dollars to help cover its prenatal, labor-and-delivery, and postpartum services. According to New York State Department of Social Welfare reports on the clinic, although paying for the services gave "the patient a feeling of self respect," "the greater proportion of cases [were] taken free of charge."[75] Clinic statistics from 1932 to 1936 show that 40 percent were "dependent upon relief organizations for support," 40 percent had incomes of less than $20 per week (less than $14,852 per year in 2006 dollars), and 20 percent had incomes of over $20 per week.[76] Clinic records from 1932 to 1939 provide a more specific breakdown of incomes, indicating that the clinic received increasing numbers of poor patients as the Depression progressed. Between 1932 and 1939, 40 percent of clinic patients "were on Home Relief or Work Relief," 10 percent had incomes of less than $10 per week (less than $7,426 per year in 2006 dollars), 34 percent had incomes of less than $20 per week (less than $14,852 per year in 2006 dollars), 10 percent had incomes of less than $30 per week (less than $22,278 per year in 2006 dollars), and 6 percent had incomes of more than $30 per week.[77] According to an MCA publication from the late 1930s, many clinic patients lived in "tenement homes, cold water flats with the most primitive facilities," and struggled with "[health] problems which arise from poor housing, from unemployment, from stark poverty."[78]

Although MCA and FNS nurse-midwifery services shared a similarly indigent patient population, a similar approach to birth, and a similar commitment to nurse-midwives as one solution to the nation's maternal and infant health problems, the services had several important differences.

While FNS served entire families, Lobenstine Clinic served pregnant women only.[79] Lobenstine operated its prenatal and postpartum clinics out of a comparatively small space: "the first floor of . . . [a] three-story basement and brownstone former residence."[80] The clinic staff was also more particular than FNS about the pregnant women they served; they turned away patients with "any abnormal condition" because they had the option of sending those patients to local maternity hospitals, with which they had cooperating agreements. Furthermore, MCA worked closely with a variety of New York City agencies, including social-welfare organizations, such as the Henry Street Settlement and the Metropolitan Life Insurance Company's Visiting Nurse Service, both of which provided Lobenstine Clinic patients with postpartum nursing care.[81] Although FNS worked with hospitals as far away as Lexington, Cincinnati, and Richmond, its remote location meant that it did not have the multitude of local options available to MCA.

A large difference between the MCA and FNS nurse-midwifery services was in their patients' race and ethnicity. FNS advertised constantly that it served the "finest old American stock," but MCA was vague about its client base. While MCA made clear that Lobenstine Clinic served indigent patients, the few publications that discussed the clinic almost never mentioned anything about patients' racial or ethnic background. MCA probably made this choice because the clinic served mostly African Americans and Puerto Ricans, a clientele no one—sometimes not even MCA staff—wanted. In the late 1930s, Corbin reported that "the district which has been served from the 113th Street [Lobenstine] clinic is increasingly made up of Puerto Ricans and a rather low level of colored folks." She hoped to open a second clinic in Washington Heights, located "in the center of an area of better class white people," to "reach a better class clientele."[82] Of course, New Yorkers who knew the clinic was located in Harlem would have assumed that the patients were African American, since by the 1930s, Harlem was known as an African-American community. That MCA literature sidestepped the race and ethnicity of clinic patients indicates that MCA administrators realized that highlighting such information could have harmed MCA.

Until 1947, the clinic was located on 113th Street between 7th Avenue and Central Park West, in southernmost central Harlem. The facility served indigent patients in a district surrounding the clinic, defined as south of 142nd Street, west of 5th Avenue to the Hudson River, and north of 86th Street.[83] Compared with FNS, which served 700 square miles in a sparsely populated mountain region, Lobenstine Clinic served a tiny geographic area, but one with a much greater population density. The clinic itself spanned both the African-American and Puerto Rican sections of Harlem, and the district included a large part of those sections, as well as parts of Morningside Heights and Manhattanville, Central Park West, and Washington Heights.[84]

Clinic statistics from 1932 to 1936 indicate that 70 percent of the patients were "colored" and 30 percent were "white."[85] As scholars have explained, the meaning of these terms constantly shifted. Corbin's comment above—that the district from where the patients came was "increasingly made up of Puerto Ricans and a rather low level of colored folks"—suggests that "colored" meant African American, and "white" included Puerto Rican. However, it is likely that some Puerto Ricans would have been classified as "white" and some as "colored"; *The WPA Guide to New York City* (1939) and economist Lawrence R. Chenault's *The Puerto Rican Migrant in New York City* (1938) both distinguish between "white" Puerto Ricans and "colored" Puerto Ricans.[86] Conversely, Chenault noted that "the entire group [of Puerto Ricans] is sometimes referred to by Americans as 'colored.'"[87] Regardless of how they were classified, the clinic always served Puerto Rican patients, and the numbers increased over the years, as seen in clinic statistics for the 1940s and 1950s and in the increased migration of Puerto Ricans to the clinic district. Even as early as 1934, Hattie Hemschemeyer told Mary Beard, an associate director of the International Health Division at the Rockefeller Foundation, that she was pleased that the foundation sponsored a nurse-midwifery student from Spain at the Lobenstine School because "her knowledge of Spanish has been of invaluable assistance to the patients and to the staff."[88]

Lobenstine Clinic patients must have struggled on a daily basis. New York City's African Americans and Puerto Rican immigrants faced even harder times than white Americans did in the 1930s. Fifty percent of African Americans were unemployed, double the rate for whites. Most decent paying jobs were closed to African Americans. Department stores, for example, hired African Americans as porters, maids, and elevator attendants, not as higher-paid sales clerks. Subways hired them as porters, not as better-paid motormen. Rents in Harlem, where African Americans were forced to live, remained higher than other places, and yet housing conditions in Harlem continued to decline. Health conditions also worsened, with African Americans having higher rates of tuberculosis and other diseases, as well as maternal and infant mortality rates double those of the rest of New York City.[89] As black medical professionals pointed out, poor living conditions and lack of access to medical resources—including discrimination and insufficient services at Harlem Hospital—caused poor health.[90] Despite such poor conditions, African Americans continued to migrate to New York City during the Depression because opportunities were fewer and conditions were worse in the rural South.[91]

In the 1930s, New York City's Puerto Ricans also faced difficult lives. Significant numbers of Puerto Ricans migrated to New York City after 1900, with the largest numbers entering the city between 1946 and 1964. As American citizens, they moved to the continental United States for a variety of interrelated reasons, which mainland companies in search of cheap labor exploited. These included poor economic conditions in Puerto Rico caused by the decline of the sugar-crop industry (the United States had forced the industry to be the basis of the Puerto Rican economy after invading and taking over the country in 1898) and the lure of jobs on the mainland. Overpopulation in Puerto Rico was also a factor and the Puerto Rican government actively encouraged emigration.[92] Before 1940, Puerto Ricans settled primarily in central and east Harlem, in the community that became known as El Barrio. They also settled in Brooklyn, and after World War II, migrated to the South Bronx.[93] Prejudice caused by their race and ethnicity, as well as their limited skills, forced them into low-paying jobs. Most Puerto Rican men worked in factories as unskilled laborers or in menial jobs in service industries, especially in restaurants and hotels.[94] Puerto Rican women often did piecework in the garment industry, where they received payment for each piece they completed, to supplement, and in some cases provide, the family income. While doing needlework at home, they worked long hours and earned extremely low wages, with payment sometimes delayed by the contractors.[95] Like African Americans, Puerto Ricans lived in substandard housing with inadequate sanitation, and they faced poor health and a lack of access to modern medicine.[96] Economist Lawrence R. Chenault found that central Harlem, which contained a large Puerto Rican population and was the location of Lobenstine Clinic, had by far the highest infant and tuberculosis mortality rates, and new cases of venereal disease, in all of New York City.[97]

If these poor Puerto Rican and African-American women did not give birth with nurse-midwives through MCA's home delivery service, where would they have been giving birth, and with whom? In the 1930s, most African-American women in New York City probably delivered their babies with physicians' help in hospitals. According to one study, in New York City between 1917 and 1923, 98.3 percent of African-American births took place in the hospital or at home with nurses or physicians. Increased efforts by public-health agencies to push women to seek medical care during pregnancy and childbirth in the 1920s and 1930s suggest that the percentage might have been greater by the time MCA's clinic opened in 1931. Another study confirms the medicalization of childbirth among African Americans in the urban North. In 1937, Elizabeth Tandy, senior statistician for the United States Children's Bureau, found that in northern cities, physicians attended 97.9 percent of all African-American births, and 61.8 percent occurred in hospitals.[98]

Traditional midwives attending births at home provided another option for African-American and Puerto Rican women, but this option was disappearing over the first three decades of the twentieth century. Across the nation, midwife-attended births decreased from 50 percent in 1900 to 15 percent in 1930, as a result of several factors. Obstetricians convinced fellow physicians and the public that midwives had set obstetrics back by decades and that reform-minded woman were demanding better obstetrical care. Other factors contributing to the decline of the traditional midwife included a decreasing birth rate and a significant drop in the number of immigrant midwives following the passage of strict federal immigration quotas in 1924. In the urban North, midwife-attended births decreased even more dramatically than they did nationwide. By 1932, midwives attended only 8 to 10 percent of births in New York City. Many of those midwives were European immigrants who attended births by women in their own ethnic communities, not black women.[99] While black midwives continued to practice in the South, many changed jobs when they migrated North; this was, in part, because northern urban black women sought professional help during childbirth. Like their white counterparts, black women in northern cities received information from public-health agencies arguing that physicians provided the best childbirth care. Plus, as the number of children they bore decreased, they wanted what they saw as the best for their fewer deliveries.[100]

However, some available literature suggests that a significant minority of northern urban African-American women continued to use midwives. One source indicates that as late as 1937 midwives attended the births of one-third of black babies in northern cities.[101] Several studies discuss the popularity of the folk healing system among northern urban blacks, including those who lived in Harlem. Black Harlemites often turned to faith healers, spiritualists, and elderly "grannies" because of a long-time belief in a mixture of African, spiritualist, and agrarian traditions. They turned away from physicians because of discriminatory practices in hospitals, lack of money, and disinterest in obtaining professional medical care. Given African-American Harlemites' devotion to folk healing practices, it would not be surprising that they also used traditional healers to help them to deliver their babies. Traditional healers offered special medicines made of dried cobwebs, rabbit brains, and "cockroach rum," as well as such folk recommendations as placing a fried egg on a woman's belly to speed labor or tying a bag of lice around a baby's neck to end teething pains.[102] Many probably combined traditional practices with care from health professionals for their deliveries.

We know much less about birth attendants and the locations of childbirth among Puerto Rican Harlemites. Most went to health department clinics to receive health care in the 1930s. At these clinics, they had access to well-baby care, dental hygiene programs, diagnosis of venereal diseases, and chest examinations for tuberculosis.[103] Staff at these clinics would have advised strongly that women seek physicians to attend their babies' births. However, language and cultural barriers, as well as negative attitudes of Anglo health professionals toward Puerto Rican patients, may have militated against patients accepting the advice of clinic staff. As one Puerto Rican writer noted, many Puerto Ricans "complain of much waiting at clinics, the abrupt or discourteous manner of the physician or nurse, the superior attitude of the North American, [and] routine treatment, which they deeply resent (being treated as they put it, 'like a machine')." In addition, clinics often lacked the resources to deal with patient needs.[104] Thus, Puerto Ricans and African Americans in Harlem who wanted professional medical assistance during childbirth faced many barriers, including high costs, discrimination, professionals' insensitivity, and inadequate services and resources. MCA provided poor families in Harlem with another option—one where the price was right and the services readily available.

## The Lobenstine Midwifery Clinic's Approach to Birth

Among the many services MCA provided was frequent prenatal care; the level of attention to the gestational period stood in stark contrast to the infrequent, or nonexistent, prenatal care provided by general practitioners and traditional midwives, who attended the majority of American births prior to World War II. Rose McNaught and her fellow MCA nurse-midwives, just like the women at FNS, encouraged patients to register early in their pregnancies at the Lobenstine Midwifery Clinic. A patient's first visit involved a thorough examination by the resident physician. If the physician found no abnormalities, nurse-midwife staff and students cared for the pregnant woman during the rest of her pregnancy, labor and delivery, and postpartum period. If the first visit uncovered an "even minor abnormality or suggested later difficulties," the physician arranged for an obstetrical consultation. From 1933 to 1952, patients averaged 7.7 prenatal visits to MCA's clinic, and nurse-midwives, nurse-midwifery students, and clinic physicians made an average of 2.3 visits to pregnant women in their homes. In normal pregnancies, nurse-midwives performed the majority of the prenatal work until the last month of pregnancy. They checked blood pressure, examined urine, and looked for metabolic problems, instructed pregnant women in "healthful living," offering prospective mothers information on diet, dress, easier ways to perform housekeeping, and information on the normal course of labor.[105]

As compared to FNS, MCA maternity patients had easier access to physicians because of MCA's urban location and design. From the beginning, MCA referred patients with medically complex conditions to hospitals, a realistic decision given MCA's location in New York City.[106] In addition, as Hattie Hemschemeyer, Lobenstine School's director, explained, MCA had to take into account "the traditional pattern of doctor-nurse relationship so firmly established in this country," in a way that FNS, a nurse-midwifery service in an isolated region with very few physicians, did not.[107]

Unlike most schools for health practitioners, MCA trained its nurse-midwives to examine all aspects of the patient's environment affecting "the health and happiness and peace of mind of each expectant mother and father," including substandard housing, unemployment, poverty, overwork, lack of proper nutrition, and lack of sunshine.[108] McNaught said that during the Depression, instead of collecting money from her patients at MCA, she and her colleagues often gave them money so they could eat.[109]

Along with regular appointments with patients, MCA nurse-midwives' broad prenatal care program included education for mothers and pregnant women. As discussed earlier in the chapter, MCA was a national leader in teaching patients about prenatal care by the time it opened its nurse-midwifery clinic and school, and the nurse-midwives continued MCA's strong prenatal care tradition in their instruction of antepartal clinic patients.

MCA nurse-midwives also educated mothers all over the world directly and indirectly through their numerous publications, maternity exhibits, and maternity institutes for public-health nurses. By 1935, half of the twenty thousand public-health nurses employed in the United States had attended a training session given by an MCA nurse.[110] By the same year, MCA had distributed 50,000 copies of its *Routines for Maternity*

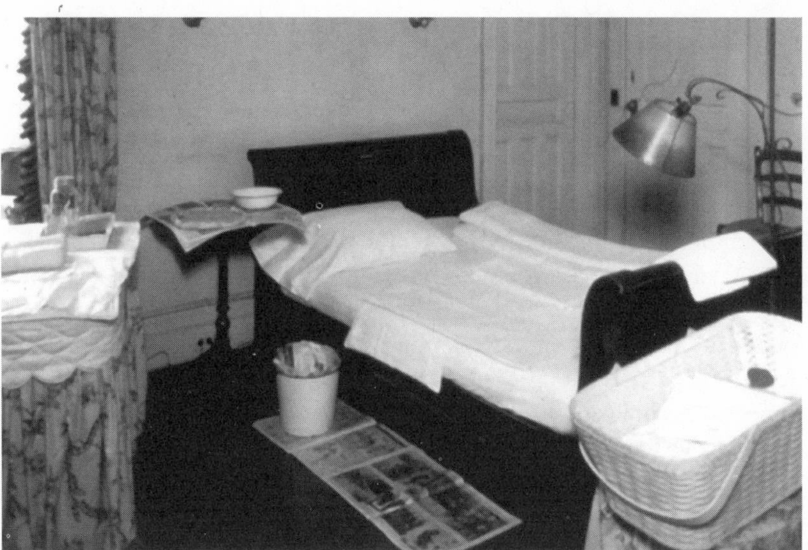

FIGURE 7. Maternity Center Association home-birth setup, c. 1930s. From the personal collection of Helen Varney Burst, CNM; originally from the Maternity Center Association.

*Nursing and Briefs for Mothers' Club Talks*, and set up a Hall of Science exhibit at the 1933 Chicago World's Fair entitled "Face Motherhood Informed—Remove All Questions."[111] Many parents ordered *The Maternity Handbook for Pregnant Mothers and Expectant Fathers*, written in 1932 by MCA's Anne A. Stevens, which presented in simple terms the major points of safe maternity care, "mak[ing] available [to] fathers and mothers everywhere the benefits of the Association's experience."[112] In 1939, MCA published *Birth Atlas*, a short, beautifully illustrated book that reproduced twenty-four life-size sculptures of fertilization, fetal growth, stages of labor, and return of the uterus to normal size and position, perhaps the most famous publication produced by MCA. Renowned obstetrician Robert Latou Dickinson designed the models that Abram Belskie sculpted.[113] MCA nurse-midwives—and thousands of public-health nurses, maternity nurses, and physicians—have used *Birth Atlas* to teach their patients, from 1940 to the present.[114]

In addition to their pioneering work in prenatal care and education, Rose McNaught and her colleagues were pioneers in labor and delivery. Like their counterparts at FNS, they generally delivered babies on their own without the interventions typical of obstetricians of this era. In the first 1081 deliveries of the Lobenstine Clinic patients (1932–1936), 84.1 percent had normal labor, with complications occurring in 15.9 percent.

However, only 7.5 percent, or eighty-one women, had complications severe enough to require hospitalization. MCA attributed the "low incidence of hospitalization . . . to the discriminating selection of patients and to the generous amount of time spent by the medical staff in the clinic and in the home. When a complication necessitating hospitalization occurred, the physician responded promptly to the midwife's call and made plans for the immediate admission of the mother."[115] Nurse-midwives used sedatives, including ether, potassium bromide with chloral hydrate, Demoral, and Seconal, "when indicated." Labors were short—the average was six hours and forty-five minutes—and nurse-midwives attended the patients for a large part of that time, an average of four-and-one-half hours. Long-time MCA clinic obstetrician Marion D. Laird suggested the short labors "may be due to the confidence engendered in the patient and her family by the satisfying personal contact in this small service."[116]

MCA's urban location and proximity to physicians and hospitals meant that compared with FNS its nurse-midwives had less autonomy and its patients more contact with physicians during labor and delivery. In fact, physicians played a larger role in MCA patients' births, despite the fact that MCA's nurse-midwifery home-birth service, the Lobenstine Clinic, carefully chose which patients it would accept. Unlike FNS, MCA's nurse-midwifery service declined to serve a number of pregnant women who wanted to deliver there. Between 1932 and 1936, the service refused a little over one-quarter of the women (379 out of 1460) who applied for their care because they lived outside the clinic district, applied almost at term, had unclean homes, were found not to be pregnant, or had complications that made a home delivery inadvisable. But MCA nurse-midwives still delivered babies under less-than-ideal conditions, often in primitive tenement homes. In fact, as Rose McNaught recalled years later, when she introduced newly graduated physician Marion Laird to home deliveries, Laird "nearly collapsed the first time she went out with me and saw what we had to do on a home delivery in some of those houses—so poor and dirty."[117] Still nurse-midwives assured patients that "no matter how lacking in modern facilities these homes are, when the time comes for the baby's arrival, the room in which he will be born is made clean and orderly by the nurse-midwife."[118] If a laboring woman needed hospitalization, the Lobenstine Clinic had an "excellent working agreement" with two New York hospitals, Sloane Hospital for Women and the Lying-In Hospital at Cornell, where patients "could be rushed right in and taken right to the labor floor with no questions asked."[119] In the 1930s, while attending patients in labor, nurse-midwives reported by telephone to the medical director who gave orders, as necessary, for "examination, medication, or treatments." Physicians visited approximately one in four MCA patients in labor. When physicians checked in on patients giving birth at home, they judged whether they or the nurse-midwife should complete the delivery. MCA staff quickly found they used "twice as much medical service as we had originally estimated to be necessary. Out of every hundred mothers who were registered for care, one in seventeen needed to be hospitalized for definite medical reasons at some time during the maternity cycle." Hospitalization resulted from prenatal and postpartum complications as well as from labor-related problems or the need for perineal stitches.[120]

Births attended by MCA nurse-midwives involved referral to and therefore intervention by physicians more often than those attended by FNS nurse-midwives. However, all women who initially saw a nurse-midwife, whether in an urban or rural location, had fewer interventions in their births and were less likely to deliver in a hospital compared with women attended only by obstetricians. In the 1920s and 1930s, an obstetrician-attended birth almost always occurred in the hospital and involved routine interventions like forceps and heavy drugs.

In addition to thorough prenatal care and innovative labor-and-delivery care, McNaught and the other MCA nurse-midwives also provided extensive postnatal care. They visited patients in the home every afternoon, and nurses from Henry Street Settlement House—sent by MCA—visited patients every morning, for the first twelve days after delivery. MCA also asked patients to return to the clinic for medical examinations at the end of one and three months after giving birth, sending any postpartum patients with abnormalities to Sloane Hospital for Women.[121]

While many physicians promoted the safety of artificial food, sometimes arguing that it was better than breast milk, and while breastfeeding was on the decline among American mothers, MCA literature assumed that mothers would nurse their babies.[122] For example, the association's handbook for pregnant mothers and expectant fathers explained how to prepare breasts for breastfeeding, and concluded that formula feeding was like thievery:

> Of course 'mother's milk' really is 'baby's milk.' It belongs to the baby. Nature has made it for him, it is his best food and it is no use at all to the mother. It is stealing from a baby not to let him have his mother's milk, unless the doctor says that nursing will hurt the mother or that her milk is not good for the baby. Nursing is the easiest, cleanest and safest way to feed a baby. Breast fed babies are sick less often than

**Table 3.2** Maternity Center Association and Comparison Groups: Maternal Mortality Rate (per 10,000 births), 1932–1936[125]

| | |
|---|---|
| Maternity Center Association (1081 deliveries, 1 maternal death) | 10 |
| New York City | 104 |
| United States: | |
| Total population | 56.8–63.3 |
| White population | 51.2–58.1 |
| Non-white population | 89.7–97.6 |

> bottle fed babies. Bottle feeding is a great help—really a life-saver—when there is some good reason why a baby should not nurse. It is always a makeshift for the baby's best food. No mother who is trying to do her best for her baby would use it if she could help it.[123]

Another MCA handbook, for public-health nurses in obstetrics who led classes for expectant parents, "assumed that every mother intends to nurse her baby"; it told nurses to explain to mothers that breastfeeding causes the uterus to contract after birth and to "urge breast feeding" in special classes for fathers. This guide did suggest that nurses demonstrate how to make formula just in case a baby needed supplementary feedings or a mother could not breastfeed, but the demonstration showed that formula making was very cumbersome. In fact, the guide advised: "After this demonstration, it is well to comment on what is very obvious that the mother who can breast-feed her baby and not bother with formula is indeed fortunate."[124] Thus, at a time that many physicians discouraged breastfeeding, MCA nurse-midwives actively encouraged it.

As at FNS, MCA's comprehensive prenatal, labor-and-delivery, and postpartum care program made a difference in its patients' lives. Table 3.2 shows very low maternal mortality rates for Lobenstine Clinic patients, compared with the population of New York City and the nation as a whole. As with FNS, these rates are particularly impressive given that Lobenstine Clinic patients were generally poor, African American or Puerto Rican, and often lived in substandard housing, had poor health, and worked long hours in difficult jobs. As scholars have pointed out, race and ethnicity did not cause a higher risk of maternal death; rather the high percentage of these women who were poor, overworked, and unhealthy put them at risk.

Like FNS, MCA compiled statistics so that it could prove to the nation that its program of maternal and infant care was successful. Prior to its founding the nurse-midwifery school and clinic, MCA hired well-regarded statistician and Metropolitan Life Insurance Company vice president Louis I. Dublin, whom Mary Breckinridge had also employed for FNS. Dublin analyzed records from 1919 to 1921 for 8,743 patients receiving prenatal care from MCA nurses and postpartum care from Henry Street Settlement House, and he and MCA director Hazel Corbin compiled statistics on an MCA demonstration project between 1922 and 1929 that showcased the association's maternity work in a square mile in Manhattan.[126] Once MCA opened its nurse-midwifery clinic, it did statistical analysis in-house. Laird, medical director of MCA's nurse-midwifery service from 1931 to 1947, analyzed statistics on mortality and morbidity for patients cared for by MCA nurse-midwives between 1932 and 1936.[127] Obviously, the fact that MCA's nurse-midwifery service staff analyzed the data themselves could call into question the findings. However, there is no reason to believe that the data are false. MCA statistical evidence did show some maternal morbidity and mortality, and as a pioneer in nurse-midwifery, MCA had every reason not to want to hurt its reputation by developing faulty data.

## Conclusion

MCA's Lobenstine Midwifery School trained nurse-midwives who then went on to perform much-needed work as supervisors of traditional midwives and nurses throughout the United States, and the Lobenstine Midwifery Clinic provided maternity services to a poor, minority population in need of better care. One could imagine that MCA administrators and supporters would have wished to promote the organization's excellent, pioneering work in nurse-midwifery, especially given its skill at using media. From its beginning, MCA used the media to carry out its goal of "popular education"—to convince women that they needed to know more about pregnancy and childbirth to make maternity safer.[128] Using connections to New York City's elite, MCA pushed its agenda in pamphlets, books, billboards, radio talk shows, and even World's Fair exhibits. But while its annual reports explained the nurse-midwifery training offered at the Lobenstine School, MCA did not publicize this in its mass-media materials. MCA helped invent a new professional, the nurse-midwife, yet chose not to advertise her. More than that, MCA's media campaign pushed prospective mothers and fathers toward obstetricians, rather than promoting the new alternative to obstetricians MCA had helped create. Ultimately, MCA made the promotion of nurse-midwifery a lower priority than pushing women to seek early prenatal care.

Why did MCA make this choice? With the deep antagonism of most physicians toward anything "midwife" and the trend toward hospitalization of childbirth, it was politically safer not to promote the nurse-midwife and the Lobenstine Clinic's home-delivery service. Yet MCA had not shied away from controversy; its media materials discussed pregnancy and childbirth in an age when doing so was seen as "bad taste" and at times "obscene." In the 1930s, some newspapers prohibited the use of the word "pregnancy," and the New York State Board of Regents banned the film, *The Birth of a Baby*, produced with assistance from MCA, as "indecent, immoral, and tending to corrupt public morals."[129] MCA was a progressive organization dedicated to breaking down barriers to maternal health care. But MCA had several priorities. The nurse-midwifery service and school, although among MCA concerns, were so novel and radical that the organization decided not to use valuable media capital promoting them.

Like FNS's Mary Breckinridge, MCA physicians and nurses had to make compromises in establishing their pioneering nurse-midwifery school and clinic. They always had to be concerned about the attitudes of New York City's physicians and nurses. Physicians feared that nurse-midwives would be competitors and that they would lower the reputation of obstetrics. Nurses worried about stepping on physicians' toes and acting too much like physicians (read: independent practitioners) and not enough like nurses (read: assistants). In addition, they were concerned that the association of nurse-midwives with traditional midwives would lower nurses' reputation. Many physicians and nurses believed that midwives—whether traditional midwives or educated nurse-midwives—should no longer exist. After years of work and criticism from opponents, MCA leaders carefully crafted the new school and clinic so that they would offend the fewest people. They opened their school in the largest city in the United States to train women who would work only in the most remote areas of the country. Those women gained experience by providing maternity care for poor women of color—patients whom other health care providers did not want to serve.

# PART II

# Active Labor, 1940–1960

CHAPTER 4

# Transitions

## New Directions, New Limitations

### Introduction

As an unmarried woman who received multiple advanced degrees, Kate Hyder was unusual for her era but quite typical of prominent mid-twentieth-century nurse-midwives.[1] Born in 1905 in Hendersonville, North Carolina, Hyder received a bachelor's degree from the North Carolina College for Women (now the University of North Carolina, Greensboro) in 1925 and a nursing degree from the Johns Hopkins School of Nursing in 1928. She stayed at Johns Hopkins Hospital to work in obstetrics for five years and then worked at the Rockefeller Institute of Medical Research for several years. At that point, Hyder was lucky enough to receive a scholarship to attend Teachers College at Columbia University. As part of her master's program there, she studied midwifery for six months at Maternity Center Association's Lobenstine Midwifery School (where she received her nurse-midwifery certificate in 1936), attended Teachers College during the second semester, and then worked in public-health nursing in North Carolina for two years as part of her scholarship requirements. She then returned to her education at Teachers College, where she supervised and taught nurse-midwives until completing her master's degree in nursing in 1941.

In the years following her graduate education, Hyder held jobs in several places. With the support of Maternity Center Association (MCA), Hyder helped found a new and short-lived nurse-midwifery school for African-American nurses in New Orleans, which I will discuss in chapter 5. Following that, Hyder supervised midwives in Guatemala for a few years, and then directed the nursing service at Chicago Maternity Center, an innovative home-delivery service that provided a team of physicians, medical students, and nurses to attend the births of poor, urban women.[2] When she arrived at Yale University in 1946, Hyder took an appointment as assistant professor of the School of Nursing, as well as an administrator of nursing in the obstetric unit at the Grace–New Haven Community Hospital. There, over the next five years, Hyder, along with psychiatrist and pediatrician Edith Jackson and obstetrician Herbert Thoms, made radical changes in the hospital's approach to childbirth and the postpartum period.

Hyder first met Jackson at a weekly Wednesday tea for staff physicians and nurses, where the doctor quickly assessed her. After exchanging brief niceties, Jackson immediately cut to the chase: "How do you feel about breastfeeding?" Hyder answered correctly: "I feel very good about it." Jackson had already begun dreaming about her rooming-in project, a groundbreaking plan for newborns and mothers to stay together in the same rooms, making breastfeeding and bonding easier, and she hoped that Hyder would join her.

In fact, as Hyder recalled years later, she was well-prepared to advance the rooming-in concept even though she had never done anything like it in the hospital setting. As a nurse-midwife, she had managed home births where rooming-in occurred naturally and where most new mothers breastfed. She had attended home births in Harlem while a student at MCA and in North Carolina while working in public health. (As Hyder remembered, pregnant black women in North Carolina were essentially forced to give birth at home since southern hospitals only allowed them to give birth by the coal fire in the basement.) Her experiences with home births made Hyder "well-attuned" to the "pleasure" of having a new mother, her husband, and younger children together for the birth of a baby. Thus, Hyder joined Jackson's crusade.

Rooming-in faced initial opposition from physicians, nursing supervisors, and nurses, yet between 1946 and 1952, the Grace–New Haven Community Hospital successfully established a small rooming-in unit. Hyder was an essential factor in the realization of the project, convincing nurses of its value and turning Jackson's dreams into a workable plan. Although her nurse-midwifery background aided the project, she knew her training would not be understood or respected and she waited several years to reveal her nurse-midwife status to many of the physicians.

Hyder left Yale when the rooming-in project ended and continued her work as a professor of nursing, this time at the graduate school of Teachers College. Five years later, she left New York City, saying it was "too big a place for me." She joined the faculty of the University of Connecticut School of Nursing, from which she retired after fifteen years. In 1991, at age 86, Hyder died in Hamden, Connecticut, just a few miles from Yale.

Hyder was one of a number of nurse-midwives in the 1940s and 1950s who were moving in new directions. In the 1920s and 1930s, leaders at Frontier Nursing Service (FNS) and Maternity Center Association (MCA) had sought to improve American maternal and infant health care by enabling nurse-midwives to attend home births and supervise traditional midwives. Starting in the 1940s and escalating in the 1950s, nurse-midwives shifted their focus to hospitals, reflecting the nationwide trend toward hospital births. In hospitals, they brought their emphasis on the physical *and* emotional aspects of a new mother's birth experience and they pioneered the nation's first demonstrations in "natural childbirth," as well as the Yale "rooming-in" project. But the majority of nurse-midwifery school graduates working in hospitals did not actually work as nurse-midwives. Rather, they found employment in obstetrics as nurses, nursing supervisors, and instructors. These women did not have any of the independence, or even semi-independence, of nurse-midwives actually practicing the profession for which they had trained. Instead they served as subordinate nurses within the hospital hierarchy.

The mid-twentieth century also saw the expansion of nurse-midwifery with the development of educational programs at some of the nation's leading universities—Columbia, Johns Hopkins, Yale, and Downstate Medical Center, State University of New York—along with the creation of nurse-midwifery services at the hospitals affiliated with these universities. The expansion occurred because nurse-midwives wanted the opportunities and recognition that came with university affiliation, and hospitals, which had a shortage of obstetricians, needed more birth attendants in the wake of the baby boom. Additionally, a growing number of women demanded that more attention be paid to the emotional aspects of childbirth; this demand was better met by nurse-midwives than by any other type of practitioner. The expansion in educational programs translated into an increase in nurse-midwives. By 1963, approximately 750 women had graduated from American nurse-midwifery schools, a dramatic increase from approximately 225 in 1946.[3] Affiliation with major universities represented a modicum of mainstream acceptance of nurse-midwifery as well as an opportunity for a small group of women to practice hospital-based nurse-midwifery, but it also meant that nurse-midwives had to work within the confines and follow the dictates of university-affiliated hospitals.

## Moving into the Hospital

To understand why nurse-midwives moved to hospital employment, it is important to understand American childbirth in the 1940s and 1950s. As seen in table 4.1, the number of American births occurring in hospitals increased dramatically between 1935 and 1945 and continued to jump in the postwar era. Women increasingly wanted to deliver in hospitals, the growing centers of American medical care. As discussed in chapter 1, in the 1920s and 1930s, more and more white middle- and upper-class women went to the hospital to give birth, despite the fact that hospital births were more dangerous than home births. Hospital births only gradually became safer starting in the late 1930s and continuing into the 1940s and 1950s, with the introduction of new medical discoveries and techniques. The establishment of hospital blood banks, blood typing and transfusions decreased the risks associated with postpartum hemorrhage. The newly discovered oxytocin (a drug which hastened birth) counteracted anesthesia, which often slowed labor and asphyxiated the fetus. Heart monitoring machines detected fetal distress. X-ray pelvimetry led to early detection of pelvic deformities and other problems.[5] During and after World War II, widespread availability of penicillin and sulfa drugs, which inhibit bacterial infections, dramatically decreased the danger of puerperal infections.[6]

By World War II, hospitals and physicians were gaining increased prestige and authority. World War II strengthened the notion that the hospital was a place of science, with the latest technologies, diagnostic, preventive, and curative medicine, and specialized physician scientists. The wartime Office of Scientific Research and Development and its Committee on Medical Research funded and coordinated the development and production of penicillin in the United States, by connecting universities,

**Table 4.1** Percentage of American Births in Hospitals, 1935–1960[4]

| Year | Percentage of American Births in Hospitals |
|---|---|
| 1935 | 35.4 |
| 1945 | 78.8 |
| 1950 | 88 |
| 1960 | 96.6 |

government laboratories, and the pharmaceutical, chemical, and distilling industries. Widespread production and disbursement of penicillin effectively curbed infections caused by war wounds. Such nationally coordinated medical research to develop and produce penicillin was not unique; the war years saw an increased emphasis on scientific research in all aspects of pharmacology and medical practice. The need for hospital services to treat infectious disease decreased as a result of sulfa drugs and penicillin, but increased for chronic illnesses, such as heart disease, cancer, and strokes. Hospitals increasingly became places for the upper and middle classes to seek treatments and cures (often without success) for chronic disease, in hopes of prolonging life. General hospital admissions grew by nearly 32 percent between 1941 and 1946, and by 26 percent between 1946 and 1952.[7] In the postwar years, hospitals grew further as a result of the Hospital Survey and Reconstruction Act (known as the Hill-Burton Act for its two sponsoring senators, Lister Hill and Harold Burton), signed by Harry Truman in 1946. Hill-Burton provided federal assistance to states for the renovation or construction of hospitals and health centers, reinforcing the belief that the more hospital services Americans had access to, the better off they would be.[8] The program resulted in a massive growth of public hospitals, especially in rural areas and small towns that lacked voluntary or proprietary hospitals. The bill, both indirectly and directly, dramatically increased hospital services to the indigent.[9]

As access to private health insurance increased from the 1930s through the postwar period so did use of hospital services. Prior to the 1930s, very few Americans had private health insurance. This changed with the development of two provider-controlled health plans, or insurance controlled by hospitals and physicians: Blue Cross, hospital insurance, in 1929, and the less popular Blue Shield, medical (or physician) insurance, in the late 1930s. Whereas Blue Cross resulted from rising costs of hospital care and the inability of patients to cover these fees, Blue Shield evolved in response to physicians' desire to prevent adoption of government-controlled health insurance.[10] The postwar period saw the expansion of employer-provided private health insurance as a way to recruit and retain employees. This expansion also occurred because labor unions won the right to bargain collectively for health benefits and because commercial insurance companies grew rapidly.[11] In 1946, one-third of Americans had some kind of private hospital insurance, the most common type of insurance; 50 percent had coverage by 1950, and 75 percent by 1960. Thus, during the postwar era, more Americans, especially the middle class, gained access to the new technologies and therapeutics found in modern hospitals.[12]

During World War II, the federal Emergency Maternity and Infant Care (EMIC) program, which was created to pay for the births of servicemen's babies, also encouraged hospital deliveries. This wartime service provided maternity care for over 1,203,500 military wives, and medical, nursing, and hospital care for their infants through age one.[13] The federal government funded EMIC, and state and local health departments administered it. The program did not require either physicians or wives to participate, and the patients could choose which physicians to use.[14] The EMIC program paid fifty dollars for prenatal, intranatal, and postnatal care to general practitioners, less than the going rate in large cities but more than in some smaller cities and rural areas; the program paid more to obstetricians.[15] EMIC enabled many women to deliver in hospitals, who otherwise could not have afforded to do so. A wartime anthropological study of maternity care in a rural New Mexican community found: "With World War II came the EMIC program providing many Spanish-American mothers with their first experience of a hospital delivery. For many it proved a happy one and carried with it prestige, making a subsequent delivery at the hospital imperative, even without the aid of federal funds."[16] Thus hospitals drew in parturient women, through wartime government funding of maternity care, the expansion of hospitals and health insurance, and women's own desires for safety and access to the best of medical science.[17]

At the same time hospitals were attracting women, creating a need for more personnel in hospital obstetrics, the number and use of practicing traditional midwives declined, reducing the need for nurse-midwives as supervisors and trainers. The number of midwives in the rural South decreased after 1950 due to several factors: state efforts to promote professional rather than lay attendance at birth, African-American migration to urban areas, and African-American women's lessening desire to use traditional midwives when public hospitals and welfare were available.[18]

The war caused a shortage of health-care personnel, "with doctors and nurses being plucked from our civilian ranks like petals off a daisy," explained Hazel Corbin, MCA's director.[19] Corbin's colleague, Hattie Hemschemeyer, director of MCA's Lobenstine Midwifery School, discussed the specific problem of wartime obstetrics in a 1942 issue of the *American Journal of Nursing*, stating that "most of [the] obstetricians were located in and around big cities, and the war has made an already poor distribution of medical service even worse." Hemschemeyer concluded: "the idea that every mother should have her personal obstetrician doesn't hold water when we look at the figures."[20] After the war, the United States continued to experience a shortage of health-care providers, created by hospital expansion, the growth of chronic care, and increases in Americans' visits to providers due to economic prosperity and popular and medical optimism about cures for disease. Expanding technologies and services especially prompted the need for more nurses.[21] This factor also contributed to nurse-midwives' move to the hospital.

Some obstetricians wanted nurse-midwives to work in hospitals, both to help patients have what they viewed as better birthing experiences and to allow obstetricians to pursue other interests. Recording the previous year's accomplishments and coming year's goals, the MCA's Medical Advisory Board's annual report for 1958 recommended increased use of nurse-midwives as part of the hospital "obstetric team" to make possible the provision of "educational and emotionally supportive facets of maternity care which are acknowledged to be desirable but are for the most part unobtainable for lack of qualified personnel." According to the Board, "with the steadily rising birth rate, there are not, and will not in the foreseeable future be enough obstetricians to provide continuous, comprehensive maternity care to the expectant mothers of this country, particularly those cared for on overtaxed ward services." Male obstetricians' "combined work load of private practice and hospital duties often makes it impossible to give each patient the time and continuous personal attention conducive to the best possible results, in terms of mental and physical health, on both an immediate and a long term basis." The Board argued that female nurse-midwives could provide that attention, thus "reducing the obstetrician's work load" and "releas[ing] him for the teaching and clinical research needed to ensure a continued improvement in maternity care."[22]

The postwar baby boom also contributed to a need for more hospital personnel. During the Depression and the war, many Americans had postponed marriage and childbearing. This changed dramatically in the postwar years with the "baby boom," which reached its height in 1957. Between 1945 and 1960, the United States population increased by around forty million, or 30 percent, creating enormous strains on hospital obstetrics departments.[23]

Finally, women's frustrations with the hospital birthing experiences helped create a place for nurse-midwives. Seeking safety and the benefits of scientific progress, increasing numbers of women during the war and postwar years had given birth in the hospital. Yet, many of these women found hospital births alienating. Removed from their homes, parturient women missed the traditional support systems their family members and friends provided, and they often disliked analgesics and forceps, which hospitals commonly used. Women felt safer delivering their babies in hospitals, but missed the "tender loving care" that was such an integral part of delivering at home.[24] According to Hazel Corbin, the "mechanization of maternity care" left women feeling like sick patients, rather than healthy laboring women; alone, without the support of family and the comforts of home; and as though "things were done *to* her, not *with* her."[25]

For laboring women, physicians, and nurses themselves, obstetric nurses were part of the problem. As historian of childbirth Judith Walzer Leavitt has explained, patients often blamed obstetric nurses for what they saw as impersonal, unpleasant birthing experiences.[26] Mothers found nurses more focused on hospital routines and efficient procedures than on their individual needs.[27] The tension may have stemmed from the fact that physicians and hospital administrators demanded that different nurses care for an individual woman in labor, delivery, and the postpartum period rather than the same nurse staying with a laboring woman throughout the process. Hospitals also dictated that nurses serve as physicians' assistants and follow doctors' orders, even though they might have made different decisions about a woman's care had they been acting independently as did the nurse-midwives who worked for such services as FNS with little supervision and much success. Finally, hospitals demanded that nurses focus on procedures laboring women often dreaded and which were unnecessary from a medical standpoint, such as giving enemas or shaving pubic hair, rather than on simply spending time with their patients providing moral support in addition to physical care.[28]

Due to widespread criticism of obstetric nursing, and nurse-midwives' disagreement with obstetric nurses' approach to maternity care, nurse-midwives, and their supporters, carefully distinguished their work from traditional obstetric nursing. Nurse-midwives made clear that they attended to patients from the first sign of labor through the postpartum period, taking time to stay with one patient continuously, to help family members adjust to the new arrival, and to provide support for the family and mother in dealing with the parturient woman's normal but occasionally alarming emotional upheavals.[29] Especially in the late 1940s and early 1950s, nurse-midwives emphasized that they, as opposed to typical obstetric nurses, focused on the psychological and emotional aspects of childbirth. As one MCA-trained nurse-midwife working in a major medical center explained, "midwifery education does not just develop the nurse as clinician, skillful in observation and judgment of the laboring woman's physical progress. It makes it possible for her to see childbirth in its total context of family life and human values." While obstetric nurses had to offer routinized, or what Corbin called "mechanized" care, nurse-midwives "raise[d] nursing care in labor to a creative art, always changing to meet the demands of the individuals in the specific situation."[30] Similarly, an MCA publication explained, "Great progress, as expressed in mortality rates, was undoubtedly made in American obstetrics in the past thirty years. In the stress on primary objectives of safety, however, too little attention was paid to the social and emotional aspects of childbearing and their influence on family life. The nurse-midwife is helping to restore the emphasis on patient-centered care and total health of mother and child."[31]

The publication argued that the nurse-midwife could "supply something valuable which had previously been lacking in hospital maternity care, and which the obstetricians did not have the time, nor the unprepared nurse the specialized education, to provide."[32] By 1952, Corbin claimed nurse-midwives, "though few in number," were the "torch bearers," changing maternity care from "the 'obstetrical factory'" and the "delivery room where every professional is an impersonal, masked automaton," to personal care emphasizing the individual needs of mothers, fathers, and newborns.[33] Corbin wrote numerous articles in nursing journals decrying the lack of attention paid to women's emotional needs and hoping to change nurses' and physicians' attitudes toward pregnant, laboring, and postpartum women.[34] She and other MCA staff and students believed nurse-midwives could help women reclaim support and control over their births.

Despite nurse-midwives' claims about their differences from obstetric nurses, most nurse-midwifery school graduates who worked in hospitals in the 1940s and 1950s were invisible because they were not practicing nurse-midwives.[35] Instead, they worked as obstetric nurses, obstetric nursing supervisors, or instructors of obstetric nursing. While these women applied their nurse-midwifery experience to their hospital-based nursing jobs, their patients, fellow health-care personnel, and the public rarely knew that the women staffing these positions had trained as nurse-midwives. In fact, it is difficult to find information about the typical hospital nurse-midwives of this era because most of the records do not differentiate between them and nurses who did not have nurse-midwifery training.[36]

Available records suggest that nurse-midwifery school graduates who worked in hospitals found their nurse-midwifery background provided them with broader experience in maternity care than they had received in nursing school; this experience gave them much-needed skills and confidence for their work in hospital maternity wards and nursing schools. For example, Barbara Sklar Laster, a 1948 graduate of MCA's Lobenstine

Midwifery School, said that in her job as an obstetric and general duty nurse at Detroit's Deaconess Hospital, "I worked nights by myself in [the] labor and delivery ward for 1 yr. Midwifery taught me to do rectals, determine progress and detect abnormalities in labor."[37] Mildred Disbrow, a 1950 graduate of FNS's nurse-midwifery school, found her nurse-midwifery experience very helpful in her position as supervisor of obstetric nursing at a Pittsburgh-area hospital. Because the institution had no medical interns or residents, the "supervisor assumed much responsibility for labor management." Disbrow also noted that her nurse-midwifery training augmented her teaching when she became a professor of obstetric nursing at the University of Pittsburgh. It helped her "in teaching total care since as a midwife one stays with [the patient] in her home throughout labor" and in taking a "better public health approach" with maternity patients.[38]

However, a nurse-midwifery background could also lead to frustration for women working in hospitals, since what they had come to see both as an ideal birthing experience and an ideal professional experience were often impossible to achieve in the postwar hospital setting. Hospital nurses were not in charge of new mothers from pregnancy through the postpartum period and thus could not practice their sustained, holistic approach to the prenatal, labor-and-delivery, and postpartum stages of pregnancy. Additionally, they sometimes encountered barriers while trying to use their education. As nurses and nursing instructors, they were expected to live up to and teach the traditional nursing ideals of subservience; yet they often felt such conservativism in the hospital setting did patients a disservice. For example, Aileen I. Hogan, who followed graduation from Lobenstine School in 1947 with a three-year stint as chair of maternity nursing at the Frances Payne Bolton School of Nursing at Western Reserve University (now Case Western Reserve University) in Cleveland, said that while her nurse-midwifery experience provided essential "background and authority in teaching," it was "also quite frustrating" for her to be "10 years ahead of current practice" and not be allowed to implement her training and experience with hospital patients.[39] Like Hazel Corbin and other nurse-midwives, Hogan criticized maternity nursing, believing that many hospital maternity nurses were not well rounded and well trained like nurse-midwives and that they did not provide new mothers with "a sense of continuity of care."[40] Despite Hogan's criticisms, she and other hospital nurse-midwives who worked as nurses or nursing instructors must have continued (whether by choice or dictate) at least some and perhaps many of the hospital routines that depersonalized maternity patients. And while

Hogan ultimately departed the hospital setting, too frustrated with the barriers she encountered, those who stayed may have internalized some of the more rigid maternity nursing values even as they tried to change them. At the very least, they would have had to adhere to traditional nursing practices as a way to maintain their employment in hospitals that required such obedience to protocol.

## Pioneers in Natural Childbirth

One small group of nurse-midwifery graduates who worked in hospitals made a significant contribution to hospital births by pioneering "natural childbirth" in the United States. In 1947, MCA brought British obstetrician Grantly Dick-Read (1890–1959), who invented the concept and practice of natural childbirth in 1933, to the United States for the first time.[41] According to Read, modern women had been conditioned from childhood to fear childbirth, but could be taught to undo that conditioning through education and relaxation techniques. Once a woman was fully aware of what would happen to her, she could eliminate her fear—and thereby her pain—along with the need for pain-relieving medications. Beginning later the same year Read arrived, MCA nurse-midwives instructed patients in preparation for natural childbirth, offering classes to first-time mothers who registered at MCA for home delivery and eventually to interested mothers who had attended MCA mothers' classes and planned to give birth at local hospitals. Graduates from Lobenstine School also staffed natural childbirth demonstrations in New Haven and New York City hospitals in the late 1940s and early 1950s. With extensive attention from the media, including articles titled "I Watched My Baby Born" and "Natural Childbirth: Young Mother Has Her Baby with No Fear, Little Pain," MCA staff and MCA graduates set up the nation's first "natural childbirth" classes, initiating a trend that would become significant in the 1970s and remains so in the present.[42]

Historians explain that natural childbirth's popularity among American women was related to decreases in maternal mortality that had become widespread by the mid-twentieth century. Women felt, and indeed were, safer in childbirth than ever before; thus, they and their health-care providers could concentrate on more psychological aspects of birth.[43] This new focus led to "natural childbirth," which offered an alternative to increasingly mechanized, anesthetized, and impersonal hospital births.

MCA nurse-midwives began to offer their patients prenatal education in natural childbirth for two reasons. First, nurse-midwives' long-standing values and beliefs fit well with the requirements of the natural childbirth method. Since the 1920s, nurse-midwifery organizations had espoused the normality of pregnancy and labor and valued an investment of time and close personal relationships with patients.[44] Second, the natural childbirth method appealed to nurse-midwives because it gave them a definite role in hospital obstetrics. Although nurse-midwives still attended the births of many poor women in their homes, their role as home-birth attendant and supervisor of "granny" midwives had diminished. They created a new niche for themselves: improving obstetric nursing in the hospital. Part of their improvement plan included introducing the new method of natural childbirth. Genuinely believing in the benefits of natural childbirth, nurse-midwives thought their special skills and training would enable them to be experts in and teachers of the method.

MCA nurse-midwives based their instruction on Read's *Childbirth without Fear* (1944) and on *Training for Childbirth* (1945) by Minnie Randall, a British nurse and physical therapist. In fall 1947, Helen Heardman, a British physical therapist who had worked with Read and other British obstetricians, came to MCA and helped reshape MCA's approach toward natural childbirth. Because Read's book dealt mostly with theory and not with specific ways to help patients, Heardman focused on practice. She taught MCA nurse-midwives exercises and relaxation techniques for women in the prenatal period and in labor and delivery. Beginning in fall 1948, MCA opened its natural childbirth classes to all women registered for home delivery through its nurse-midwifery service, and to those attending mothers' classes at MCA who were interested in or whose obstetricians had requested that they prepare for natural childbirth. MCA provided a series of six classes, lasting one-and-one-half hours each, for nurse-midwives to explain the principles of natural childbirth, including "the hard work required of the mother during labor," "the persistent effort she must make during pregnancy to acquire patience, self-control, and ability to relax and carry through to the end," and "the satisfactions of being awake to participate in the baby's birth progress and hear its first cry as soon as it is born." They also taught breathing and relaxation exercises.

Pregnant women wore loose clothing so they could participate fully in the exercises, designed to help women "utilize breathing in the relaxation of their bodies and minds" and "strengthen the muscles which are active in labor, to increase their elasticity, improve their tone, and use them purposefully." Women were to practice these exercises at home, preferably with their husbands, and sometimes even their children. MCA titled the last class, "Rehearsal for Labor," in which pregnant women learned about the sensations and procedures they would experience throughout the course of labor. In this last class, women practiced the breathing and exercises in the actual positions hospitals expected them to assume during the first and second stages of labor. Advocates of natural childbirth believed women must understand the natural childbirth method thoroughly to have a satisfying birth, for "upon completion of these classes, a report of each mother's participation and performance is sent to the doctor who requested her attendance at the series."[45]

Natural childbirth provided MCA nurse-midwives entrée to hospital obstetrics as nurse-midwives. The nurse-midwives created a *raison d'être* for themselves, arguing they "filled a gap in existing maternity services, helping the hospital and obstetrician to provide more complete and satisfying care to expectant mothers and their families."[46] MCA staff believed that nursing education, even graduate education in nursing, did not prepare nurses well to care for maternity patients. As an MCA publication explained, "A few leaders in obstetric nursing education recognized how inadequate the available preparation was to provide either satisfying service to the mother or professional gratification to the nurse. Those who had first-hand experience with nurse-midwifery and the use of nurse-midwives in public health work realized that here was a possible answer to some of the major problems in obstetric nursing education and patient care."[47]

In the late 1940s and early 1950s, MCA participated in two hospital demonstrations of natural childbirth, one at Grace–New Haven Community Hospital and the other at Columbia-Presbyterian Medical Center. From 1948 to 1949, MCA, in cooperation with Yale University's Schools of Medicine and Nursing and Grace–New Haven Community Hospital, participated in a widely reported demonstration of the principles of natural childbirth run by Herbert Thoms (1889–1972), chief of obstetrics and gynecology at Yale University.

This first demonstration took place outside New York City, in part because of MCA's inability to get enough obstetricians at a New York hospital to start a demonstration.[48] Eight nurse-midwives, all graduates of the Lobenstine School, served in the Connecticut hospital, two at a time for six months each, financed by MCA. Two physicians, also subsidized by MCA, worked with them. MCA nurse-midwives instructed patients in this experiment in six prenatal classes, offering one lecture and two exercise classes during the early stages of pregnancy, and another lecture and two more exercise classes on labor and delivery in the last month of pregnancy. The last class included a tour of the labor and delivery rooms in the hospital.[49]

Yale's natural childbirth demonstration coincided with its pioneering Rooming-In Research Project run by psychiatrist and pediatrician Edith Jackson and nurse-midwife Kate Hyder. Many women who used natural childbirth also tried rooming-in and breastfeeding. At first, most Yale physicians and nurses opposed rooming-in. As Hyder explained, the obstetricians opposed it because they "didn't think the mothers needed to know anything more than what they told them," and the nurses were afraid of change. Typically, obstetric nurses knew about mothers but not babies and nursery nurses knew about babies but not mothers. The rooming-in project required that nurses perform tasks that they had not been trained to do—work with mothers and newborns together, and the nursing supervisors feared that the project might necessitate the use of more nurses during a terrible nursing shortage.[50]

Despite resistance to rooming-in, Hyder and the physicians opened a small unit from 1946 to 1952. As Grace–New Haven Community Hospital's director during this era suggested, Hyder may have been the key to the project's success. She succeeded in convincing the nursing supervisor and the nurses in maternity and nursery services—all of whom were originally opposed to this seemingly radical idea—of its advantages. Hyder completed a time study showing that one nurse spent less time caring for four mothers and babies together than did separate obstetric and nursery nurses working in the more typical manner. She also began the rooming-in unit with a graduate nurse and Yale nursing students who supported the idea, so that the unit's first employees were people unused to traditional hospital routines and therefore not afraid of change.[51]

In addition, Hyder served as a bridge between Jackson's rooming-in ideals and the reality of hospital routines. For example, Jackson wanted the mother to nurse her baby whenever the baby needed to be fed, even if a nurse had just brought the mother a tray of food. But Hyder explained to Jackson that this could not work because if the mother did not eat right then, the tray would be taken away because no staff member was available to reheat it. So Hyder came up with that she saw as a solution: "the nurse on the ward would come and pick up the baby and pat it and try to placate it until [the mother] had finished eating." Hyder believed that this was the way "to keep the mother happy but liv[e] within the routine of the hospital."[52] She was more realist than revolutionary, making an unorthodox project work within conservative hospital routines and among staff afraid of change, while subtly refusing to push for Jackson's true goal: total priority placed on the breastfeeding relationship between mother and newborn.

Unlike the MCA-Yale demonstration, MCA's second attempt to promote natural childbirth did not coincide with a rooming-in project. From 1951 to 1952, MCA sponsored a natural childbirth demonstration in conjunction with Columbia-Presbyterian Medical Center at the Sloane Hospital for Women. An MCA nurse-midwife, who had spent six months at the Grace–New Haven project, conducted the study. She acquainted herself with the staff, procedures, and attitudes toward parents at the hospital, finding that many nurses had already attended MCA for instruction on preparing mothers for natural childbirth, and welcomed the opportunity for other nurses to receive this preparation. The MCA–Columbia-Presbyterian program for preparation in childbirth began with a series of six classes for mothers, each lasting an hour and a half. Later in the study, mothers and fathers received instruction together. The nurse-midwife in charge analyzed the deliveries of three different groups: randomly selected registrants in the prenatal clinic who were asked if they wanted to attend natural childbirth classes and did so; randomly selected registrants in the prenatal clinic who expressed initial interest but chose not to attend the classes because they could not find child care for their other children, were unable to speak English, or lost interest; and women who explicitly sought instruction in natural childbirth. The medical and nursing staff always offered medication "whenever the patient showed any sign of stress or increasing discomfort." They found that patients who attended the classes required fewer analgesics and smaller dosages than those who did not attend the classes, although the majority of patients in all groups used some Demerol, Seconal, and/or scopolamine.

The nurse-midwife and obstetrician who coauthored the study concluded that natural childbirth aided both the family and the hospital, strengthening parents' ties to one another and helping them "develop a family feeling about the baby." It also brought together various specialists within the hospital, creating less anxiety and "more intelligent cooperation" of patients with physicians. Significantly, many of the prepared patients were probably middle-class. The non-English speakers and those who could not find baby-sitting made up a large percentage of those choosing not to attend the natural childbirth classes.[53] At the end of the two-year demonstration, the nurse-midwife became a full-time member of the nursing faculty at Sloane Hospital for Women, "ensuring continuation of the program."[54]

MCA solicited letters from women who took natural childbirth classes at MCA demonstration sites from around 1947 to 1951. Unlike many of nurse-midwives' earlier clientele, who were poor and often from racial or ethnic minorities, most of these letter writers were middle class, and most likely white. The letters, which are an invaluable source for patients' perspectives, reveal that natural childbirth provided choices to women who were unhappy with the existing childbirth options.[55] The majority of the women who wrote to MCA about their natural childbirth expressed satisfaction with the method, saying that it gave them a sense of security and control, support during labor and delivery, an immediate connection with their newborns, and reduction or elimination of fear.

A physician's daughter explained that after reading *Childbirth without Fear*, she wanted to deliver as a "Read patient." Delivering without anesthesia or analgesia, she reported, "I honestly had no pain at all and have never been through such a miraculous experience in all my life. I watched the entire process in the anaesthetist's mirror." She followed her natural childbirth with a stay in the rooming-in unit where her baby slept in a crib next to her.[56] A nurse whose husband was a medical student also sang the praises of natural childbirth because she enjoyed "the privilege of being aware and of seeing what was taking place." Like the physician's daughter, the nurse followed her birth with rooming-in, "complet[ing] an unbelievably enjoyable hospital experience."[57] The wife of a Yale student who delivered naturally and roomed-in with her infant emphasized three aspects of her birth experience that she especially enjoyed. First, she had one nurse throughout her labor, giving her "a sense of security to have someone know just what was happening and of the progress I was making. She explained what was occurring and what could be expected." Second, she was reassured by the use of the word "contractions," rather than "pains." Third, she found "the mirror over the delivery table . . . very reassuring. It meant I could see exactly what was happening and all fear was removed."[58] The natural childbirth method appealed to these women because it offered them an alternative to the typical postwar childbirth experience, providing them with awareness during and immediately after the birth, emotional support, immediate bonding with their baby, and the promise of decreased pain.[59]

Ironically, nurse-midwives who were still delivering babies at home or supervising traditional midwives knew more about natural childbirth—if "natural" is defined as "present in or produced in nature"—than those employed at the Yale or Sloane natural childbirth demonstrations.[60] At home, birth tended to involve less technology and fewer interventions; in other words, there was less "science" and more "nature." At hospitals, pioneering nurse-midwives and physicians involved in natural childbirth tried in some ways to recreate what had been typical in other settings, cultures, and eras.

Although nurse-midwives taught natural childbirth at relatively few hospitals in the late 1940s and early 1950s and although other health professionals soon became involved in establishing natural childbirth classes, avant-garde nurse-midwives set the stage for a rethinking of childbirth practices in U.S. hospitals.[61] In the 1970s, the feminist, women's health, and consumer movements combined to produce a new interest in natural childbirth. Increasing numbers of women demanded their right to be fully awake and aware during delivery and condemned what they saw as misogynistic medical practices controlling a fundamentally important and defining event in their lives as women. Today, shifting norms and values have caused a change; women are no longer given an amnesiac whereby they forget the childbirth experience as was typical in the mid-twentieth century.[62] Now, most of the drugs given to women during labor, such as epidurals, allow them to participate consciously in the birth of their babies. Some women want their births to involve as few interventions as possible and actively seek out health practitioners who will support them in their approach.

## Hospital Demonstrations and New University Programs

In the mid- to late 1950s, nurse-midwives accelerated their move into the hospital by creating nurse-midwifery educational programs at three major university medical centers, Columbia, Johns Hopkins, and Yale, all of which had large teaching hospitals associated with them. The heads of obstetrics and gynecology departments at the large hospitals associated with these university medical centers welcomed the opportunity for nurse-midwives to attend the skyrocketing numbers of baby boom births, which obstetric residents were unable to handle on their own. Additionally, in 1958, MCA closed its home-delivery service due to women's decreased interest in home birth, and simultaneously moved its School of Nurse-Midwifery to Downstate Medical Center, State University of New York in Brooklyn, New York, using Kings County Hospital for students' clinical experience. The nurse-midwives working at these four university medical centers were unique: unlike other nurse-midwives working in hospitals in this era, these women actually worked in hospital nurse-midwifery services and practiced hospital-based nurse-midwifery.

MCA heavily influenced the four new programs. Columbia, Johns Hopkins, and Downstate Medical Center were directly affiliated with MCA, and their nurse-midwifery directors were graduates of the Lobenstine School. Although not directly affiliated, Yale's program had several important connections to the association, including the Yale-MCA natural childbirth program that laid the groundwork for the school, and Ernestine Wiedenbach, the administrator of Yale's nurse-midwifery program, who was a Lobenstine alumna and had worked at MCA. Given MCA's influence, it is no surprise that the four programs were interconnected. Nurse-midwifery students at one institution often gained additional clinical experience at one or all of the other three institutions.

The four programs had a number of similarities. Columbia, Johns Hopkins, and Yale had conducted earlier demonstrations with nurse-midwives, either natural childbirth programs or pilot nurse-midwifery services, before opening schools of nurse-midwifery and placing students in their affiliated hospitals. Nurse-midwives worried about convincing not only fellow health professionals but also expectant mothers of their value, given that by this time most American mothers expected physician management of pregnancy and birth. Thus the programs claimed that the earlier demonstrations proved the efficacy using nurse-midwife students and staff to work with normal cases, and that the nurse-midwives convinced their necessary audiences of this success. The programs trained students to stay with mothers throughout labor—which was atypical for nurses and physicians in this period (and even today)—and to emphasize emotional aspects of childbirth. They all received extensive support from chiefs of obstetrics and gynecology in their institutions. In particular, Nicholson Eastman from Johns Hopkins and Louis Hellman from Downstate Medical Center were nurse-midwife enthusiasts, believing that nurse-midwives provided excellent, personalized care and that they were essential to resolving the huge shortages in obstetric personnel.

Nurse-midwives and physicians working at these major medical centers challenged hospital routines in childbirth and assumptions about the necessity for predominantly male physician management of childbirth. They reflected frustrations with current trends in hospital-based, obstetrician-managed childbirth, and they showed that the "male medical model" of medicine and science did not go unchallenged in the mid-twentieth century. These nurse-midwives and physicians worked within the system to challenge existing norms, which meant that their challenge was fundamentally conservative. They worked and led departments at the top medical and nursing schools in the United States, they certainly

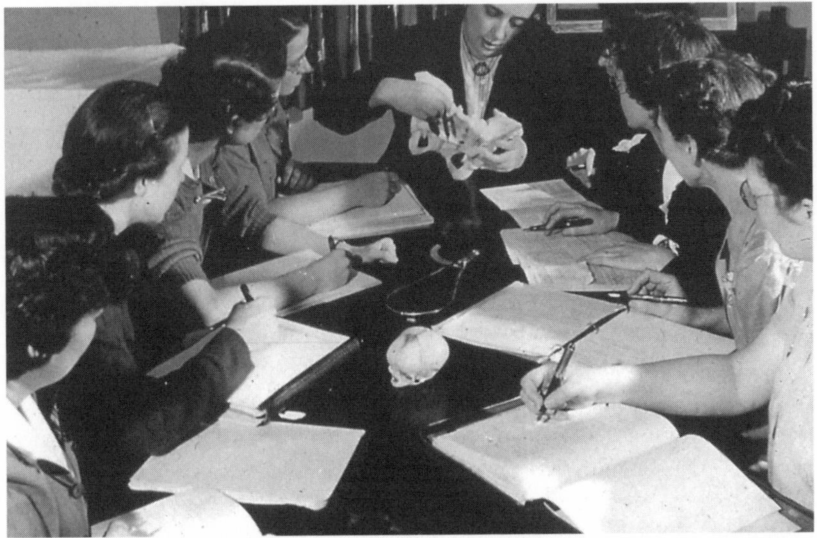

FIGURE 8. Class of student nurse-midwives at Columbia University, c. 1960. From the personal collection of Helen Varney Burst, CNM; originally from the Maternity Center Association.

believed in the value of obstetricians managing birth, and they had to make compromises in order for nurse-midwives to be accepted. But perhaps working *within* the system made the challenges offered by nurse-midwives and physicians associated with the new nurse-midwifery programs especially subversive. They challenged the rules, written and unwritten, in the very institutions that influenced larger trends in American medicine.

## *Columbia*

In 1955, Columbia University's School of Nursing established a nurse-midwifery program, in cooperation with MCA, Columbia's School of Public Health and Administrative Medicine, and the Presbyterian Hospital in New York City. This program was administered by two MCA nurse-midwives and one registered nurse. Students took either an eight-month course to receive a certificate in nurse-midwifery or a twelve-month course to receive simultaneously a master of science in nursing and a certificate in nurse-midwifery. Master's students majored in public health or hospital nursing.[63] Students received clinical experience at Sloane Hospital for

Women (which was part of the Columbia-Presbyterian Medical Center), as well as at MCA before it closed its home-delivery service in 1958, and at Kings County Hospital once MCA transferred its work to that location.[64]

Columbia laid the groundwork for its nurse-midwifery educational program in two ways. First, as discussed earlier, it conducted a demonstration in natural childbirth classes. After the demonstration ended in 1953, Margaret Hogan, Lobenstine alumna and coordinator of the Sloane demonstration, became a full-time faculty member at Columbia's School of Nursing. Then, "with the cooperation of the medical and administrative staffs," she worked with two nurse-midwives from MCA to develop a nurse-midwifery program and advanced maternity nursing at Columbia.[65] Second, in January 1954, Columbia tried a pilot nurse-midwifery service at Sloane. Nurse-midwives staffed prenatal clinics for women whose pregnancies were expected to be normal and who received approval from an attending or resident obstetrician. Obstetricians saw the expectant mothers in the sixth and ninth months of pregnancy and if any abnormalities appeared. Deemed a success, "these [prenatal] clinics fitted in well with the hospital's clinic and educational program." The "medical results were comparable to those in the rest of the service," and "not one mother refused" the program once it was explained—in fact, "many who were passive at the start evinced interest and satisfaction as their care progressed." Later that year, MCA registered twelve expectant mothers to deliver at Sloane with a nurse-midwife. However, "instead of allowing the nurse-midwife to assume full responsibility under the supervision of the medical staff as long as progress remained normal, the resident assumed full responsibility, wrote all of the orders, and scrubbed in with the nurse-midwife for delivery." By spring 1955, though, the obstetricians must have decided that they trusted the nurse-midwives because they allowed the nurse-midwives to deliver the babies of ten of the twelve mothers registered.[66]

In September 1955, after slowly paving the way, the Columbia-MCA program began granting master's degrees in maternity nursing and certificates in nurse-midwifery. According to its 1957–1958 course catalogue, students learned to be "specialist[s] on the obstetric team," managing all phases of pregnancy and childbirth, "with medical guidance," in normal cases, and providing and supervising care of newborns. Students provided "not only expert obstetric care, but [also] education of the expectant parents for their role, preparation of the mother for the labor experience, skilled attendance and emotional support throughout labor, and integration of maternity care with good family living." Program sponsors believed that nurses needed nurse-midwifery education if they intended to perform certain jobs, such as teachers of expectant parents, consultants in maternal and child health, supervisors of public-health nurses or hospital maternity departments, obstetrics instructors in nursing schools, instructors and directors of nurse-midwifery schools, and supervisors and teachers of traditional midwives.[67] The master's program, which some students took in conjunction with the nurse-midwifery certificate, required students to take a wide array of classes to gain a broader knowledge of the administration of hospitals or public-health agencies. Located in one of the nation's premier nursing schools, this program was innovative because it taught student nurse-midwives in a university setting and provided them with practical experience at a major urban hospital.

## *Johns Hopkins*

In 1956, MCA helped establish another university-affiliated program at Johns Hopkins University, administered in partnership with the Department of Obstetrics of the Johns Hopkins University School of Medicine and Johns Hopkins Hospital. This program's international focus made it unique. For the first three-and-one-half years, the Johns Hopkins Hospital received funding from the China Medical Board of New York "to train as many foreign students as possible, as well as American nurses planning to serve abroad," to work in maternal and child health in underdeveloped countries.[68] After that time, the hospital received funding from the United States Children's Bureau.[69] By April 1961, forty-six of the first eighty students who had completed the Hopkins program worked outside the United States, mostly in Africa.[70]

Like Columbia, Hopkins conducted a pilot program with nurse-midwives prior to establishing a nurse-midwifery school. In this program, nurse-midwives were called "obstetric assistants." Although the title seemed to link them tightly with obstetricians, they were no more or less independent than nurse-midwives in other programs. At the prenatal clinic, the obstetrics professor was always present, but the obstetric assistants "assumed complete responsibility" for the prenatal care of mothers whose pregnancies and deliveries were expected to be normal. The obstetric assistants also handled deliveries of these patients, with "medical consultation and supervision . . . available as needed," and they took responsibility for postpartum care as well. The pilot program worked; after the first six months, only two of 114 mothers refused to register with the obstetric assistants.[71]

After this success, Hopkins founded a nurse-midwifery educational certificate program under the direction of Nicholson Eastman, chief of obstetrics at Johns Hopkins Hospital, Sara Fetter, Lobenstine alumna and director of the Hopkins nurse-midwifery program, and Hattie Hemschemeyer, associate director of MCA.[72] All Hopkins students took courses and received clinical experience at both MCA and Hopkins—with four months spent in New York City and four months in Baltimore; thus in the early years they learned about both home and hospital deliveries, until MCA discontinued its home-delivery service.[73] Students took courses in medical issues—Normal Obstetrics, Problems and Complications in Obstetrics, and Anesthesia and Analgesia. They also learned to work with parents—Preparation for Group Work with Parents and Marriage Counseling, and in different employment settings—Midwifery in Developing Countries, Administration for Nurse-Midwifery Education, Introduction to Public Health, and Maternal and Child Health Service. At Johns Hopkins Hospital, a team of three, which included the director of the nurse-midwifery program, a nurse-midwife instructor, and the assistant resident, met every month to decide which expectant mothers should be transferred to the nurse-midwifery service for their maternity care. Patients were then given an option between the nurse-midwifery service and the medical service (conducted by obstetricians and medical residents), with the fees being the same for both. At the nurse-midwifery service, nurse-midwife students, under the supervision of a nurse-midwife instructor, managed all aspects of prenatal care; patients saw the assistant resident if complications developed (and were transferred to the medical service for the remainder of the pregnancy, if necessary). Once a patient in the nurse-midwifery service went into labor, she was admitted to the labor-and-delivery suite, met by the nurse-midwife student, and then examined by the assistant resident and the nurse-midwife student. The nurse-midwife student, "under the supervision of the nurse-midwife instructor and with medical guidance available from the assistant resident," managed the labor and delivery, staying with the patient the entire time. Nurse-midwife students then visited their postpartum patients and newborns at least twice each day until they were discharged on the third or fourth day after delivery, and then several visits once the mother and baby left the hospital. At the six-week postpartum visit, the nurse-midwife student examined the patient, and the obstetrician reviewed what she did with her.[74] Thus, Johns Hopkins nurse-midwives managed most of the prenatal, labor-and-delivery, and postpartum care of their patients, using medical guidance and intervention only when necessary

.

## *Yale*

In 1956, Yale University's School of Nursing established a master's of science in nursing program in maternal and newborn health nursing, with an optional elective in nurse-midwifery. Although not affiliated with MCA, this program was directed by MCA alumna Ernestine Wiedenbach, who was known as the "relaxation lady" by doubting physicians. Fellow MCA staff had paved the way for the Yale nurse-midwifery program with the natural childbirth demonstration, "convinc[ing] the medical directors associated with Yale that nurses with specialized knowledge of obstetrics could improve hospital maternity care and contribute to the education of nurses and physicians."[75] After working at the natural childbirth demonstration, Wiedenbach joined the Yale School of Nursing faculty in 1952. When the School of Nursing decided to include graduate programs, Wiedenbach, influenced by her "friend, counselor and advisor" Hazel Corbin, promoted a specialized master's program in nurse-midwifery.[76]

Yale's maternity nursing program focused on the psychosocial aspects of birth management. Its curriculum "provide[d] an opportunity for the nurse to broaden her understanding of people and of relationships through the social and behavioral sciences and to deepen her knowledge of her chosen clinical area through the nursing, medical and public health sciences." Courses included a Patient Centered Seminar, Psychodynamics, Marriage and the Family, and The Nature of Culture. Students received experience in the maternity out-patient department, labor-and-delivery unit, and rooming-in unit of the Yale–New Haven Medical Center.[77]

However, Yale was unable at first to grant nurse-midwifery certificates to master's students who wanted them. The place where the students gained clinical experience, the University Service of the Grace–New Haven Community Hospital, did not allow them to develop the independent thinking skills nurse-midwives needed. With few mothers registered for the service, and medical students and first-year residents seeking similar field experience, the nursing students gained "meaningful experience in maternity nursing," including "counseling and conducting a complete visit with a mother in clinic, testing her blood and urine, teaching classes in preparation for childbirth and parenthood, supporting mothers-in-labor, delivering them with guidance from the resident obstetrician, and meeting needs for . . . mothers and their newborn presented during their postpartum-postnatal stays in the hospital." This experience, according to Wiedenbach, was "an introduction to skills implicit in nurse-midwifery," but not "an experience in nurse-midwifery practice per se" because "it was too medically dominated." Wiedenbach explained,

> The nurse-midwife instructor and her student, for instance, could not, because of medical policy, act on their evaluation of a mother's normal obstetric progress or need, without first obtaining the approval of the resident obstetrician. The policy required that he make his own evaluation of every situation and his decision was final. In relation to nursing, this policy was appropriate. The fact, however, that responsibility for management of a mother's normal labor could not be delegated to the nurse-midwife instructor and her student, impeded the student's ability to develop judgment essential for the practice of nurse-midwifery.[78]

Beginning in 1958, Yale provided interested maternity nursing students an opportunity to get a certificate in nurse-midwifery by providing summer field experience at other institutions, including Johns Hopkins, Sloane Hospital for Women, Kings County Hospital, and Chicago Maternity Center. According to Wiedenbach, nurse-midwifery training gave the master's level maternity nurse new skills, deeper knowledge about childbirth, and the ability to take fuller responsibility for the health of mothers and children. By 1961, nine of the thirteen students who had received a master's of science in nursing and a nurse-midwifery certificate held faculty positions in schools of nursing, three worked in nurse-midwifery services, and one directed patient care in a hospital.[79]

Wiedenbach was determined that student nurse-midwives should learn to take full responsibility for expectant mothers and women in labor and delivery. However, Yale did not allow students or nurses to oversee completely the birthing process. Changing such policies would have threatened female nurses' "second-class citizen" status in the hospital hierarchy, a role that dictated nurses should not take charge of childbirth—a medical procedure, and therefore one that only physicians should perform.[80] When Yale refused to alter its policies to fit the needs of nurse-midwives' hands-on training, Wiedenbach sometimes asked students to leave the institution and work elsewhere in order to gain the experience she believed necessary to a nurse-midwife's education.

## *Downstate Medical Center, State University of New York —Kings County Hospital*

By helping establish several hospital-based university-affiliated nurse-midwifery programs, MCA was finally participating in (and one might argue even facilitating) the long-term American trend wherein childbirth was moving out of the home and into the hospital. However, this trend and MCA's ultimate participation in it had a detrimental effect on the organization's ability to train nurse-midwives, no matter where they would eventually practice, because nurse-midwives were rarely allowed to deliver babies in the hospital setting. In 1958, MCA closed its home-delivery service and set up a nurse-midwifery service in Kings County Hospital in affiliation with Downstate Medical Center, State University of New York. Since 1931, MCA had operated a successful home-delivery service staffed by nurse-midwives, but by the late 1950s, fewer patients used the service. In the year it closed the home-delivery service, only .5 percent of births in New York City occurred at home.[81] As MCA director Hazel Corbin explained: "By this time there were very few home deliveries. Most of them wanted to go to the hospitals, and they had insurance of one kind or another. Their husbands had insurance, the unions had insurance. The thought of going into the hospital and having a rest for a week or two weeks sounded wonderful to them. And so there wasn't an adequate number of women [giving birth at home] to provide experience for a school."[82] MCA also faced another problem: obstetricians did not like the fact that some middle- and upper-class women, who were seeking an alternative to routinized hospital births, had recently begun using the home delivery service, and they feared that nurse-midwives were entering their turf. At the same time MCA was losing patients and, in suspicious obstetricians' view, attracting the "wrong kind" of patients (in other words, patients obstetricians wanted for themselves), Kings County experienced an obstetrician shortage, which led to substandard care for patients.

Louis Hellman, chief of obstetrics at the hospital, offered Corbin a potential solution to the problems both MCA and Kings County faced: move MCA's nurse-midwifery service and school to Kings County.[83] Beginning in 1957, several conferences between MCA and nursing and medical representatives from Kings County explored the possibility of this merger. After many conversations, the two institutions hammered out policies and plans for the new nurse-midwifery education program and service. MCA agreed to fund both the school and the service, which it did until 1974.[84] With the finances settled, the focus of conversations among the two institutions' administrators often centered on one contentious question: What exactly should medical supervision of nurse-midwives entail? For prenatal care, MCA and Kings County decided to continue a practice used at MCA's home-delivery service: physicians took a pregnant woman's prenatal history and conducted a physical examination on her first visit. Then, if a physician determined that the woman was expected to have a normal pregnancy, she or he assigned the woman to the nurse-midwifery service. Nurse-midwifery students managed labors and deliveries, and then held postpartum teaching rounds with their nurse-midwifery instructors' supervision. However, compared with MCA's original home-delivery service, the MCA–Kings County service included much more physician management in the labor-and-delivery and postpartum periods because physicians were always nearby in the hospital maternity ward.[85]

Before MCA's nurse-midwifery service moved to Kings County, nurse-midwives expressed concerns about what the hospital environment would do to "patient-centered maternity care"—something nurse-midwives felt they had created in the home-delivery service.[86] Their concerns were well founded. Since physicians were present at all times in the hospital (and thus did not need to be summoned on horseback or on a late-night city street), they were more able to intervene in childbirth, even when nurse-midwives were given responsibility for the process. Additionally, Kings County nurse-midwives did not provide the continuity of care that they had at MCA. They did not cover the hospital labor floors every hour of every day, and therefore could not always be attentive to patients' needs. Furthermore, many of the patients nurse-midwives delivered had not received prenatal care through the nurse-midwifery service.[87] However, according to a Kings County nurse-midwifery instructor, the service provided a much more personalized kind of care than the regular medical service. Certainly, staff physicians and residents quickly realized and accepted that nurse-midwives offered something different.[88] The hospital environment also allowed Kings County nurse-midwives to expand their practice to include performing and stitching episiotomies, repairing lacerations, and by the mid-1960s, inserting intrauterine devices. In addition, nurse-midwifery students gained broader clinical experience because they worked with many more patients than they had in the small, declining home-delivery service.[89] The expansion of nurse-midwives' services and increased number of patients they served benefited both nurse-midwives and physicians: nurse-midwives developed expertise in new areas and the students were able to train with more patients; physicians were freed to focus on less routine practices and procedures, and they carefully supervised and controlled nurse-midwives on their turf—the hospital.[90]

More than any of the other university programs, the Kings County nurse-midwifery program represented the end of one era and the beginning of another. MCA moved its service to Kings County Hospital because it had no other choice. For most Americans—and certainly most residents of New York City, home birth represented a thing of the past. Reflecting this trend, MCA's nurse-midwives stopped delivering babies at home and entered large mainstream hospitals where they faced both new restrictions and new opportunities.

## Obstetrician Allies

Nurse-midwives' move to the hospital could not have succeeded without the support of prominent obstetricians. Of course, back in the 1920s and 1930s, obstetricians like Lobenstine, Watson, and Kosmak had been essential partners in the creation of MCA's educational program and service, and obstetricians played an important supporting role in the founding of FNS. In the 1950s, the two most influential and vocal obstetrician proponents of nurse-midwifery were Nicholson Eastman at Johns Hopkins and Louis Hellman at Downstate Medical Center, Kings County Hospital.

Eastman was chief obstetrician at Johns Hopkins Hospital when Hopkins's nurse-midwifery program began. He believed that nurse-midwives provided "superior" maternity care, arguing that nurse-midwives could improve American maternal health care and lift a burden from overworked physicians. According to Eastman, small rural hospitals needed nurse-midwives because uneducated nurses' aides handled many deliveries (despite the fact that physicians, mostly general practitioners, signed the birth certificates), and large urban hospitals needed well-trained women to assist in birth. Eastman always emphasized, however, that he thought nurse-midwives should serve as assistants to obstetricians, as part of an "obstetric team."[91]

Even before Hopkins had a nurse-midwifery program, Eastman had been a supporter of nurse-midwifery. In 1952, he praised a Maryland State Health Department film, *Nurse-Midwifery—Education and Practice*, which depicted a nurse-midwife working for a county health department.

He found "especially noteworthy . . . the joyful attitude toward childbearing which permeates the whole picture. This happy atmosphere, which stems from the approach of the nurse-midwives, provides spiritual and emotional support for the mother and in so doing illustrates one of the advantages of home delivery and midwifery care. To any young woman who is choosing a vocation, or to any nurse who is considering post-graduate training, this film will tell a heartwarming and inspiring story."[92]

After Hopkins piloted a nurse-midwifery service under Eastman's supervision, he praised nurse-midwives even further:

> Having observed rather closely the work of our Obstetric Assistants [the term Eastman used for nurse-midwives] for almost a year, and having imposed upon them a good many times to follow private patients in labor along with me, I have almost wondered sometimes if they did not mesmerize these mothers. The secret of their success with parturient women is, of course, the constant, sympathetic and encouraging attention they give, plus the hundred and one little things they do, such as positioning, pressure on the small of the back, and the like. I have watched all this with my own eyes and am convinced that the meticulous type of care they give is the answer to the greatest weakness in American obstetrics, namely, lack of emotional support both in pregnancy and labor.

Eastman continued, arguing that "by training, temperament and outlook" nurse-midwives are "singularly fitted" to offer "a unique, personalized form of attention throughout pregnancy, labor and the puerperium."[93] Eastman's critiques of American obstetrics and praise for nurse-midwives, although common today, were revolutionary at the time.[94]

Eastman's motivation for using nurse-midwives was practical. He believed that nurse-midwives were necessary to meet the huge and growing shortage of obstetric personnel in a time of rising birth rates. "Who is going to deliver all these babies and provide the desired teaching and emotional support for mothers during pregnancy, labor and the puerperium? . . . Will not obstetricians need all the skilled assistance they can get over the next decade?"[95] According to Eastman, nurse-midwives brought something special to hospital birth—a willingness to spend time with their patients and to offer them personalized care in a way that obstetricians, by training, temperament, and outlook, could not. Most importantly, obstetricians *needed* them in the wake of a physician shortage.

Louis Hellman was just as enthusiastic as Eastman in his support of nurse-midwifery. Hellman was chair of the Department of Obstetrics and Gynecology at Downstate Medical Center, Kings County Hospital, and later held positions on President John F. Kennedy's panel on mental retardation and as the Deputy Assistant Secretary for Population Affairs in the Public Health Service. In a 1964 article in the *Saturday Evening Post*—"Let's Use Midwives—To Save Babies"—Hellman passionately argued for widespread use of nurse-midwives. His concerns about the state of American maternity care sounded like those from earlier in the century. Hellman began his article:

> The state of maternity care in the United States is astonishingly inferior—and getting worse. In our affluent society, with its vast medical centers, the average layman may think he can take it for granted that such an elemental procedure as birth would be carried out with the highest medical standards. The truth is that in many cases there are no medical standards because there is no medical care.

He explained, as had Eastman, that there were not enough physicians to care for pregnant women. He also pointed to the uneven distribution of obstetricians, who rarely practiced in places where the poor were concentrated—the centers of cities and rural areas. Hellman went on to say that many patients ended up preferring nurse-midwives due to the personalized care they provided.[96] Some of Hellman's comments, like Eastman's, provide an echo to discussions today. Like their predecessors, many early twenty-first-century reformers are concerned about the uneven distribution of health professionals, point to patient dissatisfaction with modern obstetrical care, and suggest that nurse-midwives might solve both problems.

Like Eastman, Hellman carefully positioned nurse-midwives vis-à-vis physicians, showing the need for nurse-midwives and the ways in which obstetricians would benefit from having them. In an article in the *American Journal of Obstetrics and Gynecology*, Hellman pitched his support of nurse-midwives to his obstetrician audience from his very first statements: "One cannot gainsay the common sense fact that the mothers of America would be better off if each at the time of labor and delivery were continuously attended by a board-certified obstetrician. A brief glance at the logistics of the situation will show that this goal is not now attainable and that the future holds no hope for its achievement." Hellman added though that logistics were not the only problem; in fact, many women were unsatisfied with obstetric practices. He argued that the nurse-midwife could "extend the hand of the obstetrician immeasurably," so that the obstetrician "could well double his activities with no loss of personalized or meticulous care of his patients." Hellman also asserted that nurse-midwives "would encourage better and more thoughtful personalized care."[97]

While many physicians continued to be threatened by nurse-midwives in the 1950s, Hellman and Eastman advocated nurse-midwifery as solutions to two problems: a physician shortage and depersonalized maternity care. They, of course, had an enormous impact on the nurse-midwifery programs associated with their institutions: Downstate Medical Center, Kings County Hospital, and Johns Hopkins. They also tried to convince their peers and the public that nurse-midwives were both needed and valuable.

## Conclusion

In 1960, Hattie Hemschemeyer pointed out a great advantage to nurse-midwives' new hospital homes. In hospitals, nurse-midwives worked closely with physicians, who would then understand their value, and this understanding would lead eventually to "the establishment and wider distribution of the services of the nurse-midwife in other hospitals and institutions." But she also acknowledged the great trade-off that came with working in hospitals: some of nurse-midwives' "cherished convictions" would have to be altered to fit into mid-twentieth century hospital obstetrics.[98]

Hemschemeyer was right about both the advantages and disadvantages of nurse-midwives' entrance into hospitals. However, their role in hospitals developed more slowly than she had anticipated. Nurse-midwives who worked at the hospitals affiliated with Columbia, Johns Hopkins, Yale, and Downstate Medical Center did the actual work of nurse-midwives, providing, in most cases, prenatal, labor-and-delivery, and postpartum care to their patients. But other hospitals did not give nurse-midwives the chance to practice nurse-midwifery, nor did they give nurse-midwives any degree of autonomy. Instead, these hospitals employed nurse-midwives to be in more subordinate positions as maternity nurses and maternity nursing supervisors. In their nursing roles, they responded to the widespread criticism of obstetric nursing and the bureaucratization of medical institutions by offering obstetric patients personalized care, within the limits the hospital setting imposed, and taught the new "natural childbirth" method. But they did not manage their patients' maternity care, or come anywhere close to doing so. In addition, the number of nurse-midwives in any hospital was small, so they had little impact on hospital policies and practices.

Yet the expansion of nurse-midwifery into hospitals, and especially into major medical centers associated with universities, was very important. Nurse-midwives practiced their profession in medicine's leading institutions, and received enthusiastic support from some of the nation's top obstetricians. While their numbers were small, their symbolic importance was large. Their presence challenged the notions that childbirth, even among elite women, required physicians, and that major hospital procedures required physicians. Nurse-midwives' entrance into hospitals also highlights the problems inherent in mid-twentieth century American obstetrics and medicine. First, the United States did not have enough medical personnel, at least not in all places and with all races and classes of people, to meet patient needs. Second, many women expressed deep dissatisfaction with hospital maternity care, a fact of which some of the leading physicians were aware. Third, nurse-midwives had trouble pushing their way into hospitals because they subverted the health-care hierarchy, which had always placed physicians above nurses.

CHAPTER 5

# Traditions

## Home Birth in a High-Tech Age

### Introduction

Born in 1907 in rural Missouri, Hannah D. Mitchell took a long and winding road to becoming a registered nurse.[1] Her family had been financially comfortable, but that changed when her father, a carpenter, printer, and farmer, died in a construction accident while she was still a young woman. The hardships brought on by her father's death prompted Mitchell, the oldest of six, and her eldest brother to attend a college where students worked part-time to pay their way, John Brown University in Arkansas. A little older than the other women there, Mitchell earned her keep by serving as a residence-hall matron during the school year, and as a Boy Scout and Campfire Girls' leader for a university-run summer program. After receiving a bachelor of arts degree, she chose not to return to accounting work, which she had done prior to university and found unsatisfying, but instead taught history for awhile. Then, Mitchell decided to go to nursing school. Although years later she recalled that she had always been interested in taking care of ailing people or animals, she also noted that her financial responsibilities to her family limited her options and encouraged her to choose nursing.

A year after graduating as a registered nurse from the nurse training school at St. Luke's Hospital in Kansas City, Missouri, Mitchell, then thirty-two, entered the Frontier Nursing School of Midwifery. In 1940, she became the first American nurse to graduate from and teach courses in the midwifery program. For the next four years, Mitchell was a district nurse-midwife, caring for women and families first in the Bull Creek district and later in Red Bird. To get around the districts, she rode Lady Ellen and Traveler (horses that Mary Breckinridge had also ridden), something her girlhood on the farm in Missouri had prepared her to do. In 1944, officials from Washington, D.C., who visited FNS witnessed Mitchell do something remarkable. She successfully diagnosed a very rare and often fatal condition for mothers and babies, with the result that the mother's life was saved. After watching Mitchell, the officials specifically requested her to help start a nurse-midwifery school in Panama. Despite the honor, she hesitated to leave a life and job she loved until Breckinridge herself encouraged her: "Mitch, this is making nurse-midwifery history. You have to go." In 1946, after serving in Panama, Mitchell returned to the United States to get a bachelor of science in public-health nursing at Columbia University. While she was at Columbia, the Georgia State Department of Health recruited her to create demonstration nurse-midwife programs in rural areas where local midwives, often African American, delivered most of the region's babies. Under Mitchell's leadership, nurse-midwives in rural Georgia delivered babies in homes and local hospitals, supervised and trained traditional midwives, and provided prenatal care clinics for midwives' patients.[2] After three years of leading the nurse-midwife programs, Mitchell took a leave in 1949 to get a master's degree in public health at the University of Michigan, returning to her work in Georgia until she retired in 1967 due to ill health.

Mitchell worked on many important projects while serving as a leader in maternal and child health for the State of Georgia. She helped create a guide for pregnant women, the *School Health Guide* for school health programs, and *Birthright,* a documentary film on venereal diseases.[3] Her most well-known project was as a nurse-midwife consultant for *All My Babies*, an educational film completed in 1952 which was designed to instruct traditional midwives, health-care personnel, and expectant mothers in Georgia and throughout the South.[4] The Georgia State Department of Health commissioned George C. Stoney, later seen as a pioneer in documentary film, to write, direct, and produce the film.[5] The health department provided two nurse-midwives, including Mitchell, to serve as advisors, and Stoney relied heavily on Mitchell to make sure that the film met the 118 requirements established by the film committee, such as demonstration of proper sterile techniques and evidence of the midwife's understanding of the tests conducted at the prenatal clinic. Mitchell also helped choose the film's star. She asked nurses from around the state whom she supervised to tell her about the best "granny" midwives. She then chose "Miss Mary" Coley, an African-American woman whom she described as both "bright" and "home folksy." According to Stoney, "Miss Mary" was five feet, two inches tall and 280 pounds, yet "for all her squat bulk, she was truly graceful." Of a higher socioeconomic class and more talented than many of her midwife peers (at least according to Mitchell and Stoney), Miss Mary owned a car, as well as a nice home, and charged thirty dollars, almost double the typical fee, for her services. As Mitchell explained, she had the love of her patients, as well as the respect of the physicians and nurses in her hometown of Albany, Georgia. Stoney came to admire "Miss Mary" and her midwifery skills, citing in particular her graceful hands, her "ingenious way . . . of persuading mothers—and grandmothers!—to abandon . . . harmful superstitions," and the standards of cleanliness she upheld. *All My Babies* was used by the Georgia State Department of Health, as well as in other places in the South, and later around the world through UNESCO and the World Health Organization.[6] The film won the prestigious Flaherty Award for documentaries, and in 2002, the Library of Congress selected this "landmark film" for inclusion in its National Film Registry.[7] Hannah Mitchell helped create a film that showed what she and other nurse-midwives believed to be possible: an African-American "granny" midwife who was successful because she worked within the medical system and under proper supervision of (mostly) white nurse-midwives and public-health nurses.

While many of Mitchell's peers moved into hospitals in the war and postwar years, she and her colleagues did, for the most part, what nurse-midwives had been doing since they first began their work in the United States in the 1920s: home deliveries, and supervising and educating "granny" midwives. Increasingly nurse-midwives' approaches to home-based prenatal, intranatal, and postnatal care, and their oversight of traditional midwives, came to be viewed as unusual, because most Americans were now giving birth in hospitals and had more access to medical care. Yet the two original nurse-midwifery services, FNS and MCA, continued to care for their low-income patients at home (although MCA leaders believed they had no choice but to move their nurse-midwives to a hospital in 1958). On a fundamental level, FNS and MCA nurse-midwives continued to believe in the value of home birth. Their students' experiences with home deliveries prepared them to supervise traditional midwives and to work abroad as missionaries in areas where home births were more typical than in the United States. American nurse-midwives during this time even *expanded* their traditional work to new locales, establishing nurse-midwifery home-delivery services and schools in New Orleans, Louisiana, Tuskegee, Alabama, and Santa Fe, New Mexico, as well as demonstration sites in other places, like Hannah Mitchell's Georgia.

In this age of scientific medicine, why did nurse-midwives like Mitchell *begin* something that seemed to look to the past? According to nurse-midwife Marian F. Cadwallader, Mitchell's colleague in Georgia, her consulting partner for *All My Babies*, and a fellow FNS graduate, Hill-Burton hospitals and attempts to get young physicians to practice in rural areas had failed to meet patient needs. The unequal distribution of physicians, combined with poverty and the desire for midwives among African Americans, indicated a continuing need for traditional midwives. Although midwives attended only 14 percent of births in Georgia, Cadwallader maintained it was impossible "to supplant the lay midwives in this state by more professional practitioners [obstetricians, general practitioners, or nurse-midwives] at a very early date," and she called for nurse-midwives to train traditional midwives.[8] In other words, Cadwallader made some of the same arguments for using nurse-midwives, and keeping traditional midwives, in the 1950s that reformers had made in the 1910s.

Although traditional midwifery had decreased dramatically in the Northeast and the Midwest over the first half of the twentieth century, midwives had continued to play an important role in the rural South, especially among African Americans. In the 1940s, they attended more than 75 percent of births in Mississippi, Alabama, Louisiana, South Carolina, Florida, and Georgia.[9] In Mississippi alone, midwives attended the births of 80 percent of African-American babies.[10] Given these percentages, the U.S. Children's Bureau, Julius Rosenwald Fund (a private philanthropic organization dedicated to helping African Americans), and other groups opened the Tuskegee School of Nurse-Midwivery in Tuskegee in 1941 and the Flint-Goodridge School of Nurse-Midwivery in New Orleans in 1942 to train black nurses to be nurse-midwives and supervise the "grannies." Both programs, associated with black universities, survived for only a few years due to problems with racism, funding, and the recruitment of black nurses. While their numbers were small and the programs specifically for black nurses were short-lived, understanding the experiences of these black nurse-midwives provides a fuller and more nuanced picture of the profession.[11] Black nurse-midwives provided a bridge between black traditional midwives and white physicians and public health officials.

A third new nurse-midwifery home delivery service and school, Catholic Maternity Institute (CMI), attempted to address the problems Cadwallader outlined. Founded in 1944 in Santa Fe, CMI provides a case study of women who self-consciously bucked the childbirth trends in the postwar era. Until it closed in 1969, CMI trained nuns and laywomen to become nurse-midwives to poor Latinas. These nurse-midwives practiced in an area with high maternal and infant mortality rates, a lack of access to modern medicine, and the presence of many *parteras*, or traditional Latina midwives. At CMI, as with the other nurse-midwifery services, female nurse-midwives, rather than male physicians, attended the bulk of births, which primarily took place at home or in the first out-of-hospital birthing center in the United States. The nurse-midwives at CMI also emphasized both religion and science in their practice, and they promoted natural, family-centered childbirth. Although CMI differed in some ways from the other mid-twentieth-century nurse-midwifery home-delivery services, its presence and mission, like those of FNS and MCA, demonstrated that the "male medical model" of science and expertise did not go unchallenged.

## Frontier Nursing Service

During the war and postwar years, FNS nurse-midwives continued to provide maternity and general nursing care to Appalachian patients at their homes, with public-health clinic appointments supplementing home visits if necessary. The nurse-midwives advised only "potential problem cases" among the expectant mothers to deliver at Hyden Hospital, the small hospital run by FNS.[12]

In recognition of its efforts, FNS received an "honorable mention" for its "Home Delivery Technique" exhibit at the American Congress of Obstetrics and Gynecology in 1952. Two nurse-midwives staffed the exhibit, which resembled a simple eastern Kentucky home, with a kerosene lamp, fireplace, bed, baby crib, and the delivery equipment and trademark FNS saddlebags in which the nurse-midwives placed their supplies while riding horseback to their destinations.[13] As in an earlier era, FNS continued to emphasize home births to promote their unique work, explaining that they stayed through the night with parturient women, waiting patiently for them to deliver.[14]

Statistics suggest, however, that by the early 1950s, many FNS patients delivered in the hospital. Records of pregnancies and births at FNS between 1952 and 1954, as tabulated and analyzed by the Metropolitan Life Insurance Company, reveal that 52.8 percent of the women delivered in Hyden Hospital. In 1940 (the previous time Metropolitan Life analyzed

FNS records), only 12.3 percent of women delivered in Hyden Hospital.[15]

However, we must analyze these statistics carefully. The increase in hospital births resulted in great part from the increased number of maternity patients receiving care from outside the regular FNS area. According to an article on FNS in a nursing journal in 1955, "provided they are willing to attend the antenatal clinic regularly and make the journey into the hospital for delivery, patients are booked from a wide area. The nearest alternative in-patient accommodation is twenty-five miles away. Potentially normal patients who live in the F.N.S. territory are encouraged to have their confinements at home, so as to save the hospital beds for the abnormal cases, and those living in more inaccessible places."[16] Statistics support this last statement. For example, in fiscal year 1951–1952, of the 421 women FNS nurse-midwives attended in childbirth, 173 (41 percent) were from outside the area. Nurse-midwives attended ten of those 173 at home, with the remainder delivering in the hospital. As the report for that fiscal year explained, "most of our outside-area patients move into our districts or our Hospital for delivery."[17] (In fiscal year 1939–1940, when only 12.3 percent of patients were delivered in the hospital, outside-area maternity patients made up a small fraction (twenty-seven out of 413, or 6 percent) of the total maternity patients.[18]) This suggests that the FNS move to hospital births was practical, to serve patients who lived far from the service's outpost centers. Eastern Kentuckians continued to experience difficulties traveling from place to place, however. Although a state road came to Hyden, and WPA built roads in eastern Kentucky, even many of the areas in the service's large territory could not be serviced by jeeps, due to rough trails, steep mountains, and rocky creek beds.[19] Nurse-midwives' convenience, and the realities of their work days and Appalachian topography, took precedence over any rhetoric about the benefits of home births.

Despite this shift, FNS continued to focus on home births, not hospital births, in its publications. First, FNS nurse-midwives continued to attend the majority of births for women inside the FNS territory at home. Second, they were not interested in promoting themselves as part of the mainstream, but rather in portraying their work in a romantic fashion; thus, nurse-midwives were typically depicted riding horses through the mountains to attend women in simple Appalachian homes. The service's niche was not in moving toward the hospital and greater professional status, but in its special outsider status. Outsider status had its benefits: since FNS did not present a threat to physicians or traditional nurses in the hospital environment, they did not try to hinder FNS nurse-midwives' work in the rural setting.

Whether attending births in the home or hospital, FNS nurse-midwives continued to buck American birthing trends in the 1940s and 1950s. They used fewer drugs and interventions in childbirth than most physicians and hospitals, but they did not offer natural childbirth classes as some of their contemporaries did at major university medical centers. The service's childbirth approach resulted from nurse-midwives' frequent attendance at births in the home, and their willingness to spend extended periods of time with their patients. Breckinridge believed in the normality of childbirth, but appeared unfamiliar and unconcerned with the specifics of prenatal education in the natural childbirth method. In 1949, she explained to a friend:

> Yes, we do have a copy of Dr. Grantley [*sic*] Read's 'Childbirth Without Fear' over in the library of the Frontier Graduate School of Midwifery for the use of the nurse students. My assistants have read it but I have not read it myself. I gathered from my assistants that the principles of the book were those in which [FNS] midwives were carefully trained. We have often been told outside the mountains that it is too bad that our normal maternity cases cannot have anaesthetics because they are delivered in the homes and by nurse-midwives. We have always replied that the mountain women did not want anaesthetics for normal childbirth and didn't need them; that it was the duty of the nurse-midwife to stay by them and so to handle them that they went through childbirth as a normal process that they could accept.[20]

Breckinridge viewed "natural childbirth" through her racist prism, insisting that her patients already instinctively practiced natural childbirth methods and had an extraordinarily low rate of forceps deliveries and Caesarean sections because of their superior heredity. According to Breckinridge, the reason Kentucky women "can deliver their babies themselves is because both belong in a homogeneous population," where "the baby's head is racially designed to go through the mother's pelvis." This situation had come about, in Breckinridge's opinion, because Appalachian women had had "a complete lack of ancestral obstetrical care—a lack going back to the dawn of time," which "by a severe process of natural selection," had eliminated those women who were unable to bear children naturally. Finally, she believed that breastfeeding, common to the Appalachian region, caused future mothers not to have flattened pelvises, allowing for natural childbirth.[21]

While FNS continued to focus on home delivery and the "natural," the service had a brush with one of the most important medical inventions of the twentieth century, oral contraceptives. Although none of the nurse-midwifery services and schools in the early to mid-twentieth century had a stated mission to provide birth control, FNS participated in one of the first clinical studies of oral contraceptives in humans. These trials began in the 1950s, first on a small scale at two Massachusetts hospitals and then on a large scale at several locations in Puerto Rico, and later Haiti.[22] In 1958, G. D. Searle & Company, a Chicago-area pharmaceutical corporation, and the Worcester Foundation for Experimental Biology chose FNS as another trial site, and FNS nurse-midwives began administering the oral contraceptive Enovid (the trade name for norethynodrel) to 100 patients.[23]

That FNS got involved in these trials is quite amazing given Breckinridge's views on birth control. She had opposed birth control for Appalachian women in most circumstances, claiming that it was impossible to educate them in family planning and that they "would have nothing to do with it," anyway.[24] (Additionally, Breckinridge argued that birth control was not the cure for overpopulation among the poor, and suggested that reducing poverty among eastern Kentuckians was more likely to expand their options and lead them to have fewer children.[25]) In the early days of FNS, nurse-midwives always referred patients who inquired about birth control to the FNS medical director, as laws dictated that only physicians could prescribe birth control and distribute contraceptive information.[26] But, before the advent of oral contraceptives, FNS was stingy in its contraceptive offerings. The staff only offered women who had at least five children contraceptive choices, such as condoms, sponges, diaphragms, and jellies. Although the staff also offered tubal ligations to women who had at least eight live children, Breckinridge opposed the procedure unless it was a medical necessity. (The service's policies and Breckinridge's position on tubal ligations were typical of this era.[27]) Despite Breckinridge's views on birth control, FNS seems to have become involved in the trials because of her close relationship with the Worcester Foundation's John Rock, an obstetrician and gynecologist who conducted the first human contraceptive trials, and his wife Nan with whom she had worked in a post–World War I relief program in France.[28] FNS decided to use the trial to learn whether nurse-midwives, rather than physicians, could effectively administer and supervise oral contraceptives.[29] While both Rock and the FNS staff saw the trial as a success, the results were not published with those of the other large-scale trials in Puerto Rico and Haiti, and both contemporaries and historians have almost entirely ignored the study. Yet the trial's results had an impact both on the Food and Drug Administration's ultimate approval of Enovid in 1960 and on the future orientation of FNS.[30]

After the Kentucky oral contraceptive study began, family planning became an important part of FNS; a significant percentage of nurse-midwives' visits were devoted to family planning, the birthrate of FNS patients slowed, and the Frontier Graduate School of Midwifery began to include lectures on family planning.[31] The service's important place in the early history of oral contraceptives shows the complexity of institutions and individuals. While FNS seemed to reject technological innovations, and Breckinridge seemed to reject birth control, the institution and its founder chose to play a part in what became one of the major symbols of the "high-tech" age. In addition, the service's participation in this trial should be seen in light of changing attitudes toward birth control in the 1960s, and in nurse-midwives' expansion into family planning starting in the mid- to late 1960s.[32]

## Maternity Center Association

In the 1940s and 1950s, FNS emphasized home births and the "natural," while simultaneously sending more of its patients to the hospital and entering into an early human trial on oral contraceptives in 1958. During the same period, MCA continued and even extended its home-delivery service, begun in 1932 in Manhattan. In 1942, MCA opened a second nurse-midwifery clinic called the Berwind Branch on East 103rd Street. The Berwind Corporation loaned the clinic building to MCA. This loan of a building formerly "operated by Cornell Medical School and the New York Lying-In Hospital, [was] to provide experience for medical students in the art of home delivery." World War II and the resulting "changes in the medical curriculum and the heavy draft on civilian physicians for the armed forces" had caused a physician shortage.[33] According to Hattie Hemschemeyer, the school's director, "To the nurse-midwives, this was an opportunity that we had long hoped for in New York City—an extension of the Lobenstine service."[34]

In fact, the second clinic dramatically increased the number of patients, and "nearly swamped" the nurse-midwifery staff. As a result, MCA rushed to train more nurse-midwives, aided by scholarships from the United States Public Health Service. After the war, the Berwind Corporation gave MCA the Berwind clinic building, along with $10,000 toward its upkeep, and MCA transferred patients there from the Lobenstine Clinic, which it closed. In 1952, MCA purchased the former residence of a deceased board member, and moved everything—home-delivery service, school, prenatal clinic, parents' classes, and institutes for health professionals—to East 92nd Street.[35] Although the clinic moved into a grand building on the Upper East Side, Hattie Hemschemeyer noted that the Berwind Branch retained its location "in the heart of the Puerto Rican district" from whence a large percentage of its clientele came. From 1952 to 1958, 65 percent of the newborns who were born at the clinic had native Puerto Rican parents.[36] Regardless of its location, the association's nurse-midwives remained committed to home delivery and to patients of color.

In 1955, an MCA publication acknowledged the trend toward hospitalization but suggested that "it created new problems[,] as deeply rooted emotional values were subordinated to administrative routine." While this report carefully indicated the impossibility and undesirability of maternity care at home for most American women, it suggested that "for normal women with suitable family situations, home delivery may sometimes offer a satisfactory answer to familial needs, personal desires, and overcrowded, understaffed wards." The report also found that "ninety per cent of the mothers confined at home . . . said they would choose to repeat the experience if they had additional children. They enjoyed having their husbands with them and being with their families."[37] Although the data do not indicate how many women registered with MCA for home delivery each year, statistics indicate that 6,884 women applied for home-delivery with the service between 1932 and 1951, and 1,548 women between 1952 and 1958. Between 1932 and 1951, MCA dismissed 16.5 percent of the women who registered for home delivery during their pregnancy because their poor social and economic conditions did not qualify them for the service even though they were medically approved; 14 percent were dismissed for the same reasons between 1952 and 1958. Patients hospitalized for medical reasons comprised 11.3 percent of patients in the earlier period and 13 percent in the later period. In sum, 72.2 percent of patients in the earlier period and 73 percent of patients in the later period delivered at home.[38] MCA discontinued its home-delivery service in 1958 because by then so few New York City women were choosing home birth and because Corbin and other MCA staff wanted to upgrade and expand nurse-midwifery education by placing it in universities, accompanied by the wide range of clinical experiences available at university-affiliated hospitals.[39]

The stories of Elizabeth (Betty) Berryhill and Gabriela Olivera, women who became friends while attending the MCA nurse-midwifery school in the early 1950s, provide a window to understand the association's home-delivery service, as well as the lives of MCA nurse-midwifery students, in the postwar era.[40] Born in London, Ontario, in 1923, Betty Berryhill was the only child of a farmer and his wife. Six-feet tall and athletic, she played basketball for a local technical institute, where she took a business law course while waiting for acceptance into a nursing school. During her nursing education, Berryhill developed a passion for obstetrics and public health, and for home visits and home deliveries. Those interests prompted her to enter the MCA nurse-midwifery school in 1951.

Gabriela Olivera, born in Valparaiso, Chile, in 1914, was the second of thirteen children of a British import-export company employee and his wife. She had always wanted to work with mothers and babies, inspired by her grandmother who had assisted a British physician in delivering the babies of British businessmen living in Chile. But Olivera's father disapproved of his daughter's plans, so she waited. Although her father died young at age forty-five, Olivera could not immediately pursue her dreams because she had to support her family. Finally, she attended nursing school. For a year after graduation, she worked for a maternal- and child-health clinic run by the Presbyterian Church, which sent her to MCA in 1950 so she could gain the experience necessary to return as director of the clinic.

The Canadian Berryhill and Chilean Olivera lived at International House, a Columbia University dormitory that housed foreign students. With only a small amount of money on which to live (the Presbyterian Church gave Olivera just two dollars a day as a stipend) and no refrigeration at the International House, they were grateful to Marian Strachan, educational director at MCA, for sharing food with them and the other students. Every weekday morning the two women attended classes, although Olivera could not understand the lectures because she spoke so little English. To learn the material, Olivera translated the medical texts at night, and to learn English, she chose not to spend time with other Latin American students living in her residence hall. Although her fellow Latin Americans thought she was snobby, she learned English quickly, and her Spanish proved helpful on visits to the many Spanish-speaking patients MCA serviced.

In addition to morning classes, Olivera and Berryhill gained clinical experience by seeing patients at the MCA clinic every afternoon, and by attending home deliveries. Most of their patients came from Harlem or the Bronx and could not afford to pay for physician care. A few of their patients, usually the wives of graduate students, had enough money for private physicians but came to MCA because they specifically wanted the type of maternal health care the nurse-midwives provided—home delivery and natural childbirth, rather than heavy sedation in labor and delivery with forceps in a hospital.

Two students and an MCA instructor typically attended each birth. The more advanced student attended the mother and managed the delivery; the less advanced student monitored the fetal heart rate and helped as needed; and the instructor observed, assisted, and offered suggestions. In rare cases of serious difficulties, students telephoned the on-call physician and summoned an ambulance to take the woman to the hospital. Olivera and Berryhill traveled to many poor, sometimes dangerous, neighborhoods to see their patients. Yet they maintained that they always felt safe because everyone recognized their blue public-health uniforms. They traveled by subway or bus, or in urgent cases, taxi, and brought with them a black bag filled with essential supplies for the delivery, including medications to stop hemorrhage, a local anesthetic, silver nitrate drops for the baby's eyes, and newspapers to make pads for equipment or the bed to prevent the spreading of germs.

Home deliveries were structured, but they always involved a certain amount of adventure. Nurse-midwifery students had to be prepared for whatever occurred. For example, Olivera was surprised to see a large cockroach climbing on what she called "my so-called sterile apron" as her patient began pushing out her baby. Since few of their patients' homes had phones, the students also carried dimes to pay for phone calls. With money in hand, they would go down the hall or to the nearest bar, making frequent reports about the patient's progress to Hattie Hemschemeyer, associate director of the nurse-midwifery program, or to the nurse-midwife on duty.

Berryhill and Olivera were typical MCA graduates of the 1950s in many ways. Before they were accepted into the nurse-midwifery program, they had proved that they had no desire to engage in private practice and compete with American physicians. Both wished to return to their home countries. After a couple of years of work in Canada and Chile respectively, Berryhill and Olivera became Presbyterian missionaries and together went to remote Tabacundo, Ecuador, high in the Andes mountains, where they, along with eight others, worked to improve indigenous people's standard of living. They then moved on together to missionary work in Colombia, but separated in 1964 when Berryhill returned to North America to pursue further education and Olivera stayed on as a missionary in a different Colombian location. By 1970, both women were in North Carolina doing public-health projects and university teaching.

## Flint-Goodridge and Tuskegee

FNS and MCA were not the only places in the country where nurse-midwives like Betty Berryhill and Gabriela Olivera attended home deliveries in the 1940s and 1950s. In close cooperation with MCA, two new nurse-midwifery home-delivery services and schools began in this period in the Southeast. These services provided care for low-income African-American patients and training for African-American nurses who planned to supervise traditional midwives.

Before analyzing the two African-American nurse-midwifery schools and services, it is necessary to examine the traditional midwives they supervised. African-American traditional midwives in the South were known as "granny" midwives, or "grannies," among white officials and sometimes among themselves. Black southern midwives were among the most highly regarded members of their communities. Most became midwives because they believed God had called them to do this work, or because they followed mothers, aunts, and grandmothers into it.[41] African-American southern women learned about midwifery from older women in their families and communities, rather than through formal schooling. Sometimes midwives learned their skills through state health department programs. In the 1910s and 1920s, when southern state midwifery laws began to require midwives to pass exams and register with the state health departments, those departments provided courses for "grannies," where public health nurses taught basic hygiene (along with an emphasis on cleanliness), the importance of calling physicians if complications occurred during deliveries, and domestic work, like preparing food and giving baths.[42] African-American midwives did not focus on prenatal care because they saw pregnancy (and childbirth) as natural states. They used medicinal plants, like gingerroot and tread sash tea, along with other substances like castor oil, to induce labor; they used massage to move babies in the correct position for birth; and they drew on magic and religion to guide them in all aspects of their work.[43] "Grannies" also offered tremendous comfort and support throughout labor, staying with women until their babies were born.[44] During the postpartum period, black midwives not only cared for mothers and new babies but also provided valuable domestic help, such as cooking and cleaning, while the new mother recuperated.[45] Midwives continued to give advice and folk remedies for children to mothers long after the babies were born.[46] Because so much of the contemporary literature, written by physicians and nurses, blamed African-American midwives for high infant and maternal mortality rates, it is difficult to evaluate their actual performance in delivering both mother and child safely. Yet, statistics show that the record of midwives was no worse, and sometimes better, than that of early twentieth-century physicians.[47]

Nurse-midwives (and the physicians and nurses who supported their efforts) hoped that the two new schools for black nurse-midwives would bring scientific medicine to these traditional midwives. Founded in 1942, the Flint-Goodridge School of Nurse-Midwifery at Dillard University in New Orleans received funds from the U.S. Children's Bureau and the Julius Rosenwald Fund. Albert W. Dent, superintendent of the Flint-Goodridge Hospital, developed the six-month midwifery course for nurses to decrease the influence and power of "granny" midwives and promote the status of the hospital.[48] The school's faculty consisted of two MCA alumnae, Kate Hyder, director of the program (who, as discussed in chapter 4, played an important role a few years later in Yale's natural childbirth demonstration), and Etta Mae Forte, a Jamaican nurse-midwife, and Wesley Newton Segre, a black obstetrician from Birmingham, Alabama.[49]

Students at the school attended lectures on obstetrics and labor management, and they participated in prenatal and postpartum care in the hospital and at least twenty home deliveries.[50] In 1943, the school graduated its first class of two nurse-midwives, who went on to work for the health departments of Louisiana and Mississippi.[51] Immediately after graduation and just one year after it had opened, the school closed. According to the new hospital superintendent, the "temporary" closure was due to the "war emergency"; however, the school remained closed.[52] Although the reason the school did not reopen remains unclear, opposition by local physicians may have been at least a partial cause. While the chair of the Medical Advisory Board and two obstetricians at Flint-Goodridge Hospital supported the opening of the school, some local obstetricians and the state and city health departments did not.[53]

The Tuskegee School of Nurse-Midwifery in Tuskegee, Alabama, founded in 1941, and directed by two MCA graduates, operated in conjunction with the John A. Andrew Memorial Hospital, Macon County Health Department, Georgia State Department of Health (which allotted funds from the U.S. Children's Bureau), and the Julius Rosenwald Fund.[54] Two years prior to the school's founding, the Macon County Health Department opened a home-delivery service for African-American women, staffed by MCA-trained African-American nurses. When the Tuskegee School opened, the home-delivery service provided a clinical site for Tuskegee students.[55] Although the school was only in operation for five years, it graduated thirty-one nurse-midwives and had a substantial positive impact on the health of mothers and infants in Macon County where the school was located.[56] After two years of operation, the county fetal death rate dropped from 45.9 to 14 per 1,000 births, and the maternal death rate declined from 8.5 to zero per 1,000 live births.[57]

The Tuskegee School was short-lived for a variety of reasons, most notably its difficulty recruiting African-American nurses to assume leadership in the development of the school. First, African Americans lacked nursing preparation and experience. Second, the white-controlled health department resisted raising the salaries of African-American nurse-midwives. Finally, racism in this rural area meant that only the poorest housing and living conditions were available for the black nurses. In 1946, as a result of these problems, the school discontinued its operations. Neither the Tuskegee Institute nor the John A. Andrew Memorial Hospital School of Nursing provided enough institutional support to maintain the school. After the school closed, the U.S. Children's Bureau used its funds to provide medical care to maternity patients in the region.[58]

Upon graduation, Tuskegee alumnae worked at southern public-health departments and nurse-midwifery services, and a few stayed to teach at the Tuskegee School of Nurse-Midwifery.[59] Maude E. Callen and Mamie O. Hale were typical Tuskegee graduates. Mamie O. Hale, or "Nurse Hale," as "granny" midwives and white public-health nurses and physicians respectfully called her, was a 1943 graduate.[60] Prior to entering the school, she had worked with traditional midwives for an Arkansas county health department. In 1945, Hale became the midwife consultant for the Maternal and Child Health Division of the Arkansas Department of Health, helping public-health nurses educate, supervise, and register traditional midwives. She developed a seven-week midwife training program, covering completion of birth certificates, appropriate selection of cases, prenatal visits (Hale encouraged midwives to make a minimum of three prenatal visits), medical supervision (Hale urged midwives to obtain physician supervision, and to get patients to receive a medical exam), labor and delivery, and postpartum care. Midwives who attended Hale's program and met certain state requirements received midwife permits at special graduation ceremonies where they heard local public-health officials reaffirm the importance of cleanliness, medical supervision, and following public-health regulations. Hale not only created the midwife training program but also accompanied midwives to patients' homes to teach them. In addition, she explained the training program to groups of parents.

Hale, who was in her mid-thirties when she graduated and began her public-health work in Arkansas, was widely admired by many groups. The

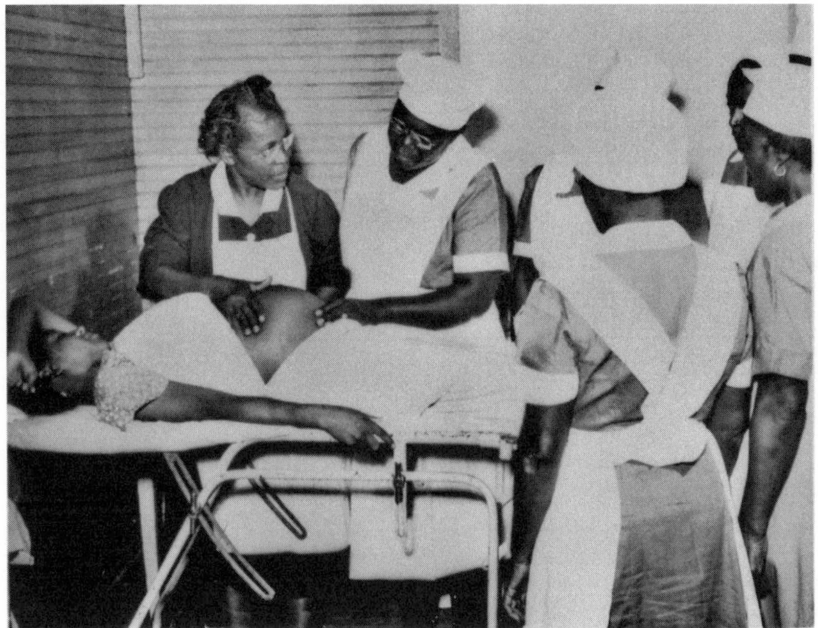

FIGURE 9. Nurse-midwife Maude Callen, a graduate of the Tuskegee School of Nurse-Midwifery, conducts a class at the State Board of Health's Midwife Institute at Frogmore on Saint Helena Island, South Carolina, c. 1950. Callen and a group of her students—traditional midwives—surround a pregnant woman on a stretcher. Courtesy of the National Library of Medicine.

black midwives with whom she worked, who were mostly in their sixties and seventies, regarded her highly despite their age and educational differences; and, despite the prevalence of racism, white public-health nurses and obstetricians also highly valued the young African-American professional woman's work. In fact, out of deference to Hale, white public-health nurses, when traveling throughout Arkansas with her, did not eat in restaurants that refused to serve African Americans. Hale's reputation was well deserved and her work directly contributed to the betterment of African Americans' lives in the South in many ways: increasing the number of black women receiving prenatal care, raising the number of counties with maternity or child health clinics run by public-health nurses, ensuring the greater availability of obstetricians who could consult with the maternity clinics, increasing the number of state-certified midwives overall, and, most importantly, decreasing African-American maternal mortality.

Another 1943 graduate of Tuskegee's nurse-midwifery school, Maude E. Callen, known as "Miss Maude," was born in Florida in 1900 and

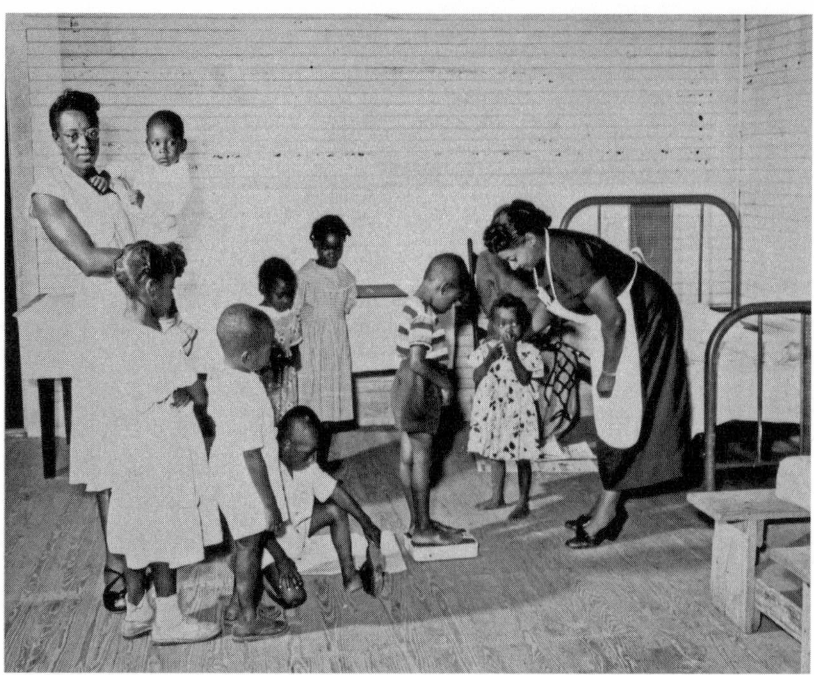

FIGURE 10. African-American children in 1949 at the school clinic in Cainhoy, South Carolina, wait their turn to be weighed by nurse-midwife Eugenia Broughton, a graduate that year of Maternity Center Association's Lobenstine School of Midwifery who worked closely with Maude Callen. Courtesy of the National Library of Medicine.

moved to Berkeley County, South Carolina, in 1923 as a missionary nurse.[61] In that position, she taught children to read and write, held nutrition classes for poor mothers, provided vaccinations for children, and educated local midwives and accompanied them on deliveries. In 1936, when Social Security Act funds created the position of public-health nurse with the Berkeley County Department of Health, Callen jumped at the job. With increased financial support, she could put a more formal midwifery training and supervision program in place. Along with seven other nurse-midwives and Dr. Hilla Sheriff, director of the state Division of Maternal and Child Health, Callen eventually ran two-week Midwife Training Institutes every summer on Saint Helena Island. Callen was instrumental in creating a setting where midwives took control over and pride in the institutes. As historian Patricia Evridge Hill explains, these institutes were "an effective partnership between two groups of medical women: white public health officials who provided supplies, funding, and training and African-American nurse midwives and peer leaders, most significant,

Maude Callen, who contributed their expertise, experience, and cultural awareness."

In addition to midwifery work, Callen developed Berkeley County's first prenatal and venereal disease clinics, and provided immunizations and care to tuberculosis patients. She dedicated herself to improving all aspects of patients' health. In 1951, *Life* showcased her good work in a photographic essay by W. Eugene Smith titled "Nurse-Midwife: Maude Callen Eases Pain of Birth, Life, and Death."[62] *Life* readers responded so strongly to Callen's story that they sent her a total of $27,000, which she used to build Berkeley County's first permanent health clinic. "Miss Maude" retired from her position with the county health department in 1971, and died in 1990, just before she was inducted into the South Carolina Hall of Fame.

Tuskegee graduates Hale and Callen shared a desire not to eliminate traditional midwives but to educate and support them with access to medical and nursing resources. These black professional women knew that midwives served a valuable function in the Jim Crow South where most black women did not have access to medical care. They bridged black female folk tradition and white male scientific medicine by resuscitating (and improving) a dying approach to childbirth in the United States.

## Catholic Maternity Institute

Like FNS, MCA, Tuskegee, and Flint-Goodridge, Catholic Maternity Institute in Santa Fe, New Mexico—another early nurse-midwifery service and school in the United States—continued nurse-midwives' tradition of attending births at home.[63] But CMI nurse-midwives' approach toward childbirth was different from that of other mid-twentieth-century American health professionals in a variety of ways. CMI's unusual approach is illustrated by the following story, depicted in a 1948 film produced for the Medical Mission Sisters by Pauline E. King, *Nurse-Midwife*.[64]

In 1948, Rosita and José, a poor Latino couple living near Santa Fe, New Mexico, began preparing for the birth of their first child.[65] During the early stages of her pregnancy, Rosita saw the nurse-midwives at CMI's clinic once a month. As she entered her seventh month, her visits increased.[66] Recognizing that "motherhood is more than a physical experience," Rosita gained a "richer and fuller appreciation of what it means to be a mother" by attending the institute's classes for prospective mothers.

José also attended "special classes for fathers so that he ha[d] some idea what to expect." When Rosita's labor began, José rushed to the local grocery store to call Sister Theophane, the attending nurse-midwife. Sister Theophane then joined José and Rosita's mother, offering Rosita support and praying for her. Carefully, Sister Theophane watched the progress of labor, interfering as little as possible. She encouraged Rosita to relax, gave her no anesthetic, and did not restrain her in any way. Eventually they all welcomed a healthy baby into the world. Sister Theophane's services did not end with the delivery; she visited the family every other day for the first twelve days, and Rosita and her newborn then went to the clinic for checkups.[67] Like the other nurse-midwives at CMI, Sister Theophane offered patients a mix of religion and science.

Founded in 1944 by the Medical Mission Sisters (MMS), CMI trained nuns and laywomen to become nurse-midwives, and then provided prenatal, labor-and-delivery, and postnatal care to poor Latina women in the Santa Fe area. CMI represented a blending of public and private health initiatives and religious and nonreligious motivation. The institute was developed in cooperation with the archbishop of Santa Fe, New Mexico State Department of Health, and the U.S. Children's Bureau, but was staffed and maintained by the MMS. Like other early nurse-midwifery services, CMI offered an alternative to hospital births attended by male obstetricians. Unlike the other services, however, CMI challenged what they perceived as the false opposition between science and religion. Despite the scholarly emphasis on the triumph of the "male medical model" of science and expertise after World War II, my research on CMI demonstrates the continuing importance of faith and religion in childbirth. It also shows the error of equating religion with tradition and science with modernity (since CMI nurse-midwives valued both religion and professionalism), and emphasizes the role of religious orders in the provision of "modern" health services.[68] Finally, by demonstrating that there were female medical "experts" who rejected the medicalization of motherhood before the women's movement in the late 1960s and 1970s, CMI challenged conventional understandings of "natural childbirth." Religion, and not simply feminism, psychological theories, or women's frustrations with depersonalized hospital births, stimulated much of natural childbirth's popularity.[69]

CMI began for two major reasons. First, the Catholic Church wanted to reduce the influence of Protestant missionaries, government agents, and family-planning advocates at Santa Fe's Maternal Health Center, a clinic founded by nationally known birth control activist Margaret Sanger. Second, the Medical Mission Sisters wanted to perform useful and professional work in accordance with their beliefs. By establishing CMI in 1944, the sisters created the first Catholic obstetrical educational program, training sister-nurse-midwives to serve patients in New Mexico and in missions around the world. Prior to 1936, the Catholic Church had prohibited nuns from engaging in surgery and obstetrics or performing medical work perceived to be harmful to their chastity. The Medical Mission Sisters, a Philadelphia-based order with mostly foreign missions, became the first order to minister officially to childbearing women and infants. During World War II, though, wartime restrictions circumscribed their ability to travel abroad. As a result, MMS opened two "home missions" (CMI in Santa Fe and another in Atlanta, also founded in 1944), which fulfilled the desire of medical missionary women to serve poor patients.[70] In addition to supplying opportunities for education and satisfying work, CMI gave nuns an opportunity to promote Catholic values by providing a family-centered and natural childbirth experience. While increasing numbers of American women gave birth in isolated and sterile hospital rooms with expensive and increasingly technological obstetrical care, the staff at CMI viewed birth as a natural, normal family event, requiring few, if any, medical or surgical interventions.

## *Choosing Northern New Mexico*

Northern New Mexico provided an ideal site for the mission for several reasons. First, the area's high rates of maternal and infant deaths were of concern to the state health department, U.S. Children's Bureau, local Catholic Church, and medical missionary women. New Mexico had the highest infant mortality rate and the second highest maternal mortality rate in the United States.[71] The death rate among Latino infants and children was almost three times that of the Anglo population in the area.[72] Latinos made up 60.4 percent of the population of Santa Fe County in 1950, and 54.3 percent in 1960.[73] Low-income Latinos, who made up the majority of CMI patients, had little or no access to professional health care, and tended to use *parteras* (local midwives) to deliver children. Missionaries, like New Mexico public-health authorities, believed *parteras* were unprofessional and even dangerous, and efforts to improve and regulate midwifery before and during the time CMI was in operation helped bring a statewide decline in the number of *parteras*. However, many families in northern New Mexico, the area with the state's largest Latino population, continued to seek out traditional Latino birth attendants.[74] Native Americans comprised another significant minority population in the area CMI served, but because they had the option to receive health-care services from a government-sponsored Indian hospital in Santa Fe, the nuns believed Native Americans did not need CMI.[75]

Another factor making this site ideal was the presence of threats to Catholic views of religion and family. Historically, Protestant and Catholic missionaries had competed throughout the American Southwest. Protestants were more successful than Catholics in proselytizing after the Civil War, and had developed a separate women's missionary movement in the Southwest. Protestant women sought to convert Latino Catholics and assimilate them into American culture in northern New Mexico and southern Colorado, first through their schools, and later through their health-care programs. While most Latino Catholics did not convert to Protestantism, they did take advantage of the education, health care, and other services the Protestants provided.[76] Although the Protestant threat may have diminished by the post–World War II period, the Catholic Church was determined to provide Latino Catholics with health care within a Catholic setting.[77]

The Catholic Church also wanted to offer an alternative to the Santa Fe Maternal Health Center (MHC), founded by Margaret Sanger. When MHC opened in 1937, Santa Fe's archbishop denounced its distribution of birth control information and devices and warned his flock to stay away from the new clinic.[78] The opposition of the Catholic Church, along with the needs of the center's poor patients, caused MHC to deemphasize its contraceptive services, and focus more on providing comprehensive maternal and infant health care and social services.[79] But Catholic leaders continued to view the center as a threat.

Condemnation of birth control was a major impetus for CMI's maternity work. Sister Catherine Shean, a CMI nurse-midwife, argued that the founding of CMI was necessary more to combat "those who desir[ed] race suicide" than to provide birth attendants or lower the high maternal and infant mortality rates.[80] CMI nurse-midwives praised Latino Catholic families, which seemed "to achieve far greater success in rearing large families, and in trying to live according to the laws of God and Church, than many families in the middle and high income brackets in the large cities."[81] A 1953 Catholic magazine article on the Medical Mission Sisters' work at home and abroad argued: "Limiting the family to a few children, as advocated by Mrs. Sanger and her ilk, may seem the obvious path to better health all around, more prosperity, easier living and less unhappiness.

Strangely enough, it doesn't work out that way."[82]

The expansion of government-run maternal and child health services may have provided another impetus for CMI's creation. In the 1920s and 1930s, county, state, and federal health-care personnel, workers from New Deal agencies, agricultural and home demonstration agents, and literacy program teachers visited northern New Mexico to help poor Latino villagers.[83] These secular missionaries seemed to threaten the Catholic welfare programs. As the founder of MMS explained about the mission in Santa Fe, although "the Government has inaugurated rehabilitation and housing projects and the Public Health Department has given its services," "there is plenty of room for improvement, and what is more important, opportunity and urgent need for Catholic initiative to extend the Church's social program to these peoples."[84]

## *Nuns, Health Care, and Obstetrics*

Essential to understanding the Catholic Maternity Institute's work is understanding of the role of nuns in health care and the history of the Medical Mission Sisters. Within the Catholic Church, the order's work was innovative. Until 1936, the Catholic Church prohibited nuns from providing for "the immediate care of children in the cradle or of women who . . . have children in the houses called maternities and all other works of charity which do not seem fitting for virgins consecrated to God."[85] Although a few nuns worked in obstetrics and surgery despite the Church's prohibition, none publicly challenged canon law.[86] However, nuns had cared for the sick since ancient times. Women religious established the first Catholic hospital in the United States, Mullanphy Hospital in St. Louis, in 1820, and administered at least 265 hospitals during the nineteenth century. Nuns nursed soldiers, new immigrants, and victims of cholera, small pox, and yellow fever. Yet, papal prohibitions forbade them to work in obstetric units—"*even assisting* at obstetrical cases," or to work in nurseries, venereal wards, and other places where their sexual purity could be threatened. It also discouraged women religious from learning anatomy and surgical procedures.[87]

Changes to papal law came only after much prodding. In the early 1900s, Agnes McLaren, an older Scottish physician and Catholic convert, and her protégé, Anna Dengel, a young Austrian physician, wanted nuns to staff a new Catholic hospital in India, where Muslim rules prohibited male doctors from attending women in childbirth. However, they encountered continual resistance from papal authorities. In 1925, Dengel finally decided to circumvent the canon law on women religious and medicine by founding the Medical Mission Sisters; these women had to take vows of obedience, poverty, and chastity privately, rather than publicly.[88]

In 1936, after McLaren's and Dengel's repeated requests to change papal rules and after eleven years of Medical Mission Sisters bringing medical aid to mission countries, Pope Pius XII allowed nuns to work in obstetrics. According to the papal instruction, mission lands needed nuns to provide "more suitable safeguards for the health of mothers and infants." In places such as Africa, mothers and babies were dying in large numbers, yet only "the civil authorities and non-Catholic sects are giving closest attention to these conditions." Pius XII encouraged the development of new congregations of women religious devoted "to help[ing] both mothers and infants whose lives are endangered" and explained that "these new tasks demand both an adequate knowledge of the medical art and special training of the soul." Thus, nuns should obtain medical or nursing degrees from Catholic hospitals and universities, and receive special spiritual training.[89]

Catholic Maternity Institute directly answered the 1936 papal instruction. CMI provided maternity services in homes and local clinics and established a school of nurse-midwifery, "*the only Catholic school of this kind in the United States*."[90] Affiliated with the Catholic University of America in Washington, D.C., the CMI School of Nurse-Midwifery filled a real need by offering sister-nurse-midwives and other interested women clinical instruction and fieldwork in nurse-midwifery. After six months, students became certified nurse-midwives.[91] Not only did "they save the baby" in New Mexico—as the title of one article in the Catholic press claimed, students also saved souls in impoverished areas throughout the world.[92] Although the school admitted women who were not nuns and not Catholic, many trained at CMI were sister-nurse-midwives who lived and worked in medical missions in developing countries.[93]

Catholic writers, pleased that the Church's long-standing prohibition against nuns working in obstetrics was over, had high hopes for the sister-nurse-midwives. As one commenter explained, "Catholic Medical Missions could not develop because there were no Catholic doctors for the missions. The care of the sick for the most part was in the hands of Religious Sisterhoods, who were not allowed to study and practice medicine, surgery and obstetrics until recently."[94] A sister-physician writing in the Catholic medical press argued that "professional medical aid in Catholic missions has been, and still is, singularly backward." Conversely, she noted, Protestants had a long history of trained physicians, nurses, and midwives doing mission work.[95] With the advent of MMS, Catholics could now compete with Protestants not only in the growing area of *professional* health care but also for the bodies and souls of their patients. As one sister-nurse-midwife explained, "medical work in the missions makes Christ's love for the sick a visible, tangible action that even the most ignorant can understand and appreciate."[96] For this nun, medical missionary work was a loving wedge into the culture and religion of the people she served.[97] In addition, in an era of medical professionalization, both the Catholic Church and its nuns wanted the opportunity to offer health care based on scientific training to Catholic patients and potential converts.

## *Faith in Religion and Science*

Sister Theophane Shoemaker and Sister Helen Herb, two of the first nurse-midwives to work at CMI, had trained at Maternity Center Association, the nurse-midwifery school that helped pioneer the natural childbirth method. Supporters of natural childbirth, as discussed in chapter 4, advocated minimal use of drugs so that women could participate fully in the central event of their lives. According to its promoters, natural childbirth was an ecstatic experience requiring education and preparation. Developed in Britain in the early 1930s and popularized in the United States during the mid-1940s, the natural childbirth method promulgated the idea that a woman's happiness with her birthing experience was the basis for a happy family, and by extension a stable society. Informed by a postwar emphasis on motherhood, family, and home and by new psychological theories, natural childbirth advocates argued that laboring women who used this new method felt pleasure and a sense of accomplishment. However, supporters also believed that natural childbirth was suitable for only some women—those with no medical or psychological complications, and those who asked for natural childbirth in advance; this latter group was usually limited to the upper and middle class.[98] The select group of women who used natural childbirth often also chose to "room-in" with their newborns rather than be separated from their babies during the postpartum period, as was the norm at American hospitals. Both "rooming-in" and natural childbirth were attempts to personalize for women the often impersonal (and in the mid-twentieth century, with the use of heavy anesthesia, almost disembodied) process of giving birth in the hospital.[99]

Unlike most natural childbirth advocates, CMI also tried to make religion an essential element of family-centered and natural childbirth. These

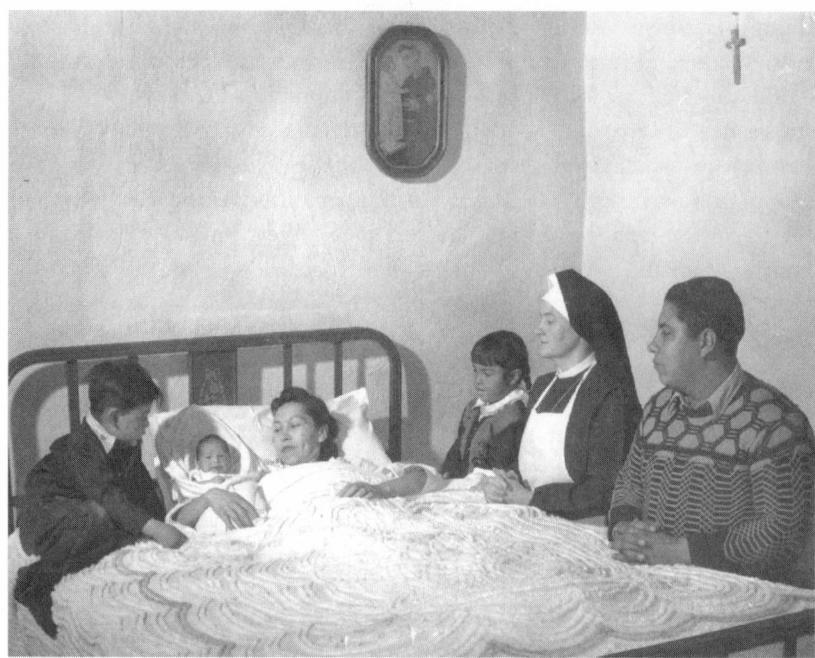

FIGURE 11. Catholic Maternity Institute's Sister Catherine Shean with a family after delivery, 1953. The custom was to offer a prayer of thanksgiving following the birth. Courtesy of the Medical Mission Sisters Archives.

approaches to childbirth fit with CMI's desire to promote birth as both a manifestation of God and the most important event in a woman's life, to be shared by the whole family. According to CMI staff and students, witnessing and participating in the miracle of birth was necessary to solidifying the Catholic family.

For CMI nurse-midwives, birth was a moment of exhilaration, the revelation of God's work. One woman who accompanied a CMI nun on a delivery explained, "At the moment of birth of a baby (of a new soul) every woman is exalted. Feeling herself closer to creation, she remembers her secret pact with God somewhere in the depths of her spirit. All I can say, is that the feeling at that time was akin to joy and yet was above joy. Perhaps it was a sort of ecstasy which comes with the completion of birth—at the end of creation as at the beginning."[100] One Catholic magazine told the story of Adalina Montano, "a typical patient at the Catholic Maternity Institute," who was expecting her sixth child. Montano used the techniques she learned in CMI classes and thus "suffered no fear or tension during labor, but simply worked calmly to bring forth her child. During the whole time, her husband stood by, occasionally speaking softly to her and joining her in the Rosary. This seemed to give her a great deal of comfort. In a very short while, she gave birth to a healthy, beautiful little boy. After the baby was laid in his tiny bed, everyone joined together around Mrs. Montano's bed to offer a simple prayer of thanks."[101] In a family-centered home delivery, God and family came together. As Sister Paula D'Errico remembered: "With home deliveries, I was always deeply impressed when the family got together bedside after birth. And mom and junior were at center stage. All the family knelt down and said a prayer of welcome to the baby and thanksgiving to God."[102]

CMI nurse-midwives' approach to childbirth challenged the distant professionalism common to modern medical practice.[103] Both CMI nurse-midwives and writers in the Catholic press favorably compared the institute's approach to childbirth with those found in more technological settings. After attending a home birth with one of the nuns, a CMI student-nurse-midwife "could not help marveling at the wonderful occurrence we had just witnessed. What a remarkable difference in this type of warm, personal consideration of the total family health picture, to the usual hospital delivery of a large city, with its marked impersonal professional team, its expensive equipment, and scientific explanations for 'rigid procedures, surgery, analgesia, anesthesia, and technique.'"[104] Another witness to a CMI home birth maintained, "I was seeing what birth was meant to be—a family affair—not just another late night for an obstetrician, a headache for an over-worked student-nurse, and the pacing of ether-smelling halls for the father, with nothing to do. No, this father had plenty to do and might still have. He had an important part in this lovely, mysterious drama. Thank God! I thought to myself, Christ was not born in a modern hospital. Could anything have been more horrible!"[105] For CMI's nuns, even a manger was preferable to a bleak, sterile hospital bed.

Prior to 1950, almost all CMI deliveries were conducted in patients' homes. This differed dramatically from national trends in childbirth; by 1950, 88 percent of all American births took place in hospitals.[106] In 1951, CMI opened La Casita, the nation's first out-of-hospital birth center, a maternity in-patient unit with a home-like atmosphere, to provide for patients who lived far from Santa Fe, or whose homes were deemed inadequate for deliveries. As a result, home births declined. Despite the attempts of CMI staff to present "an adequate home environment as the ideal setting for a normal delivery," increasing numbers of women asked to be delivered at La Casita, rather than at home. Patients argued that they rested better at La Casita following their deliveries, but CMI staff felt that giving birth at

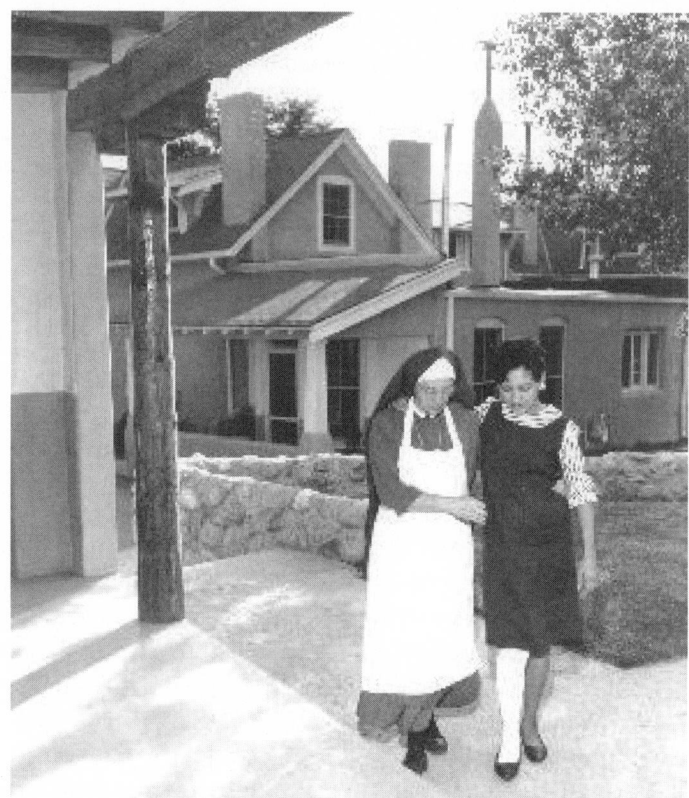

FIGURE 12. Sister Betty Dougherty assisting a pregnant woman into La Casita, the United States's first out-of-hospital birth center, at Catholic Maternity Institute, Santa Fe, New Mexico (date unknown). Courtesy of the Medical Mission Sisters Archives.

La Casita might also have been a status symbol to some women.[107]

Evidence suggests that patients liked what CMI had to offer. Whether deliveries occurred at La Casita or in their homes, CMI patients seemed to appreciate the nurse-midwives' commitment to personalized, home (or home-like) care at a low price. The patient caseload grew by word of mouth. In fact, CMI nurse-midwives often delivered several generations of babies in one family.[108] Women who chose CMI were too poor either to afford maternity care in Santa Fe's only hospital (Saint Vincent's, run by the Sisters of Charity) or to pay one of Santa Fe's limited number of general practitioners. In addition to prohibitive cost, CMI patients may have avoided physician and hospital care because they preferred female birth attendants.[109]

CMI provided a middle ground between scientific "male medicine" and the traditional *partera*. Not formally educated, *parteras*, like traditional African-American midwives, learned mostly from other midwives, often older female relatives and neighbors, as well as through occasional contact with physicians and midwives' classes arranged by state health departments. Highly esteemed in their own communities, *parteras* performed their work as neighbors and friends, not only as wage laborers. The care they provided varied, depending on their skills and experience, as well as their contact with scientific medicine. Some knew safe hygienic practices, while others did not. Many used folk practices passed down through generations, with little theoretical understanding of why those practices worked. Traditionally, *parteras* provided no prenatal care; many Latinas often did not see the necessity of prenatal care because they viewed pregnancy and childbirth as a natural physical process. *Parteras* delivered babies in the mothers' homes using medicinal plants to hasten the delivery or deal with such problems as postpartum hemorrhage. They also provided a comfortable environment for birth, and said prayers as part of their services. In the postpartum period, *parteras* advised new mothers to stay in bed for eight days and to eat a special diet for forty days following the birth. After taking health department midwives' classes and receiving a midwifery license, some *parteras* became well respected in both Latino and Anglo communities. They mixed Latino and Anglo healing practices and worked with local nurse-midwives, public-health nurses, and physicians.[110]

Unlike many *parteras*, CMI nurse-midwives placed great emphasis on prenatal care. Months before her delivery, a patient would register with CMI, where a nurse-midwife took her medical history, and the medical director, a certified obstetrician, performed a complete medical examination. She would visit the prenatal clinic once a month through the seventh month, and every two weeks thereafter until the ninth month, when she was examined weekly by a nurse-midwife. Pregnant women also attended six mothers' classes, which included instruction on normal childbirth; those who could not attend received individual instruction. In the last month, the medical director performed another medical examination. As a CMI nurse-midwife explained: "When a patient is in labor and a normal delivery is anticipated, she calls the Institute and a certified nurse-midwife attends her in her home, giving support, maintaining nutrition, coaching her through the labor and, ultimately, delivering the infant." The nurse-midwives prepared patients for natural childbirth, but gave analgesics, such as Demoral, when necessary. If complications arose, patients were sent to the institute's medical director and/or to nearby Saint Vincent's Hospital.

The nurse-midwives also made postpartum and newborn visits on the first, third, fifth, seventh, ninth, and twelfth days after delivery.[111]

For CMI nurse-midwives, who mostly spoke only English, the language barrier was undoubtedly a problem with some of their patients. While nurse-midwives assisting at home deliveries found that many of the men spoke English and most of the women knew at least some English words, few nurse-midwives or nurse-midwifery students spoke or understood Spanish (although they generally learned some Spanish words on the job). In the prenatal clinic, CMI used volunteers to translate. Reflecting on the attitudes she and her fellow CMI staff members held in the mid-twentieth century, Sister Catherine Shean explained: "The thinking [at the time CMI opened] was that the Spanish-American people were American citizens and so they should learn to speak English. . . . Looking back now I think it would have been wonderful if we'd all spoken Spanish."[112]

Unlike *parteras*, CMI nurse-midwives did not share their patients' Latin American heritage or language skills. However, nurse-midwives, like *parteras*, spent extensive time with patients and their families, and, because they shared the Catholic faith, supported Latino families' emphasis on prayer and religious rituals.[113] The fact that many CMI nurse-midwives were nuns surely helped CMI attract and retain Latino patients. Indeed, CMI's mostly Catholic patients seem to have felt an immediate trust for the sister-nurse-midwives because they were nuns. Furthermore, patients transferred that trust to any laywomen students accompanying the nuns.

The religious, ethnic, class, and regional backgrounds of CMI nurse-midwifery students varied; included among the students were nuns from different religious communities as well as laypeople from throughout the United States and abroad. Despite the heterogeneity within its student population, the institute's approach and its association with nuns continued to dominate, indicating that the commitment to natural childbirth and the shared religion created a powerful bond among the diverse staff, students, and patients.[114]

CMI's nurse-midwives offered patients an opportunity to combine their own view of birth as a natural, religious event occurring in the home, with the promise and status of safe, modern, scientific professional care at low cost. The sisters also believed natural childbirth appealed to their patients and was one of the reasons they chose CMI. CMI nurse-midwife, Sister Michael Waters, argued that an emphasis on "the *mother's own idea*, that childbirth is a natural function of the body, normally uncomplicated," helped convince Latina women of the need for medical supervision during pregnancy.[115] Judging by the popularity of CMI, its patients preferred nurse-midwives to healers within their own communities.[116]

## *The Closing of Catholic Maternity Institute*

CMI ceased operations in 1969 for a number of reasons. First was decreased funding for the institute from MMS. MMS, which had always focused on foreign missions, decided to refocus their limited resources to areas outside the United States, which appeared to have greater needs and fewer health professionals than the American Southwest and Southeast, where its two domestic institutes had been located. As the number of sister-nurse-midwives called to work domestically declined, the lay staff at CMI expanded. Yet CMI was unable to pay adequate wages to these new employees. Second, by the late 1960s, with CMI's help, mothers and children in the region CMI served enjoyed more health-care options than they had in 1944. In Santa Fe County, the infant death rate per 1,000 live births had decreased from 87.6 in 1939 to 15.1 in 1967, compared with an overall decline in the United States from 48.0 to 22.1. In that same period, the maternal death rate per 1,000 live births in Santa Fe County decreased from 4.67 to zero.[117] Third, low-income families could now choose hospital care for their deliveries because New Mexico passed a bill paying for hospital service for the medically indigent, and because Santa Fe's Saint Vincent's Hospital expanded to service all of the area's maternity needs. With greater access to health care available to women in New Mexico, MMS began to consider CMI a luxury service. While the sisters at CMI might have seen thirty to fifty patients per day, those working in India might have seen 500 patients per day. Finally, CMI was facing increased opposition from local physicians and decreased enthusiasm from the School of Nursing at Catholic University of America. As a consequence of all these factors, MMS decided to turn CMI over to the community.[118]

In August 1969, CMI was transferred to a local lay board of directors and became the *Community* Maternity Institute. Investigations in 1969 and 1970 concluded that the institute's "serious financial troubles" were a result of having served low-income families unable to pay their bills. The investigations indicated further that local financial support for CMI had waned and that it would need outside funds to continue. Additionally, they found that CMI lacked the backing of Santa Fe's medical profession. Despite these problems, the investigations revealed that the institute had received "enthusiastic endorsement" from patients and that there was a continuing need for the maternity services CMI provided. Between late 1969 and mid-1970, Community Maternity Institute operated a limited program with prenatal and postnatal care performed by its staff, and with the actual deliveries made by physicians at a local hospital. However, after exploring several possible roles for the new CMI, the Board of Directors finally voted to close existing services in June 1970.[119]

By then, CMI had satisfied the missionary goals of the Catholic Church and the Medical Mission Sisters. First, through its work, CMI had offered an alternative to the services of Protestant missionaries, government agents, and family planning advocates in the area. Second, the institute's nurse-midwifery staff had reinforced Catholic family values through its personal, family-centered, and natural approach to childbirth. Although similar to that of other early nurse-midwifery services, this approach differed from the care most American women received in hospitals. Finally, CMI allowed nuns, for the first time, to receive an obstetrical education in a Catholic setting. Thus, CMI provided a place for the Catholic Church to do good work by providing health care within a Catholic environment and keeping Catholic families in its fold. CMI also offered the Medical Mission Sisters an opportunity to serve the poor, promote their values regarding childbirth, birth control, and the family, and openly do work which had until then been forbidden for Catholic nuns.

## Conclusion

During and after World War II, nurse-midwives opened services in and schools affiliated with hospitals, since that is where the majority of women gave birth. However, some nurse-midwives continued the tradition of home deliveries and of supervising traditional midwives who attended births at home. FNS and MCA preserved their home delivery services, even though the percentage of hospital births at FNS increased and MCA eventually had to cease providing its unique service. In addition, in this era, a number of public-health departments set up nurse-midwifery demonstration sites, such as those established by Hannah Mitchell in Georgia, where nurse-midwives attended home births and oversaw the work of traditional midwives (although Mitchell also participated in colleagues' moves that more closely followed national trends, supervising nurse-midwives who managed hospital deliveries). Finally, three new nurse-midwifery schools and services opened in the Southeast and Southwest.

The programs at Flint-Goodridge and Tuskegee, although short-lived, point to the continuing importance of black "grannies" in the Southeast—and the role that black nurse-midwives played in reshaping the grannies' work to combine science with tradition. Catholic Maternity Institute nurse-midwives, drawing on their deep commitment to both religion and science, offered patients the advantages of medical science without the disadvantages of depersonalized, assembly-line care. The history of CMI clearly shows that health-care providers and patients sought to mix faith in religion with faith in science. The nurse-midwifery services and schools discussed in this chapter thus force us to reassess the dominance of the "male medical model" in the years following World War II. They demonstrate that the bureaucratization found in twentieth-century hospitals and childbirth was neither all-pervasive nor undisputed.

CHAPTER 6

# Don't Push

## Struggling to Create a Political Strategy and Professional Identity

### Introduction

Born in 1899 in Ottawa, Ontario, Aileen I. Hogan grew up in a middle-class family, with two older and two younger siblings.[1] After high school, Hogan completed a secretarial course and worked for Canada's War Department during World War I. After both of her parents died within the same year, Hogan and three of her siblings ventured off to New York City, where she found work as a medical secretary. In her late thirties, she decided to attend nursing school at the Columbia-Presbyterian School of Nursing. There, she became interested in maternity nursing. After graduation, Hogan worked as a staff nurse, and eventually head nurse, on the labor-and-delivery service at Sloane Hospital. During World War II, she went to Britain and France in a special Presbyterian Hospital unit. Although she did not work with mothers and babies during those years, Hogan learned about parent education from talking to young soldiers who were about to become fathers. When she returned to the United States after the war, she used the GI Bill to attend Teachers College, Columbia University, to get a bachelor's degree in nursing. At Columbia, she took classes from Hattie Hemschemeyer, director of Maternity Center Association's nurse-midwifery school. Impressed by Hemschemeyer's lectures on nurse-midwifery's focus on continuity of care during pregnancy, childbirth, and the postpartum period, Hogan "had to see if it worked," so she enrolled in MCA's program in 1947.

Referring to her nurse-midwifery education as "a joy," Hogan remembered that "in one way it was too ideal a situation . . . not one that could be duplicated." As Hogan explained, a nurse-midwife graduate felt "secure in her service skills, and educational ability," but was frustrated because she had "few opportunities to actually be in midwifery." Although Hogan avoided this problem for a year after graduation from MCA by returning to Teachers College for a master's degree, she certainly faced it when she became chair of maternity nursing at the Frances Payne Bolton School of Nursing at Western Reserve University (now Case Western Reserve University) in Cleveland, Ohio.[2] Hogan found herself at "the center of surgical obstetrics, which meant heavy medication during labor, spinal anesthesia for delivery . . . delivery by high forceps as soon as the cervix was open; a baby in need of resuscitation by hot and cold baths, and usually in oxygen for the first day." Despite an open-minded chief of obstetrics, an understanding dean, a great faculty, and wonderful students, Hogan faced one barrier after another as she tried both to implement what she had learned in nurse-midwifery school and to respond to what many parents were asking for: "a different type of maternity care." Although Hogan created successful programs in natural childbirth, she resigned after three years, realizing that she "could not teach a health-oriented program in a surgically oriented hospital." Once free from her problematic job, she accepted a position as a consultant for MCA and, for the next fifteen years, engaged in "fascinating, delightful, and rewarding work" creating parent-education programs with nurses all over the United States and Canada. Looking back, Hogan explained that she was "typical of the nurse-midwifery graduate of the 40s . . . using my midwifery experience as a background for teaching, spreading the gospel of midwifery."

While working for MCA, she also got involved in the politics of nurse-midwifery. She tried working within several nursing associations to organize nurse-midwives, but kept coming up against obstacles. Years later, Hogan understood why the national nursing organizations refused to "make room for us." "They themselves were in the process of organizing a new nursing set-up. The problems were enormous, and to them we were probably just an annoying minority group that should have had the good sense to be patient, and wait till the mother organization was set up, and ready to go." But to Hogan and her colleagues, nurse-midwives could not afford to wait. They felt that for years, they had done good work and now needed to create coherent plans for the education and practice of nurse-midwifery so that it could have a recognized place in the American health system. By 1955, they had decided that "if there was not a place for midwifery in nursing, then we'd have to establish our own place," and they formed the American College of Nurse-Midwives (ACNM).

By the year ACNM was established, nurse-midwives had been practicing in the United States for three decades, yet they remained misunderstood and were not respected. Invented to serve as a stopgap until all women had access to well-trained physicians, nurse-midwives were never expected to be at the center of American health care. However, by the 1950s, they seemed even less necessary than they had in the 1920s for several reasons. Most births now took place in hospitals, and very few hospitals had, or saw the need for, nurse-midwifery services. Obstetricians, now part of a prestigious specialty, attended the births of more American women. Shifting trends in American culture and medicine, such as a decline in immigration, the growing prestige of both physicians and hospital births, campaigns by health professionals against midwives, and changes in laws related to midwifery, had, for the most part, killed the traditional midwife. Maternal mortality was no longer the terrible problem it had been earlier in the century. So, what place would nurse-midwives have? Would they work closely with physicians or independently of them? Would they work within the mainstream health-care system or outside of it? Would they practice in hospitals or outside of them? Overall, nurse-midwives answered these questions by pursuing a strategy of accommodation; in other words, they made a conscious decision to work within the health-care establishment. However, they disagreed among themselves about exactly how accommodating they should be.

It would be easy to conclude that nurse-midwives sold out, or that internal disagreements weakened their resolve, but those conclusions would ignore the very difficult climate in which nurse-midwives functioned and the different paths they chose to take. Nurse-midwives had to cope with a health-care system and with other medical professionals that often rejected them and what they represented. Political scientist James C. Scott has argued that underdogs—and in the health care hierarchy, nurse-midwives were underdogs—have rarely made direct political attacks on their superiors because doing so would be "dangerous, if not suicidal."[3] If we apply Scott's theory here, we see that American nurse-midwives could not simply have rejected the mainstream medical establishment. They needed physicians and nurses as allies in order to survive; they needed physician backup for their home delivery and hospital services, and they had to work with doctors and nurses in hospitals. Nurse-midwives would have committed professional suicide had they directly confronted physicians, nurses, or hospitals. Moreover, many of them had no desire to reject

American medicine; indeed, nurse-midwives defined themselves in part as *not* like traditional midwives, but as modern professionals and collaborators with physicians. Thus, they tried to make inroads into American obstetrics by subtle, rather than direct, methods of resistance—through calculated forms of accommodation—by using the "weapons of the weak," as Scott called them.[4] But nurse-midwives had different approaches to accommodation, as seen in two sets of documents from the mid-1950s: 1) the rank-and-file's range of responses to a proposed definition of "nurse-midwife," and 2) the leadership's arguments about the formation of a national nurse-midwifery organization. Given that most mid-twentieth-century health professionals—and Americans—associated midwives and women with a past best forgotten, nurse-midwives fought an uphill battle as they tried to find a place for themselves in the American health-care system and to change the American way of birth.

## The Profession in the 1950s: Misunderstood, Unrecognized, and Rejected

To understand why nurse-midwives disagreed about the best ways to carve out a piece of the health care pie, it is important to consider where nurse-midwives worked, and what others thought about them. By the mid-1950s, most worked in hospitals or government bureaucracies where either administrators or institutional policy (or both) dictated to a great degree what they did and how they did it. Although all nurse-midwives practiced direct clinical midwifery—providing prenatal and postpartum care, and managing births—while in school, few did so after graduation. In one survey, 20 percent practiced clinical midwifery, mostly providing prenatal and postpartum care only, and 7 percent managed labor and delivery.[5] A small number continued what nurse-midwives had traditionally done, staffing home-delivery nurse-midwifery services in select locations, as discussed in chapter 5. In the mid- to late 1950s, other pioneers, discussed in chapter 4, worked at a handful of major university medical centers, where they staffed hospital nurse-midwifery services and offered an unusual, and more personalized, option for postwar maternity patients in hospitals. But few hospitals had nurse-midwifery services, and as more women wanted to give birth in hospitals, there seemed to be little need or desire for home-delivery nurse-midwifery services. Therefore, most nurse-midwives did not practice direct clinical midwifery but instead worked as maternity nurses or supervisors, as Aileen I. Hogan did at Case Western, or as administrators of maternal and child health programs where they often taught and supervised traditional African-American and Latina midwives.

Wherever they worked, nurse-midwives felt misunderstood and unappreciated. These feelings became clear when a group of leading nurse-midwives in 1954 questioned all known nurse-midwives as part of their efforts to organize a national nurse-midwifery organization. In response to the question, "In what ways do you think . . . [a national nurse-midwifery] organization could help you?" nurse-midwives frequently answered by saying that an organization might help other health care professionals and the public to know and understand what nurse-midwives did. One Frontier Nursing Service (FNS) graduate wrote that she hoped a national nurse-midwifery organization could "bring . . . the practice of nurse-midwifery to the attention of the American public, particularly doctors."[6] Another thought such an organization might "help to give nurse-midwifery the recognition it deserves."[7] Another nurse-midwife believed a national organization could "help me translate to other professional personnel the value and work of nurse-midwives."[8] Yet another nurse-midwife hoped an organization could "help clarify the meaning of nurse midwifery to the public."[9] Two nurse-midwives, writing from the South, expressed particular frustrations with the views held of nurse-midwives in their region. Virginia Lamb Chrestman from Baton Rouge, Louisiana, believed that only "maybe [a national nurse-midwifery organization] could help change the attitude of people in the South about nurse midwives."[10] Jane McAllaster Burr explained that she "would like to see Nurse-Midwives be recognized to be more than Grannies," but doubted that a national nurse-midwifery organization could help her "out here" because Oklahoma did not recognize midwives to begin with.[11]

The answers nurse-midwives throughout the United States gave to the question, "What comments do you have on the suggested definition of nurse-midwifery?" provided nurse-midwives an opportunity to air their exasperation with common misperceptions about their occupation. One nurse-midwife said that "I have only one suggestion. It is not about the definition but that nurse midwifery not be made so much fun of but publicized more."[12] Similarly, another nurse-midwife, originally from England, suggested: "I feel that with more publicity, the general public, would not look upon [us] . . . as 'odd.' I feel that more should be made known in the U.S. to the nursing and medical profession as to what a nurse-midwife really is. . . . [In my] recent experience in a maternity hospital, I felt that all but one doctor out of five felt the [nurse-midwife] was a real asset."[13]

Another nurse-midwife complained about physicians' lack of knowledge about her profession: "I think Doctors in general should be informed what a nurse midwife is. They have no idea that a nurse midwife even knows how to tie a cord."[14]

In fact, the young profession had faced problems with terminology and publicity for a long time. As far back as the 1910s, before nurse-midwives practiced in the United States, health-care providers debated what this new type of birth attendant should be called. In 1914, physician Frederick J. Taussig, the first American to use the term "nurse-midwife," anticipated the problems that would surround it. He suggested that nurses might object to the new term, fearing that "the public may identify such nurses with the objectionable type of women engaged in midwifery here in America."[15] In 1927, Mary Breckinridge, founder and director of FNS, explained that she liked the term "nurse-midwife," *because* it incorporated "midwife," which she saw as an ancient, important calling, still highly regarded in European countries. She noted that in continental Europe, midwives "kept abreast of modern developments" and therefore their position remained "dignified and assured," and that English women had standardized and improved midwifery, creating the Central Midwives Board in 1902. Although midwife was "a name in disrepute" in the United States, Breckinridge and her FNS staff chose to call themselves "nurse-midwives" because local people used the term midwife and "any other, such as 'obstetrical nurse,' would only confuse them."[16] In 1943, a nurse-midwife working in rural Georgia wrote to a colleague about the confusion surrounding their occupation's name. She hoped a professional organization of nurse-midwives would "find a different name which implies interest in the whole maternal and infant cycle, rather than the present name which indicates someone interested in the delivery alone. . . . And besides the 'grannies' have forever received the name 'midwife' for use—at least in the South."[17]

In the mid-1950s, nurse-midwives were still arguing over what they should be called. In 1953, Nicholson J. Eastman, professor of obstetrics at the Johns Hopkins School of Medicine and director of Johns Hopkins' experimental nurse-midwife training program at its obstetric clinic, insisted that nurse-midwives be called *obstetrical assistants* because this term "more nearly connotes than any other the main function which we would envisage for such nurses, namely, the rendering of skilled assistance to obstetricians." He elaborated: "In vast rural areas of this country and in understaffed hospitals, this skilled assistance may also include the conduct of normal deliveries but never without the supervision and control, *in absentia*, of a readily available obstetrician."[18] Sister Theophane sympathized with Eastman's professional position, but reaffirmed the need for the term "nurse-midwife." In a letter to the dean of Catholic University's School of Nursing Education, she wrote: "In principle, I believe he [Eastman] is not opposed to calling us nurse-midwives but he thinks it expedient or diplomatic to use a name his confreres are more apt to accept. We cannot let the obstetricians *supervise and control* our practice. They could accept or throw us out at their wish. [Nurse-midwifery] has to be a self-governing body."[19] At an American Nurses Association Convention in 1954, nurse-midwives "generally agreed that the title 'nurse-midwife' is the only one that is understood on an international level and that this title was preferable to any other so far proposed." They also agreed that "any prejudice that is a hang-over from granny-midwife days *and ways* could be outlived with a moderate amount of determination on the part of nurse-midwives."[20] Yet they were wrong; even in twenty-first-century America, that prejudice still exists.

In the mid-1950s, nurse-midwives faced rejection even by people who, at least theoretically, should have been their allies. From the beginning, nurse-midwives had faced resistance from nurses, but the resistance became more formalized during the 1950s. When a group of nurse-midwives discussed organizing themselves in 1954, they first approached national nursing associations, hoping they could "set standards for education," "standardize practice to some extent," "define functions," and "provide for official status and legislations as well as a tool for official publicity."[21] Sister Theophane Shoemaker, chair of the Committee on Organization and director of Catholic Maternity Institute (CMI), explained why the committee wanted to organize within a national nursing organization. First, the survival of nurse-midwifery depended on it. Second, nurse-midwives would be perceived as more professional if they were part of "a well organized and recognized group," in other words, by becoming a subsection of a national nursing organization.[22] Finally, anticipating future debates, Sister Theophane said that nurse-midwives might leave nursing if not more closely associated with the profession: "It is a pity to allow the few hundreds of nurse-midwives who are now actively engaged in their professional capacity and the larger and ever increasing number to follow, to be torn away from nursing. And if we do not organize and become unified in our thinking, this is what will happen, I am afraid."[23] Thus, Sister Theophane implied that nurse-midwifery *needed* nursing—to provide political backing and safety in numbers—and that nursing would also benefit from increasing their members by adding nurse-midwives, as well as through exposure to nurse-midwives' different perspectives on health care.[24]

In addition, nurse-midwives had previous successful experience organizing within a national nursing organization. From 1944 to 1952, the National Organization for Public Health Nursing (NOPHN) included a nurse-midwifery section, comprising nurse-midwives, nurses, and physicians.[25] Once the NOPHN dissolved in 1952, nurse-midwifery leaders tried to find a new home for the nurse-midwifery section in either the National League for Nursing (NLN) or the American Nurses Association (ANA), both prestigious organizations interested in nursing credentials and professionalization.[26] The NLN and ANA responded with tentative suggestions about forming groups to study nurse-midwives' function. This response frustrated nurse-midwifery leaders, who decided to form a separate nurse-midwifery organization, believing the bureaucratic, cumbersome approach of the NLN and ANA would not allow nurse-midwives to accomplish their purposes.[27] As Sister Theophane explained, the officers of the national nursing organizations rejected nurse-midwives because they "believed nurse-midwifery was equivalent to medical practice and thought it impossible to encompass us within a nursing organization."[28] In other words, they thought that nurse-midwives were too independent to be considered "real" nurses, and therefore, might disrupt the nursing organizations' all-important relationships with physicians.

## Different Approaches to Accommodation

### *Example 1: The Rank-and-File Debate the Meaning of Nurse-Midwifery*

Feeling misunderstood, unrecognized, and rejected, nurse-midwives in the mid-1950s debated among themselves: What is a nurse-midwife? What does she do? Where does she fit into the health care system? In 1954, a group of leading American nurse-midwives in attendance at that year's American Nurses Association annual meeting formed a Committee on Organization to develop a formal way to bring nurse-midwives together and set standards for their education and practice. The committee struggled to develop an official definition of "nurse-midwife" and agreed upon the following:

> The Nurse-Midwife combines the knowledge and skills of professional nursing and midwifery, enabling her, in addition to the usual nursing functions, to assume full responsibility for the education and care of mothers throughout the maternity cycle so long as progress is normal. With this combined background of preparation, she is prepared by education and experience to meet the needs of the mother and her baby for skilled care and emotional security as well as to contribute in a constructive way to the changing pattern of maternity care and education.[29]

Although this definition seems simple, it created controversy among nurse-midwives. The Committee on Organization sent out approximately 400 questionnaires to nurse-midwives trained in the United States and working all over the world to gauge whether they agreed with this definition, the extent to which their education prepared them for their job responsibilities, and whether and how a professional organization could help them. The 156 responses they received to these questionnaires provide an excellent opportunity to understand rank-and-file nurse-midwives' concerns about their role and status; the complicated, sometimes ambiguous, relationships among nurse-midwives, physicians, and nurses; and the differences in nurse-midwives' approaches to defining and carving out their place in the American health-care system.[30]

To respondents, the most controversial part of the committee's definition of "nurse-midwife" was the explanation that nurse-midwives "assume full responsibility for the education and care of mothers throughout the maternity cycle so long as progress is normal." A number of nurse-midwives expressed concern that the definition did not mention that nurse-midwives worked under a physician's supervision. In a strong critique, Helen Marie Fedde, who trained and worked at FNS and then served as nurse supervisor at an Oklahoma hospital, wrote: "I would suggest the insertion of the clause 'under the direction of a qualified physician' after the word 'assume.' In all we have ever learned or taught we have felt that the nurse who will take any such responsibility without definite and planned medical direction will hurt the cause of midwifery far more than she will help it." In an attached letter to the head of the Committee on Organization, Fedde continued her line of thought: "The minute we set ourselves up as experts we are lost. In the United States we will always be directly responsible to a doctor and no matter how high-flown our name or how rigid our requirements we will never be more than nurses—nurses with a special skill."[31]

Others who critiqued this part of the definition held a different opinion about the role physicians should play vis-à-vis nurse-midwives. Some saw the physician's role as a consultant to or supervisor of the nurse-midwife; these nurse-midwives saw the physician as more responsible for patient care than the committee had outlined, but perhaps less responsible than Fedde's preferred wording. Emma Lois Shaffer, for example, noted that "a medical examination and consultation during pregnancy seems important when possible."[32] Sara Elizabeth Fetter asked whether "medical approval or in cooperation with the medical group" should be included in the definition.[33] Rachel Pierce Schottin argued that the definition needed to state more explicitly that the nurse-midwife cooperated with a physician who took over the case if progress was abnormal.[34] Reva Rubin wanted the definition to explain that although nurse-midwives had "full responsibility" for the care of mother and baby, they were "under medical orders in terms of care."[35] By this, Rubin probably meant that the nurse-midwife followed physician-established medical routines, not that physicians were present to give orders to nurse-midwives.

A few nurse-midwives who felt the definition should include the physician gave him/her only the task of performing an initial physical exam. For example, Peggy Helen Brown suggested that "each midwife assumes responsibility of the patient, after the latter has had a full examination by a doctor"[36] Anne Fox agreed.[37] Sister M. Elizabeth Dunbaden Hosford suggested that nurse-midwives wanted to mention physicians' involvement in their patients' care to avoid potential public relations problems. "Should not mention be made," she wondered, "that the assumption of care of normal mothers and babies is under medical guidance—for instance, the initial physical examination would still be a medical responsibility—we know what is meant, but would allied professions and the lay public?"[38] Nurse-midwives struggled to overcome the perception that they worked alone—and outside of the medical mainstream.

Still others complained that the committee's definition stopped short of explaining the real responsibility of nurse-midwives for their patients. They suggested the nurse-midwife was responsible for recognizing abnormal developments during gestation and labor, as well as the normal. Some made no mention of physicians taking over in abnormal situations, while one added that the nurse-midwife would help "secure adequate care in such cases."[39] Writing from India, Eunice LaRue noted that although the definition was "Good for U.S.A. . . . Those of other countries must also handle abnormal cases."[40]

The responses from rank-and-file nurse-midwives to the Committee on Organization's questionnaire provide one lens through which to understand the different degrees nurse-midwives believed they should accommodate physicians and hospitals. They show that while some nurse-midwives highlighted their independence and almost complete responsibility for their patients' care, others emphasized their subordinate status, arguing that "we will never be more than nurses—nurses with a special skill."[41]

### *Example 2: The Leadership Debate How Much Nurse-Midwives Should Challenge the Medical Establishment*

A second set of documents, showcasing internal disagreements among the nurse-midwifery leadership about the best way to organize, provides another useful lens through which to view nurse-midwives' range of political strategies. Rejected by nursing, nurse-midwives were left on their own to form standards and a professional organization. They then had to decide how to proceed. The leaders of the three existing services and schools, Frontier Nursing Service, Maternity Center Association, and Catholic Maternity Institute, shared a passionate belief in the good work nurse-midwives did to help women and children, along with a desire to see the profession of nurse-midwifery expand. However, each had her own idea about how that should happen. FNS's Mary Breckinridge wanted to take one path, one that was cautious and avoided any possible conflict with physicians, yet which seemed to encourage nurse-midwives' autonomy. CMI's Sister Theophane Shoemaker and MCA's Hattie Hemschemeyer, however, wanted to take another path, one that advocated gaining acceptance for nurse-midwifery as rapidly as possible and which focused on teaching and administration in public-health agencies and hospitals, rather than on more autonomous work in isolated settings.

FNS leaders had formed their own nurse-midwifery organization, the Kentucky State Association of Midwives, in 1929, a few years after the founding of FNS. The association's purpose was "to raise the standard of midwives and nurse-midwives, who are or have been or may hereafter be engaged in the active practice of midwifery, to a standard not lower than the official standards required by first class European countries in 1929." In 1939, all but one of the forty-four nurse-midwives in the association were or had been on staff at FNS, and as an FNS article admitted, "no great task has been required of its members" since the association's inception (the association held annual meetings but did little else).[42] In the early 1940s, the association was enrolling more members, many from outside Kentucky. By 1943, membership had jumped to eighty-one, 20 percent of whom had no association with FNS.[43] Increasing diversity led leaders in 1941 to change the name to the American Association of Nurse-Midwives (AANM) to reflect this more national composition of the organization's membership.[44]

When the Committee on Organization met in 1954 to consider the best way to organize nurse-midwives, FNS leaders suggested that the AANM be reorganized to attract a wider variety of members.[45] Sister Theophane agreed that if nurse-midwives could not organize within a national nursing organization, the next best option was to build on the AANM.[46] However, despite an initial display of goodwill among the leaders of FNS, MCA, and CMI, the Committee on Organization ultimately rejected the AANM proposal because of ideological differences between FNS, on the one hand, and MCA and CMI, on the other.

Personality differences also hindered the two camps' ability to work together. Although FNS leaders initially suggested building the AANM into the national organization, they later gave a "cool reception" to the idea, at least according to the members of the Committee on Organization. One committee member, Ruth Boswell, an alumna of the FNS Frontier Graduate School of Midwifery, expressed her frustration with the people at her alma mater: "people at Wendover [the town in which FNS headquarters and Mary Breckinridge resided] . . . are a tight little group and you have to be a certain kind of person to fit in. I can truthfully say that I have no nostalgic feelings for the place. The work there was hard, it was not easy for me to pay 'court,' having never been exposed to the European traditions [many of FNS nurse-midwives were British], nor was it easy for me to espouse what I felt was the hypocritical attitude then prevalent among the more religiously-inclined and the missionaries in the group."[47] Conversely, Breckinridge was frustrated at what she saw as false compliments by MCA and CMI leaders to get FNS help in forming a national nurse-midwifery organization.[48] Louis Hellman, director and professor of obstetrics and gynecology at Kings County Hospital in Brooklyn, who established midwifery instruction at his hospital in the late 1950s and had great respect for Mary Breckinridge's work, nonetheless noted later in life that Breckinridge "thought that [the] only [midwifery] education and midwifery [practice] in the United States happened in Wendover, Kentucky."[49]

Race played yet another divisive role in the FNS and the MCA/CMI camps. AANM's rejection of African Americans as members, during at least some of its history, was a major reason why MCA and CMI leaders ultimately decided that the AANM would not be a suitable national nurse-midwifery organization with which to align. In 1944, MCA invited local nurse-midwives to discuss the question: "Will a national organization of nurse-midwives help us to do a better job?" Although they answered in the affirmative, the MCA nurse-midwives decided they could not join the AANM because it did not allow African-American members, and thus the eight African-American graduates of MCA's school could not join the association.[50]

In the early 1940s, extensive discussion occurred among members of the AANM about whether African Americans should be included in the association. Year after year, the AANM decided against African-American membership, yet leaders continued to discuss the issue and sometimes modified the association's policies. This repeated discussion of African-American nurse-midwives, forty-one potential members (less than 20 percent of the entire profession at that time), suggests that race remained a contentious issue for the AANM, and whiteness was central to the AANM's conception of the nurse-midwife.[51]

Breckinridge's racial attitudes very likely affected AANM policies on African Americans. Breckinridge spoke with kindness about the slaves her family finally freed and with whom she was raised, but she would never dine with an African American. Helen Browne, FNS assistant director before Breckinridge died and director afterward, who was British, did not understand Breckinridge's racist attitudes and always wanted to accept applications from African-American nurses. But as late as the 1960s, FNS never did so, although it accepted African, not African-American, obstetricians as its guests.[52]

Personality and racial differences undoubtedly divided the FNS and MCA/CMI camps. However, the most conflicts among the two arose over strategies for how best to create a strong organization of nurse-midwives and approaches toward nurse-midwifery education and practice. Breckinridge and other leaders of FNS approached organization more cautiously than Sister Theophane and Hemschemeyer, emphasizing nurse-midwives' work in isolated, rural areas rather than hospitals, and encouraging measured organizational development and support from physicians and laypeople. Breckinridge wished to keep the AANM as the national association because it had an "old tradition which is beyond price for a young and experimental branch of nursing." She also wanted to keep the AANM articles of incorporation because they caused "no bad feeling" with other professional organizations, such as the American Medical Association or American Nurses Association. In particular, the article of incorporation stating that nurse-midwives worked "with special reference to rugged, difficult and economically poor areas," helped nurse-midwives' relationships with these organizations because working in such areas was "non-controversial."[53] Breckinridge believed "slow growth" was the best strategy to organizing nurse-midwives, because "the profession is still young in this country and could so easily incur opposition which would retard its growth by many years."[54] She and FNS assistant director Browne also wanted to continue to include lay members interested in nurse-midwifery in their organization, while MCA and CMI leaders wanted to restrict a national organization to nurse-midwives. Finally, Breckinridge felt strongly that the AANM should not have high dues because many members earned small salaries; nor should it have too many committees because members generally had little free time to serve on them.[55]

Breckinridge's ideas about organizing nurse-midwives frustrated Sister Theophane and Hemschemeyer. They worried that Breckinridge did not want an "alive, progressive, dynamic, and growing" organization. The CMI and MCA leaders hoped for an organization to promote educational standardization and coordination and to act as an "official mouthpiece," as well as a forum to share ideas, all of which would require committees and sizable dues. Sister Theophane indicated to FNS leaders that she held out hope for expanding the AANM, but to the Committee on Organization, she admitted that she had given up on this FNS-based organization.[56] Sister Theophane noted in a 1954 letter to Hemschemeyer that only three responses to the committee's questionnaire "even mentioned the American Association of Nurse Midwives although many of them are from F.N.S. Maybe they have not been sufficiently impressed to remember it exists."[57]

A second major ideological division between Breckinridge, and Sister Theophane and Hemschemeyer, stemmed from their different approaches to nurse-midwifery education. FNS trained its students to practice midwifery, while MCA and CMI trained their students to serve as teachers and administrators for traditional midwives and obstetric nurses. To some extent, nurse-midwifery leaders from FNS and from MCA and CMI accepted their different emphases, but each camp believed it knew the best way to serve patients and the profession. From the FNS camp, Helen Marie Fedde, an FNS graduate and dean of the school for two years, explained:

> The F.N.S. is bound to differ somewhat from both MCA and CMI in outlook and in aim. I cannot think that that is bad. Most of our students are taught with the primary purpose of preparing them as fully as possible for the actual practice of nurse-midwifery in remotely isolated areas of this country or on the mission field. I feel that in any consideration of functions or of educational standards that this basic purpose should be kept firmly in mind. The training for administration, in my opinion, will always be secondary to this.[58]

From the MCA and CMI camp, Hemschemeyer agreed that nurse-midwives needed regular contact with patients, but felt "midwives should become more articulate about their work and devote more of their time and energies to administration, teaching, and interpretation."[59] She believed her suggestions would elevate the professional status of the nurse-midwife.

An even more dramatic ideological conflict concerned two MCA/CMI and FNS approaches to nurse-midwifery practice. As CMI director and MCA-educated Sister Theophane explained, first, a student trained at MCA only accepted normal patients "delegated to her by the obstetrician" after completion of a physical examination. Second, "the nurse-midwife [trained at the Lobenstine School] would not be a private practitioner as was the principle of work in Kentucky." Nurse-midwives trained at MCA, Sister Theophane concluded, prepared primarily to supervise and teach, and could only work where medical services were available, while FNS graduates prepared to practice and had less contact with and supervision by physicians.[60] MCA and CMI leaders thus believed, somewhat incorrectly, that FNS promoted nurse-midwives as autonomous health professionals.

Both the FNS and CMI/MCA approaches to nurse-midwifery possessed some radical and some conservative elements; in limited ways each approach undermined the modern American notion that male physicians would dictate patient care and, more specifically, childbirth. The FNS approach directly challenged medically supervised births, but reached relatively few people because FNS focused on its eastern Kentucky demonstration site, and trained students primarily to be direct practitioners.[61] Also, its approach did not seem to accept the reality of childbirth in the mid-twentieth century: most women wanted to deliver their babies in the hospital. The MCA/CMI approach was in some ways more threatening because it reached more people. These institutions trained students to teach nurse-midwifery to nurses and traditional midwives, who would then teach their patients. In addition, as discussed in chapter 4, MCA helped expand nurse-midwifery to new places (university hospitals) and in new directions (university education). However, MCA and CMI's strategy emphasized the need for obstetrician involvement in nurse-midwives' work, thus offering a less direct challenge to obstetricians.[62]

## The Formation of the American College of Nurse-Midwifery

The leaders of MCA and CMI ultimately succeeded, both in their approach to nurse-midwifery and in the creation of a new national nurse-midwifery organization. On November 7, 1955, in Santa Fe, New Mexico, five nurse-midwives signed papers to incorporate the American College of Nurse-Midwifery (ACNM). A few days later, the ACNM held its first convention in Kansas City, just before the American Public Health Association convention so that nurse-midwives could attend both; Aileen Hogan and Hannah Mitchell, whose stories I told at the beginning of this chapter and in chapter 5, respectively, participated in this first gathering.[63] The following month, the ACNM published its first journal, *Bulletin of the American College of Nurse-Midwifery*, a continuation of the short-lived broadsheet, *The Nurse-Midwife Bulletin* (May 1954–October 1955).[64] By 1955, nurse-midwives had created both a national professional organization and a professional journal.

The first executive board of the ACNM was composed of seven women; four, including president Hattie Hemschemeyer and president-elect Sister M. Theophane Shoemaker, were MCA alumnae, two were FNS alumnae, while the seventh had completed her midwifery education in Britain and later worked at both FNS and CMI. FNS leaders and staff did not join the new organization.[65]

The ACNM focused on gaining recognition for nurse-midwives and regulating the entry of nurse-midwives into practice. In 1956, as part of this focus, the organization formed a committee charged with formalizing the profession's philosophy and practice, as well as nurse-midwives' functions, standards, and qualifications. The committee, reinvented several times with different members, did not get its recommendations approved by ACNM membership until 1966. The membership disagreed about how to avoid alienating their obstetrician supporters and how to recognize the many different kinds of roles that nurse-midwives played—from direct clinical practitioners in midwifery to obstetric nurses to maternity consultants in federal, state, and local departments of health.

The first configuration of this committee, in existence from 1956 to 1960, moved away from the Committee on Organization's emphasis on nurse-midwifery as an independent profession and toward nurse-midwifery as a clinical specialty within nursing under medical guidance. A later configuration of the committee stressed medical supervision, but suggested that once nurse-midwives received approval from physicians for their plans, they took care of patients on their own unless complications occurred. This approach to nurse-midwifery alarmed even diehard obstetrician supporters like Louis Hellman, who was concerned that nurse-midwives would become independent practitioners and that the ACNM as an organization was trying to be too independent. Thus, the committee's final list of nurse-midwifery functions, published and approved in 1966, stated clearly that nurse-midwives worked under the direction and supervision of physicians. It also acknowledged the realities of the profession in the 1950s and 1960s, stipulating that nurse-midwives who worked as traditional nurses, as many did, had to work within the rules of practice dictated by nursing, while those who practiced clinical midwifery had additional functions, including the administration of analgesics and anesthesia, performing episiotomies, and delivering babies. In 1966, the same year the committee got approval on its list of nurse-midwifery functions, the ACNM started reviewing and approving nurse-midwifery educational programs, although it was not recognized as the accrediting agency for these programs by the U.S. Department of Education until 1984.[66]

ACNM, the MCA- and CMI-based organization, and AANM, the FNS-based organization, finally worked out their differences, merging in 1968 under the American College of Nurse-Midwives name. It is not a coincidence that the ACNM first proposed the merger just months after Breckinridge died in 1965. In 1967, when the AANM was folding into ACNM, FNS leaders wanted to ensure that their organization's history and bylaws were not lost in the process. As late as 1969, competition or conflict arose between FNS and the newly merged ACNM. In that year, Vera Keane, the president of ACNM and an MCA graduate, criticized then FNS director Helen Browne for discussing only FNS, rather than the broader topic of nurse-midwives, in a *Today Show* interview on midwifery with Barbara Walters.[67] Regardless, by this point, with many nurse-midwives working in hospitals and as nurses, rather than in direct clinical midwifery practice, ACNM leaned in favor of major accommodations with physicians and nurses in order to survive and expand their profession.

## Conclusion

In the mid-1950s, as nurse-midwives tried to renegotiate their place in American health care, they faced a series of problems: defining their profession, getting outsiders to understand who they were and what they did, and winning support for their fairly radical views about childbirth. To negotiate the rocky path to public respectability and professional acceptance these obstacles created, nurse-midwives chose the political strategy of accommodation. Given the climate in which they worked, they had little choice. Increasingly, mid-twentieth-century nurse-midwives, such as Aileen Hogan at Western Reserve (now Case Western), were not autonomous. With the exception of the home-delivery services at FNS and CMI, most nurse-midwives worked in hospital or government settings where they had to report to superiors who often had little understanding of their education or capabilities, who sometimes disagreed with their approach to childbirth, and who usually resisted nurses or women being in charge.

Despite their nearly universal decision to accommodate physicians, nurse-midwives disagreed about the degree to which they should work within the health-care establishment, as seen in debates among both the rank-and-file and leadership and in the newly formed American College of Nurse-Midwifery. To what extent would physicians actually be involved in nurse-midwives' work? To what extent would nurse-midwives work autonomously on the frontiers of health care or under the watchful eye of physicians and nurses in the center of health care? To what extent would nurse-midwives push physicians and nurses to allow them to regulate and control their own profession? The ACNM helped nurse-midwives move toward the center of the health-care establishment and gain some control over their profession, but in the process nurse-midwives compromised by agreeing to work under the direction of physicians. By definition, their strategy of accommodation, a "weapon of the weak," had its limitations.

EPILOGUE

# Afterbirth

## Learning from the Past, Looking to the Future

### Nurse-Midwifery from the 1960s to the Twenty-First Century

By 1960, nurse-midwives had followed American women into hospitals to attend births. In hospitals, they had new opportunities but also faced new barriers. A few worked in nurse-midwifery services at select academic medical centers, where they made symbolically important inroads into mainstream health care. However, the number of such nurse-midwives was small, and they now had to conform to physicians' and hospital administrators' desires much more than when they were on the frontiers of medicine. Many more nurse-midwives worked as hospital maternity nurses or supervisors because the vast majority of hospitals did not have—and did not want to have—nurse-midwifery services. Thus although many more nurse-midwives in the 1960s were working within the mainstream health-care apparatus, which provided them job security and other benefits, these women lacked the opportunity to practice clinical midwifery, for which they were trained and which most of them saw as more of a calling or a passion than simply a job.

By the mid-1960s, most of the nurse-midwives who provided direct clinical midwifery care, including attendance at labor and delivery, worked in Kentucky, New Mexico, or New York City, the only places with laws allowing them to practice as nurse-midwives. A few worked in other southern states, which allowed nurse-midwives to practice under laws that governed traditional midwives. Others participated in a state-sponsored demonstration project (1960–1963) in Madera County, California, in which a special short-lived law enabled nurse-midwives, titled "nurse obstetrical assistants," to work in a rural hospital to make up for a physician shortage.[1]

In the late 1960s and early 1970s, new federal government programs, many of them spurred by Lyndon B. Johnson's Great Society programs, positively affected nurse-midwives, encouraging their work with the poor and medically underserved. Instituted in 1965, Medicaid, a means-tested program for the poor, set caps on dollar amounts providers could charge for health-care services for eligible patients. This discouraged obstetrician participation, which in turn encouraged the development of maternal health-care programs especially for Medicaid recipients. These special programs employed many nurse-midwives and increased support for changing state laws to allow them to practice. As with the Medicaid programs, new federally sponsored family-planning services for the poor through the Office of Economic Opportunity, founded in 1965, and the Family Planning Services and Population Research Act of 1970, created opportunities for nurse-midwives because of physician shortages for these services.[2]

During this era, nurse-midwives generally served poor patients in inner-city and rural areas. In 1968, the New York City Department of Health began employing nurse-midwives at twelve hospitals affiliated with its Maternal and Infant Care projects. In 1969, a new federally funded county health improvement program for Holmes County, Mississippi, employed nurse-midwives; in order to train area nurses for the program, the University of Mississippi began to offer a certificate nurse-midwifery program with grants from the federal Maternal and Child Health Bureau, successor to the Children's Bureau. Federal funds eventually allowed the university to expand the program to prepare nurse-midwives to work all over the Deep South. Maternal and Child Health Bureau grants also funded Indian Health Service nurse-midwifery programs in Alaska, Arizona, New Mexico, and South Dakota in the late 1960s and early 1970s. Additionally, in the 1970s, nurse-midwives provided care in special government-subsidized programs, designed by state and municipal health authorities and academic medical centers, for the growing population of pregnant teenagers, many unmarried, in eastern cities.[3]

A number of laws in the 1970s classified nurse-midwives with two new types of practitioners, nurse practitioners and physician assistants, first calling this group "physician extenders," then "new practitioners," and more recently, "midlevel health care providers." Educational programs for nurse practitioners and physician assistants began in 1965 to alleviate physician shortages in rural and poor urban areas. The laws worked at creating practitioners dependent on physicians, sometimes for direct supervision and at other times for written agreements. Federal government programs in the 1970s also grouped together nurse-midwives, nurse practitioners, and physician assistants to provide funding for educational programs and stipends for students. This increased the federal financial aid available to nurse-midwife students that the Maternal and Child Health Bureau had provided starting around 1960.[4]

In the early 1970s, nurse-midwives began going into private practice, working with physicians and serving middle- and upper-class women, due to an obstetrician shortage and increased demand for alternative approaches to birth among some groups of women.[5] By 1977, 26 percent of American nurse-midwives were in some form of private practice.[6]

As part of the women's movement in the 1960s and 1970s, many women became more vocal in their criticism of routinized hospital births. Wanting active participation in their births, these women became involved in the natural-childbirth, childbirth-education, and breastfeeding movements, and demanded the right for husbands to be present in the delivery room. By the mid-1970s, some middle-class women wanted alternatives to obstetrician-attended births, and turned to nurse-midwives.[7]

At the same time, a lay-midwife movement grew because of women's frustrations with the approach of obstetricians and hospitals to maternity care.[8] Lay midwives were experientially trained and attended home births. Ironically, many lay midwives, several feminist critics, and some of the women who sought out nurse-midwives as an alternative to obstetricians, believed nurse-midwives were part of the medical establishment, oriented toward medicalized births and uncritical of hospital routines and practices.[9] Nurse-midwives' reactions to lay midwives' criticisms resulted in part from their insecure place in American health care. Although they had gained more acceptance during the 1960s, nurse-midwives in the 1970s still depended on obstetrician support and battled the widespread notion that physicians should manage maternity care. While many nurse-midwives supported the personalized care lay midwives offered their patients, most believed lay midwives' lack of regularized training and standards could cause problems for mothers and babies. In addition, nurse-midwives, like their predecessors from decades earlier, feared that the public's tendency to confuse lay midwives with nurse-midwives could damage their struggling profession. Given nurse-midwives' background, it is not surprising that they expressed concerns about lay midwives. Although nurse-midwifery leaders and older nurse-midwives of that period often received their training at Maternity Center Association, Frontier Nursing Service, or Catholic Maternity Institute, and thus had home-birth experience, nurse-midwives educated in the 1960s and 1970s received their clinical training in public hospitals serving a relatively large number of women with complicated pregnancies and births, and believed in the value and safety of hospital births. In 1973, the American College of Nurse-Midwives developed a "Statement on Home Birth" that "considered the hospital to be 'the perfect site for childbirth because of the distinct advantage to the physical welfare of mother and infant.'"[10] Later in the decade, ACNM president Helen Varney Burst argued that not all lay midwives had sufficient training to provide safe care, but also acknowledged that the presence of lay midwives helped nurse-midwives realize their frustrations with practicing within the bounds of physician supervision and hospital rules and routines.[11]

Challenging the necessity of hospital obstetric care, MCA nurse-midwives founded the first urban freestanding birth center in New York City in 1979. (Founded in 1951, CMI's "La Casita" was the first out-of-hospital birth center.) The Childbearing Center served as an alternative birth site to the home and the hospital, with nurse-midwives providing the majority of the care. Nurse-midwives had much more control over their practices in birthing centers compared with hospitals. The Childbearing Center accepted and retained only women with normal pregnancies, working with local health-care professionals to arrange for obstetric and pediatric consultation, transportation to hospitals, and postpartum home-nursing care. As in its earliest years, MCA intended its new program to serve as a model, which would help develop a quality assurance program for birthing centers around the country.[12]

By the 1980s, nurse-midwives practiced in many settings, including clinics, federally funded programs, Health Maintenance Organizations (HMOs), and hospitals. However, many physicians saw nurse-midwives as unnecessary, given the excess of physicians in the United States in the 1980s. While nurse-midwives have gained support during periods of physician shortages, the 1980s saw the opposite. Now nurse-midwives competed for the same patients, and potentially threatened the economic livelihood of physicians, especially since, in an age of skyrocketing health-care costs, many nurse-midwives provided services more cheaply than physicians. Some physicians worked against nurse-midwives, by denying them hospital privileges and by opposing state laws that recognized nurse-midwives, permitted third-party payments, and allowed nurse-midwives prescriptive authority. Other physicians supported nurse-midwives, providing consultation, collaboration, and referral.[13]

In the 1980s, nurse-midwives extended their practice in several ways. Many nurse-midwives expanded their work to caring for women during and after menopause. Also, in 1980, the ACNM changed its earlier position on home births, endorsing nurse-midwives' practice in all settings. However, the ACNM had difficulty getting adequate professional liability insurance for nurse-midwives to attend home births, and some health-insurance plans refused to pay for home births or set their payments lower than the cost of care.[14]

The late 1980s and early 1990s saw an expansion in the number of new nurse-midwifery educational programs, with fifty nurse-midwifery programs in operation by 1996, up from twenty-eight in 1984. This included the development in 1989 of the Frontier Nursing Service's distance learning program, Community-based Nurse-midwifery Education Program (CNEP), which enabled more nurses, especially those in small towns and rural areas, to become nurse-midwives. By the mid-1990s, the program had students in every state. The CNEP program continued the FNS tradition of practice outside the hospital and in rural areas, and helped solve two problems facing nurse-midwifery education since the late 1950s: 1) a lack of clinical opportunities for student nurse-midwives, and 2) the association of most nurse-midwife educational programs with university medical centers specializing in high-risk patients. The CNEP program included short intensive periods in Kentucky, clinical work supervised by a regional clinical coordinator, home-study courses, and extensive electronic and telephone communication with teachers. The program founders wanted to prepare nurse-midwives to practice in any setting, including out-of-hospital sites and rural areas, and actively encouraged students to gain experience outside the hospital.[15]

In the early 1990s, the growth of managed health care and push toward expanding the number of primary care professionals brought new opportunities and challenges for nurse-midwives.[16] Various policy makers and health-care providers proposed that all Americans should have a primary care provider as a health-care gatekeeper. This "gatekeeper" would attend to common health problems and refer patients to specialists when necessary. Many women did not have regular contact with any health-care provider other than an obstetrician-gynecologist, which meant they often received poor nonreproductive preventive health-care services. As more women saw nurse-midwives as primary care providers, the ACNM decided to push for nurse-midwifery education to include common non-reproductive health problems, such as sinusitis, strep throat, and high blood cholesterol.[17] Other groups besides nurse-midwives wanted them to move into primary care. In the early 1990s, President Bill Clinton's health-care reform plans included using nurses as primary and preventive care providers to decrease health-care costs.[18] Insurance providers also wanted nurses and nurse-midwives to expand their services. As Jane Brody of the *New York Times* explained, "Now as third-party payers, including the federal and state governments, look for ways to reduce medical costs, midwives are expected to flourish."[19] Today, a variety of government officials, insurance company representatives, and health-care providers see financial benefits in using nurse-midwives to serve women of all classes.

In 2000, the United States' nurse-midwifery journal made a significant name change. The *Journal of Nurse-Midwifery,* which was originally the *Bulletin of the American College of Nurse-Midwifery* (later *Nurse-Midwives*), became the *Journal of Midwifery and Women's Health.* The name change reflects two important recent changes in nurse-midwifery and in the ACNM. First, the journal added *Women's Health* because its editors hoped doing so would help change the incorrect public perception of nurse-midwives as caring for women only during pregnancy and childbirth. The editors hoped that the change would increase nurse-midwives' "pool of potential clients, scope of practice, employability, and breadth of public support."[20] Second, the journal changed its name from *Nurse-Midwifery* to *Midwifery* to reflect historic changes in the ACNM itself. In the 1990s, some midwives who were not registered nurses received the seal of approval from the ACNM. In 1994, the ACNM approved the accreditation of "direct-entry" or non-nurse-midwifery educational programs, and in 1997, it voted to accept non-nurse-midwives (called "certified midwives") approved by the ACNM Accreditation Council, Inc., along with student midwives enrolled in direct-entry programs accredited or pre-accredited by the ACNM.[21] The ACNM requires that a student applying to a direct-entry midwifery program must have a bachelor's degree (or receive one as part of the program). The student must have taken ten specific college courses in the sciences, as well as have mastery of a long list of health-care skills. In order to become a certified midwife, a graduate of a direct-entry program must pass the same certifying examination required of certified nurse-midwives. The first direct-entry midwifery educational program accredited by the ACNM was at SUNY Downstate, the institution to which MCA transferred its school and patients in 1958. That program has two tracks, one for registered nurses and one for non-nurse candidates. The direct-entry midwifery students take the same courses as the nurse-midwifery students, plus an additional three courses.[22]

The interest in direct-entry programs had been brewing for decades. Nurse-midwives had long received challenges from other midwives and often from their own who questioned the need for midwives to have a nursing background. Some believed that nursing education encouraged nurse-midwives to be too medicalized in their approach to childbirth, as well as too subservient to physicians, and others felt that the emphasis on disease and on men's as well as women's health was irrelevant for midwives.[23] According to Kitty Ernst, Chair of Midwifery at the Frontier School of Midwifery and Family Nursing, direct entry has been "growing in leaps and bounds, attracting bright, young people with liberal arts degrees" because as people who have been taught to challenge and question, they "see nursing education as punitive and inflexible."[24] Despite the inclusion of midwives who are not nurses in the ACNM and in the title for the nation's midwifery journal, American nurse-midwives still disagree about these decisions (in 1998, the ACNM voted not to change its name to the broader American College of Midwifery), and they remain connected to nursing.[25] As nurse-midwifery leader Judith Pence Rooks explains, leaving nursing would be very difficult, even if the ACNM wanted to, because "most nurse-midwives are licensed under state *nurse* practice laws, federal support for nurse-midwifery education comes through the Division of *Nursing,* most nurse-midwifery education programs are based in schools of *nursing,* and although nurse-midwifery students study *midwifery,* in the process most of them earn degrees in *nursing.*"[26]

At the beginning of the twenty-first century, American nurse-midwives continue to struggle with their relationships with physicians and with the meaning of "collaboration" and "independence"—in other words, with the same issues they have faced since they began practicing in 1925. In 2001, the latest joint statement by the ACNM and the American College of Obstetricians and Gynecologists tried to clarify the relationship between nurse-midwives and physicians. Nurse-midwives (and now certified midwives) have used this statement, like the original in 1971 and the two that followed, as they try to negotiate hospital privileges.[27] The 2001 statement specifies more clearly than earlier versions that a physician does not have to be in the room when a nurse-midwife is caring for a woman in labor. It continues to recommend that "the appropriate practice of the certified nurse-midwife/certified midwife includes the participation and involvement of the obstetrician-gynecologist as mutually agreed upon in written medical guidelines/protocols," but now emphasizes that "quality of care is enhanced by the interdependent practice of the obstetrician-gynecologist and the certified nurse-midwife/certified midwife working in a relationship of mutual respect, trust and professional responsibility."[28]

Letters to the editor in the *Journal of Midwifery and Women's Health* following the publication of the joint statement point to the problems that nurse-midwives face, as well as the difference between the rhetoric of a statement intending to promote collaboration and the occasional reality of physicians dictating how and whether nurse-midwives practice. Two writers expressed concern that the requirement of "participation and involvement of the obstetrician-gynecologist as mutually agreed upon in written medical guidelines/protocols" will, in the words of one nurse-midwife, "be used to perpetuate [state] laws that require a physician's signature on written guidelines before a midwife can practice. Physicians may then decide where a midwife may practice (and if she may compete with him or her) and how the midwife will practice."[29] Both writers cited examples of nurse-midwives whose practices were limited and eliminated because of physicians' decisions.

Today, approximately 6,200 nurse-midwives and 50 certified midwives practice in the United States.[30] Most nurse-midwives are white women who had extensive experience as registered nurses before they received training as nurse-midwives. Forty-three nurse-midwifery educational programs exist in the United States.[31] All nurse-midwifery programs accredited by the ACNM Division of Accreditation require a baccalaureate degree for entrance, or grant at least a bachelor's degree upon graduation. Most nurse-midwifery programs associated with universities offer different tracks to students from a variety of backgrounds and educational objectives. Many nurses come to a nurse-midwifery program with a bachelor's in nursing or some other bachelor's degree. These nurses attend programs where they can receive a master's degree in nurse-midwifery. Another track offers nurse-midwifery education to nurses who already have a master's degree in nursing. Yet another track allows registered nurses with diplomas or associate degrees to receive a nurse-midwifery education while obtaining a bachelor's degree in nursing. More than two-thirds of nurse-midwives have graduate degrees, and sixteen states require a master's degree before a nurse-midwife can obtain a license to practice.[32] Certified midwives, a special, recently created category of non-nurse-midwives who have been certified by the ACNM, are required to have a bachelor's degree prior to entering an ACNM-approved midwifery program, or to receive a bachelor's as part of the program.

Nurse-midwives (and the few certified midwives who exist) work in hospitals, with physicians in office practices (mainly as employees, but sometimes as partners), in educational institutions, for prepaid health-care plans, in private nurse-midwifery practices, and to a lesser extent for military and other federal agencies, public health departments, freestanding birth centers, and in-hospital birth centers. Their methods of practice vary based on setting. All provide prenatal care and care during labor and delivery; almost all provide postpartum care, contraceptive, and gynecological services. Some take responsibility for infant care. A significant minority provide other services, such as breastfeeding instruction and support, infertility services, preconception counseling, childbirth education, and routine physical examinations needed by women for entrance into school or sports. The ACNM defines nurse-midwifery practice as "the independent management of women's health care," but requires nurse-midwives to work within a health-care system so they can obtain medical consultation, collaboration, and referral.[33] But obtaining medical consultation can be difficult. Sometimes obstetrical collaboration is unavailable, and at other times, nurse-midwives must use backup from physicians whose practice style is incompatible with nurse-midwifery practice. In 2003, nurse-midwives attended 7.6 percent of all births and more than 10 percent of all vaginal births, mostly in hospitals; these percentages represent an all-time high for nurse-midwives in the United States since such data was first recorded by the National Center for Health Statistics in 1975.[34] Poor women and well-educated, professional women are more likely than other women to receive care from a nurse-midwife.[35]

Nurse-midwives practice legally in all fifty states and the District of Columbia, but laws regulating their practice vary. Some states require nurse-midwives to deliver babies in hospitals or licensed birth centers, and prohibit them from attending home births. The majority allow nurse-midwives prescriptive authority, although most states also limit which drugs they may prescribe (especially certain painkillers).[36] In 1995, one state ruled yes and one no as to whether nurse-midwives could perform episiotomies, a small surgical incision in the perineum to create a larger opening through which a baby emerges. Some states demand continuing education. Some allow nurse-midwives to serve as primary-care providers without referral from a primary-care physician in a managed-care insurance program. Many states require third-party insurance payers to pay for care provided by nurse-midwives. Federal law mandates that all state Medicaid programs pay for services provided by nurse-midwives.[37] Compared with nurse-midwives, certified midwives practice legally only in New York, while in other states, their status is less clear. In some states, midwives who are not nurses (there are many different kinds of midwives in addition to certified midwives) are legally prohibited, or "effectively prohibited" because "there is no mechanism for gaining the required legal authority to practice"; in other states, they are legal but not regulated; in others, they are legal and regulated; and in some, it is unclear how the statutes apply to them.[38]

## The Future of Nurse-Midwifery

Nearly a century after American public-health reformers proposed nurse-midwifery as a temporary solution to the problems of high maternal and infant mortality, poorly trained physicians, and "backward" traditional midwives, nurse-midwives are still with us. Rather than fading away when the immediate need declined, the profession has persisted and evolved, reflecting changing needs and attitudes in the United States. The problems are not the same as they were in the early 1900s. The nation's maternal and infant mortality rates are dramatically lower, obstetricians and family physicians receive excellent training in obstetrics, and traditional midwives for the most part no longer exist (and many midwives who are not nurses are well trained). However, the distribution of maternal and infant health services continues to be uneven. Despite spending more of its gross national product on health care than any other country in the world, the United States ranks twenty-second in infant mortality rates and twenty-eighth in maternal mortality rates, well behind most other industrialized countries. These statistics are related: middle- and upper-class Americans can buy access to the best health care in the world while uninsured and underinsured Americans receive few of the benefits of this care (more than 43 million Americans had no health insurance in 2002). The relatively high infant and maternal mortality rates in the United States reflect lower-income patients' lack of access to primary, preventive, and specialist health-care services.[39] In addition to inadequate access to health care, other maternal health-care problems exist today. Many women complain that they do not feel like partners with physicians and other health-care personnel in making decisions about childbirth. These women point to health-care personnel who do not listen to or spend time with them, who dismiss their needs or wants, and/or who demand that they labor and deliver according to a preestablished schedule. On the one hand, some women feel pushed to use childbirth technologies, such as epidurals and Caesarean sections, as a given, rather than as a matter for individual reflection and decision-making.[40] On the other hand, many women "are deciding that labor pain is a rite of passage they can do without and are gratefully accepting pain medicine during childbirth," as explained in a *New York Times* article reporting on a paper at an anesthesiology conference. More and more women are using anesthesia in labor, and in 2003, an all-time high of 27.5 percent of babies were delivered by Caesarean section.[41]

Given the current problems with American maternal and general health care, what place then does nurse-midwifery have in the future? History shows that nurse-midwives both face challenges and have particular strengths to help them overcome those hurdles. As stated in a joint report of the Pew Health Professions Commission and the University of California, San Francisco, Center for the Health Professions in 1999, nurse-midwives have been underutilized.[42] One of nurse-midwives' biggest problems, both in the past and today, is public relations. Most people do not understand what nurse-midwives do, the education they have received, where they practice, the extent to which they work in collaboration with physicians, and what they can offer women and newborns. Many people associate nurse-midwives with second-class care and with home births. But studies show that these associations are incorrect. First, births attended by nurse-midwives are at least as safe, if not safer, than those attended by obstetricians.[43] Second, only 1.1 percent of nurse-midwife-attended births were at home in 2003, although studies in the United States and elsewhere show the safety of planned home births for low-risk women.[44]

Not only are nurse-midwives misunderstood; they are often invisible, and their therapeutic approach contributes to their invisibility. When looking at "exemplary midwifery practice," Holly Powell Kennedy, a nursing professor at the University of California, San Francisco, and her colleagues found that certified nurse-midwives and certified midwives "were negotiators, not dictators."

> They believed that power rested with the women and not necessarily in themselves. This does not mean to imply that they were weak or compliant; in fact, they were often the opposite. Yet, their consistent approach in being a background, rather than a foreground presence may prevent them from being seen as a substantial force for change in our delivery of health care for women in the United States. In addition, emphasis on presence and relationship, rather than routine use of technology, may be misaligned with an institutional and consumer fascina-

> tion with machines as the solution to achieve optimal birth outcomes. In this study, the midwife represented the 'instrument' of care. It was the midwife's ability to communicate, engaged presence, and clinical judgment that presided, not the technology that was used. Consequently, strategies must be developed to document midwifery care and outcomes in ways that are understood from public health, consumer, marketing, and economic perspectives. Their invisibility as a strategy to help women realize their own strength is admirable, but they must work to increase their public visibility if they are going to continue to make a difference in the lives of women.[45]

Kennedy and her colleagues suggest that midwives need to translate their excellent work into a language that the public will understand, so they can gain their rightful place—given their excellent outcomes for women and babies—as the provider of health care for the majority of women in the United States.

As Kennedy and her colleagues explain, these public relations problems will not be easy for nurse-midwives and their supporters to solve. Throughout their history, nurse-midwives have challenged certain notions of progress and modernity, such as technology is always good, faster is better, and professionals must do "something" to prove their worth. But nurse-midwives were not and are not Luddites. They have embraced and, in fact, fought to have access to technologies, they are scientifically trained, and they participate in the medical mainstream, whether they practice inside or outside hospitals, but as compared to physicians, they are trained in a different conception of time and have a different definition of "productivity." As Kennedy puts it, they value, and are skilled at, the "art of doing 'nothing' well." That means that they spend a lot of time waiting and "'be[ing] present' with the woman, intervening only when necessary." The midwives in Kennedy's studies did not just blithely assume that pregnancy and birth would be easy and normal. In fact, with "vigilance and attention to detail," the midwives "carefully screened, measured, educated, and watched over" their patients, and quickly intervened if something went wrong.[46] Still in doing "nothing" so much of the time, they go against what more traditional American health-care providers and American culture have long defined as modern.

Added to the public relations problems that nurse-midwives face are other barriers, including opposition from physicians and hospital administrators. Even in states with laws granting nurse-midwives a fair amount of autonomy in birth management, some hospitals' guidelines and policies tightly restrict nurse-midwives and show physicians' and hospital administrators' skepticism about their work. Two examples illustrate this.

First, in the late 1990s, a small-town hospital in upstate New York had a scoring system that assigned points to such indications in a patient as previous abortions, obesity, and age; if a patient scored more than two points, she had to be attended by a physician, not a nurse-midwife. Other policies of this hospital also severely limited nurse-midwives' practice. For example, a nurse-midwife in group practice was not allowed to deliver any women she had not previously followed, while this was not the case with obstetricians in the practice. Additionally, nurse-midwives were not allowed to use pitocin or other medication to induce and/or augment labor, even after consulting with an attending physician. This system made nurse-midwife management of births unlikely, and in fact, as of 2006, no nurse-midwife practices at this hospital.[47]

In a second example, in 2002, two hospitals in Austin, Texas, closed their nurse-midwifery services, claiming that the services lost money, but, as a National Public Radio report stated, "critics suspect politics had much to do with why one of those facilities, Brackenridge, the city's only public hospital, kicked the midwives out." Sources in that report indicated that Brackenridge physicians wanted their own residents, rather than nurse-midwives, to attend deliveries, and that as of 2004, some are under investigation by the Texas attorney general's office for violating antitrust regulations by "colluding with doctors at another hospital in trying to control the midwives." The report noted that the events in Austin are part of a larger trend: the closing or cutting back of nurse-midwifery services around the country, in places as varied as New York City, Chicago, and Des Moines, Iowa. In the report, Susan Jenkins, an attorney in Washington, D.C., who represents nurse-midwives and direct-entry midwives, explained: "There are many, many cases around the country where the medical staff of a hospital has taken actions which restrict midwifery practice so that as a practical matter, midwives can't work there."[48]

Still another tangible problem facing nurse-midwives is the rising cost of medical malpractice insurance, which all health-care professionals face, but which hits obstetric providers especially hard. In fact, some obstetrician/gynecologists and family practitioners have decided not to deliver babies anymore and some hospitals have closed their maternity units because of the high rates of malpractice insurance.[49] According to the ACNM, in 2004, "despite the historically low incidence of lawsuits against nurse-midwives, malpractice insurance rates for certified nurse-midwives (CNMs) have risen as much as 1,000 % in the last year, forcing many qualified providers out of practice. Fewer carriers offer coverage to nurse-midwives and other obstetric providers, and many have massively increased their rates beyond what many nurse-midwives can afford."[50]

Finally, in the face of all of this opposition to and ignorance about their profession, nurse-midwives disagree with one another about what their profession should look like. Just like their predecessors in the mid-twentieth century, they argue about whether or how much they should try either to be part of the medical mainstream or to be on the margins. These arguments are best demonstrated in debates between the ACNM and the Midwives' Alliance of North America (MANA), founded in 1982 at an ACNM meeting. While ACNM is an exclusive organization, requiring its members to have a certain education in an ACNM-accredited program and pass a specific exam to join, MANA allows anyone who declares her- or himself a midwife to join. MANA includes nurse-midwives and non-nurse-midwives, and "MANA members do not accept the argument that formal, standardized education is necessary to provide safe and competent practitioners." Some MANA midwives, including the nurse-midwives among them, have criticized nurse-midwives for being too medicalized, too willing to use labor induction, epidurals, and episiotomies unnecessarily, and just as interventionist in birth as obstetricians. Most nurse-midwives now practice in hospitals where they must follow hospital rules and inevitably absorb part of the hospital culture, even as they are changing it. The MANA critics want midwives not to be bound by the dictates of the medical and nursing professions, to attend births at home, and to offer a distinctive alternative to the "medical model of care." These midwives believe that on the margins they can have more control and autonomy over their practices, and therefore be truly free to offer what has been called the "midwifery model of care," "providing the mother with individualized education, counseling, and prenatal care, and continuous hands-on assistance during labor and delivery, and postpartum support," as well as "minimizing technological interventions."[51] Yet, as former ACNM president Joyce Roberts explained at a MANA conference in 1997, in the current American health-care system, if nurse-midwives were not formally educated, did not collaborate with physicians, and did not take health insurance, they would risk "limiting [their] practice to a very narrow domain."[52] In other words, Roberts believes that nurse-midwives make a trade off: they medicalize somewhat so that they can practice in a wide variety of settings with a wide variety of clients—in other words, participate in the medical mainstream. These internal arguments among nurse-midwives (and non-nurse-midwives) are understandable given the external problems they face. Yet, they present a serious challenge for the future of nurse-midwifery by weakening the already frayed fabric of their professional cloth.

Despite facing enormous barriers in health care and in the larger society, the profession of nurse-midwifery has much to recommend it. Most notable is practitioners' history of good outcomes. Studies repeatedly show that nurse-midwives are at least as safe and often safer birth attendants than physicians, even among high-risk populations.[53] For example, one 1998 study found that "after controlling for social and medical risk factors, the risk of experiencing an infant death was 19% lower for certified nurse midwife attended than for physician attended births, the risk of neonatal mortality was 33% lower, and the risk of delivering a low birthweight infant 31% lower."[54] Another strength nurse-midwives have is their history of providing care to underserved and vulnerable populations, especially as increasing numbers of Americans lack access to health care. Historically, nurse-midwives have cared for patients in the greatest need, whether they were poor whites in Appalachian Kentucky, poor African Americans and Puerto Ricans in Harlem, or poor Latinas in northern New Mexico. They continue to care for many women who are at risk to have what health professionals call "poor pregnancy outcomes"; as one study in the 1990s noted, "70% of the women and newborns seen by nurse-midwives are considered vulnerable by virtue of age, socioeconomic status, education, ethnicity, or place of residence."[55]

Nurse-midwives are also more cost-effective than physicians, offering policy makers the chance to cut spending in an age of spiraling health-care costs. Several studies show that the reason nurse-midwives cost less than physicians is that they use significantly less technology and fewer interventions and procedures.[56] One 1997 study showed that "even after both biological and sociodemographic differences are controlled for, patients who initiate care with midwives have fewer intrapartum interventions and a lower cesarean section rate than patients who initiate care with physicians." Compared with both obstetricians and family physicians,

> Certified nurse-midwives were much less likely to use a variety of technological tools to monitor or modify the course of labor. Patients of certified nurse-midwives were less likely to be continuously electronically monitored during labor, to receive oxytocin to induce or augment labor, or to be given epidural anesthesia. Probably as a consequence, fewer of their patients have an operative delivery. A lower rate of

> cesarean sections—particularly among nulliparous women [women who are giving birth for the first time]—is associated with shorter hospital stays and small expenditures for operating room and anesthesia staff.[57]

It should be noted that the reason nurse-midwives are more cost effective is *not* that nurse-midwives' fees are lower than physicians'. While nurse-midwives generally earn less than physicians, they often charge similar fees for prenatal, labor-and-delivery, and postpartum care as physicians. Nurse-midwives, however, see fewer patients, spending more time with each patient during prenatal and postpartum visits and staying with patients throughout labor and delivery.[58]

Finally, nurse-midwives have shown "great resilience," as one nurse-midwife leader put it, for more than eighty years.[59] They constantly have found ways to adapt to new environments. In the 1920s, public-health nurses took a successful European model and adapted it to the United States in an attempt to solve maternal and infant health problems. Despite resistance from obstetricians and general practitioners, they opened nurse-midwifery schools and services, providing care for poor and minority women with excellent maternal and infant outcomes. In the 1940s and 1950s, when the great majority of births took place in hospitals and when the United States faced an obstetrician shortage, nurse-midwives reinvented themselves and worked in hospitals. Sometimes they worked in pioneering university hospital nurse-midwifery services or in special natural childbirth demonstrations, but more often they were employed as maternity nurses or supervisors, since very few hospitals allowed nurse-midwives to practice fully the profession for which they were trained. They did what they could in often hostile environments. In the 1970s, nurse-midwives reinvented themselves yet again. In new private practices, they provided a birthing alternative for middle-class women who, in the context of the women's and consumer health movements, wanted more personalized care. They also continued to work overwhelmingly with women who were poor, minority, or otherwise at risk for poor outcomes, and they continued to work in hospitals. In the 1990s, in an era of market-driven changes in health-care delivery and financing and concerns about rising health-care costs, nurse-midwives tried to reinvent themselves to policy makers as a lower-cost alternative to physicians as the primary health-care providers for women, even as managed care made it difficult for nurse-midwives to continue their time-intensive, prevention-oriented style of care.[60]

With both historical strengths and weaknesses, nurse-midwifery has entered the twenty-first century still in the process of adapting and defining itself. As a collective and as individuals, American nurse-midwives continue to ask: Who are we? How can we communicate who we are to the lay public and to other health professionals? What do we want our place in the American health-care system to be, and how can we best achieve that? What are the best ways to deal with the barriers we face? History shows that nurse-midwives have the potential to have a continuing, and even more central, role in maternal health care and in the health care of women and newborns. However, history also shows that they will likely face many hurdles, both external and internal, as they try to move forward. Today, nurse-midwives have assumed a larger role in mainstream health care than ever before, yet they are still marginalized. Their future will depend on changing American attitudes about childbirth, health care, and women professionals, as well as on nurse-midwives' ability to adapt to those changes. Most likely nurse-midwives will continue to navigate in difficult waters in a middle space between the mainstream and the margins of medicine, and between the nursing profession and midwifery traditions.

# NOTES

## Notes to Chapter 1

1. Sister M. Theophane Shoemaker, "Is Nurse-Midwifery the Solution?" reprinted from *Public Health Nursing* (December 1946), Medical Mission Sisters (MMS) Archives, Philadelphia, Pennsylvania.

2. For Sister Theophane's biography, see Sally Austen Tom, "Agnes Shoemaker Reinders: A Biographical Tribute," *Journal of Nurse-Midwifery* 25, no. 5 (September/October 1980): 9–12, and "In Memoriam—Agnes Reinders, FACNM (Sister Theophane Shoemaker)," *Journal of Nurse-Midwifery* 38, no. 6 (November/December 1993): 317. Later in her life, Sister Theophane left the religious order, married, and became Agnes Reinders.

3. Kroska, *50th Celebration Reunion,* video, 1994.

4. Kroska, *50th Celebration Reunion,* video, 1994.

5. Martin et al., "Birth: Final Data for 2003," 15, 81.

6. Reverby, *Ordered to Care.*

7. I thank Susan L. Smith for encouraging me to emphasize this point.

8. Peter E. S. Freund, Meredith B. McGuire, and Linda S. Podhurst, *Health, Illness, and the Social Body: A Critical Sociology,* 4th ed. (Upper Saddle River, N.J.: Prentice Hall, 2003), 258.

9. Mitford, *The American Way of Birth.*

10. See, especially, Dye, "Medicalization of Birth," 17–46; Leavitt, *Brought to Bed;* Leavitt, "The Medicalization of Childbirth," vol. 11, no. 4: 299–319; and Wertz and Wertz, *Lying-In.*

11. Around 1800, New England farmer Samuel Thomson created his botanical system which relied on large doses of remedies made out of vegetables as well as steaming the body. Thomson's ideas became very popular as a result of his handbook, and eventually the Thomsonian movement came to include botanical societies, journals, and national meetings. Cassedy, *Medicine in America,* 36–37.

12. Cassedy, *Medicine in America,* 25–39.

13. Ulrich, *A Midwife's Tale*; Leavitt, *Brought to Bed;* and Dye, "Medicalization of Birth."

14. Leavitt, *Brought to Bed,* 36–43.
15. Quoted in Leavitt, *Brought to Bed,* 43.
16. Leavitt, *Brought to Bed,* 43–47.
17. Dye, "Medicalization of Birth," 32.
18. Leavitt, *Brought to Bed,* 49.
19. Wertz and Wertz, *Lying-In,* 55–58.
20. Wertz and Wertz, *Lying-In,* 132–33.
21. Stevens, *In Sickness and In Wealth,* 105, 108–9.
22. Leavitt, "Medicalization of Childbirth," 309–12.
23. In 1930, obstetricians and gynecologists established a medical specialty examining board, excluding physicians who did not limit their practice to women, and thus effectively leaving out all general practitioners, even those with practices primarily devoted to delivering babies and caring for women. Prior to that time, hospitals had no method of excluding general practitioners who wanted to perform obstetrical surgery or other procedures. Leavitt, *Brought to Bed,* 171–80; Starr, *The Social Transformation of American Medicine,* 356–57; and Wertz and Wertz, *Lying-In,* 160–61.
24. Leavitt, *Brought to Bed,* 173–77, 189.
25. Gilbreth and Carey, *Cheaper by the Dozen,* 115.
26. Leavitt, *Brought to Bed,* 171–95.
27. Although the infant mortality rate decreased by nearly fifty percent between 1910 and 1930, neonatal (infants less than one month old) deaths, which accounted for more than half of all infant deaths, did not decline nearly as much. Litoff, *American Midwives,* 108.
28. Leavitt, *Brought to Bed,* 182–83.
29. The studies were New York Academy of Medicine Committee on Public Health Relations, *Maternal Mortality in New York City;* Philadelphia County Medical Society Committee on Maternal Welfare, *Maternal Mortality in Philadelphia;* and White House Conference on Child Health and Protection, *Fetal, Newborn, and Maternal Mortality and Morbidity.*
30. Joseph B. DeLee and Heinz Siedentopf, "The Maternity Ward of the General Hospital," *Journal of the American Medical Association* 100 (7 January 1933): 6–14, quoted in Leavitt, *Brought to Bed,* 185.
31. Leavitt, *Brought to Bed,* 187.
32. In the 1920s and 1930s, obstetricians used the term "meddlesome obstetrics" quite frequently. See, for example, Emery, "Meddlesome Obstetrics," 88–91. On obstetricians' condemnation of their profession, see Leavitt, *Brought to Bed,* 186–87. On pituitrin, which came into wide use after 1911, see Shorter, *A History of Women's Bodies,* 152. Shorter talks about pituitrin in the context of the damage it caused to British and American women attended by general practitioners at home. On "twilight sleep," which American obstetricians started to use in 1914, see Leavitt, *Brought to Bed,* 128–41.
33. Stevens, *In Sickness and In Wealth,* 173–74, 393n6.
34. Litoff, *American Midwives,* 50–51, 53–54.
35. Rude, "The Midwife Problem in the United States," 991.
36. Kobrin, "The American Midwife Controversy," 318–26; and Litoff, *American Midwives.*
37. Smith, *A Tree Grows in Brooklyn,* 336–37.

38. Flexner, *Medical Education in the United States and Canada.*

39. Antler and Fox, "The Movement toward a Safe Maternity," 490–506.

40. Baker, "The Function of a Midwife," 196–97; Baker, *Fighting for Life,* 111–16; and Meckel, *Save the Babies,* 175.

41. The Bellevue school closed in 1936 due to a lack of students. Baker, "Schools for Midwives," 162; Edgar, "The Education, Licensing, and Supervision of the Midwife," 129–43; Bailey, "Control of Midwives," 297; Noyes, "Training School for Midwives at Bellevue and Allied Hospitals," 417–18; Litoff, *American Midwives,* 52–53; Borst, *Catching Babies,* 26; and Tyndall, "A History of the Bellevue School for Midwives: 1911–1936."

42. Quoted in Dawley, "Ideology and Self-Interest," 110–11.

43. Van Blarcom, *Midwife in England,* 13.

44. Van Blarcom, *Midwife in England;* Van Blarcom, "Midwives in America," 197–207; and Dawley, "Ideology and Self-Interest," 110.

45. Noyes, "The Midwifery Problem," 466–71; and Dawley, "Ideology and Self-Interest," 111.

46. Noyes, "The Training of Midwives," 1051; and Shoemaker, *History of Nurse-Midwifery,* 8.

47. Frederick J. Taussig, "The Nurse-Midwife," *Public Health Nursing Quarterly* 6 (October 1914): 33–39; and Litoff, *American Midwives,* 122–23.

48. See chapter 3 for a fuller discussion of MCA's attempt.

49. Cassells, "The Manhattan Midwifery School." In 1923, the Preston Retreat School of Midwifery opened in Philadelphia to educate women to become midwives. Students took classes and, under supervision, managed deliveries at the Preston Retreat Maternity Hospital. Nurses were eventually admitted to this program, but it is unclear when this occurred. According to Sister M. Theophane Shoemaker, at least four registered nurses completed the program between 1933 and 1942. However, the program was not originally established as a *nurse*-midwifery school. Shoemaker, *History of Nurse-Midwifery in the United States,* 38; Katy Dawley and Helen Varney Burst, "The American College of Nurse-Midwives and Its Antecedents: A Historic Time Line," *Journal of Midwifery and Women's Health* 50, no. 1 (January 2005): 16–22; and Cassells, "Manhattan Midwifery School," 31–32.

50. Loudon, *Death in Childbirth,* 155–56.

51. All Western countries have had some version of the traditional midwife who learned her trade by practicing it, and all have had some version of the nurse-midwife, or qualified and trained midwife. The qualified midwives had to fight against the negative images of traditional midwives. Marland and Rafferty, eds., *Midwives, Society, and Childbirth,* 2–3, 9.

52. For historical comparisons between the status and education of physicians in Europe and the United States, see Bonner, *Becoming a Physician.*

53. Loudon, *Death in Childbirth,* 445.

54. Loudon, *Death in Childbirth,* 415–21; Raymond G. DeVries and Rebecca Barroso, "Midwives among the Machines: Re-creating Midwifery in the Late Twentieth Century," in *Midwives, Society, and Childbirth,* ed. Marland and Rafferty, 259–60; Rooks, *Midwifery and Childbirth,* 410–14; and De Vries, *A Pleasing Birth,* especially 23–47.

55. For the modern situation, see Rooks, *Midwifery and Childbirth in America,* 408–410.

56. Kosmak, "Results of Supervised Midwife Practice," 2009.

57. Kosmak, "Results of Supervised Midwife Practice," 2010.

58. Anne Lokke, "The 'Antiseptic' Transformation of Danish Midwives, 1860–1920," in *Midwives, Society, and Childbirth,* ed. Marland and Rafferty, 102–33.

59. Rooks, *Midwifery and Childbirth in America,* 406.

60. Loudon, *Death in Childbirth,* 406–7, 414–15.

61. Rooks, *Midwifery and Childbirth in America,* 409.

62. Quoted in Dawley, "Ideology and Self-Interest," 112; and Charles W. Carey, Jr., "Mary Beard," *American National Biography Online,* ed. John A. Garraty and Mark C. Carnes (New York: Oxford University Press, 2000), www.anb.org/articles/12/12–00065.html (accessed 11 June 2003).

63. Katy Dawley, "Origins of Nurse-Midwifery in the United States and Its Expansion in the 1940s," *Journal of Midwifery and Women's Health* 48, no. 2 (March/April 2003): 86–95. The Rockefeller Foundation refused to fund nurse-midwifery practice directly.

64. On British midwifery, see Donnison, *Midwives and Medical Men,* 176, 180–81, 184–86, 191; and Loudon, *Death in Childbirth,* 173, 207–9, 398–99.

65. Rooks, *Midwifery and Childbirth in America,* 406.

66. Apple, "Constructing Mothers," 161–78; Ladd-Taylor, *Mother-Work;* Meckel, *Save the Babies;* Lindenmeyer, *"A Right to Childhood";* Muncy, *Creating a Female Dominion;* and Klaus, *Every Child a Lion.*

67. More, *Restoring the Balance.*

68. Responses to Committee on Organization's Questionnaire, 1954, American College of Nurse-Midwives (ACNM) Archives, National Library of Medicine, Bethesda, Maryland, container 1; and "Membership of the American College of Nurse-Midwifery," *Bulletin of the American College of Nurse-Midwifery* 1, no. 2 (March 1956): 7–13.

69. Breckinridge, *Wide Neighborhoods,* esp. chap. 8, on how her children's lives and deaths influenced her founding of FNS. Breckinridge was married twice; her first husband died soon after they married. Her biography is discussed in chapter 2.

70. "Hazel Corbin, Health Expert, Is Dead at 93," *New York Times,* 20 May 1988.

71. Quoted in Sally Austen Tom, "Rose McNaught: American Nurse-Midwifery's Own 'Sister Tutor,'" *Journal of Nurse-Midwifery* 24, no. 2 (March/April 1979): 3–8. McNaught's biography is discussed in chapter 3.

72. Reverby, *Ordered to Care,* 80; "Graduates of the Maternity Center Association School of Midwifery," 1957[?], container 7, file: ACNM Membership, List of Graduates from American Midwifery Programs, ACNM Archives; Tirpak, "The Frontier Nursing Service," 125; "Roster of Graduates in Nurse-Midwifery, Catholic Maternity Institute," MMS Archives; Horch, "The Flint-Goodridge School of Nurse-Midwifery"; Canty, "The Graduates of the Tuskegee School of Nurse-Midwifery"; and "Analysis of 147 Answers to Questionnaire," container 1, file: Pre-Organization Questionnaire; Analysis, ACNM Archives.

73. Here, I rely on Robert M. Crunden's work in thinking about secular missionaries. Crunden argues that Progressives "groped toward new professions such as social work, journalism, academia, the law, and politics. In each of these careers, they could become preachers urging moral reform on institutions as well as on individuals." Crunden, *Ministers of Reform,* ix. I thank Debra Meyers for bringing this book to my attention.

74. MCA, *Twenty Years of Nurse-Midwifery,* 67–75.

75. A former nurse-midwife explained that FNS attracted "the missionary type person." Quoted from Molly Lee, in Lillian Bartlett and Phyllis Chisholm, interview by Dale Deaton, 790H197, FNS 196, 10 May 1979, transcript, 54, Frontier Nursing Service (FNS) Oral History Collection, Archives and Special Collections, Margaret I. King Library, University of Kentucky, Lexington.

76. Dammann, *A Social History of the Frontier Nursing Service,* 75.

77. Helen Browne, interview by Dale Deaton, 790H174, FNS 75, 27 March 1979, transcript, 65, FNS Oral History Collection.

78. Ruth Covell, Marian Moore, Lillian R. Talbott, Jeannette Veldman, Jeane Walvoord, and Anne De Young, "A Nurse-Midwife's Story," *Public Health Nursing* 44, no. 12 (December 1952): 659–62.

79. I am grateful to Susan L. Smith for help with phrasing in this paragraph.

80. Katy Dawley has written a number of articles, as well as a dissertation, on the history of nurse-midwifery, mostly focusing on the era after 1940. Helen Varney Burst, author of the first (and leading) textbook for nurse-midwives, has written about the profession's history in her textbook, as well as in articles. Wanda Caroline Hiestand's dissertation discusses the history of nurse-midwifery education from colonial times to 1965. Judith Pence Rooks offers an analysis of nurse-midwifery from 1980 to 1995, with some discussion of nurse-midwifery earlier in the twentieth century. Barbara Katz Rothman's work includes a short section on the history of nurse-midwifery with discussions about nurse-midwives' relative autonomy (or lack thereof) and the extent to which they contributed to the medicalization of childbirth. Judy Barrett Litoff, Richard W. Wertz and Dorothy C. Wertz, and Margot Edwards and Mary Waldorf include a chapter or a few paragraphs on Frontier Nursing Service and/or MCA in their larger works on midwifery or childbirth. Nancy Schrom Dye examines the creation and development of Frontier Nursing Service in the 1920s and 1930s. Anne G. Campbell discusses the American Committee for Devastated France, which Mary Breckinridge used as a model for the Frontier Nursing Service. And Carol Crowe-Carraco explains some of the intersections between Breckinridge's biography and the development of the Frontier Nursing Service. A master's thesis by Heather Harris argues that Breckinridge deliberately constructed "the mountain people's culture for the purposes of strengthening her ability to raise funds for the FNS," and analyzes birth-control trials at the nursing service in the late 1950s and early 1960s. Dawley's publications on this history are "The Campaign to Eliminate the Midwife," 50–56; "Ideology and Self-Interest," 99–126; "Perspectives on the Past," 747–55; "Origins of Nurse-Midwifery in the United States," 86–95; "American Nurse-Midwifery," 147–70; "Doubling Back over Roads Once Traveled: Creating a National Organization for Nurse-Midwifery," *Journal of Midwifery and Women's Health* 50, no. 2 (March-April 2005): 71–82; "Leaving the Nest"; and coauthored Dawley and Burst, "American College of Nurse-Midwives and Its Antecedents," 16–22. Some of Burst's publications include "The History of Nurse-Midwifery/Midwifery Education," *Journal of Midwifery and Women's Health* 50, no. 2 (March-April 2005): 129–37; coauthored Varney, Kriebs, and Gegor, "The Profession and History of Midwifery," in *Varney's Midwifery,* 3–27; and coauthored Helen Varney Burst and Joyce E. Thompson, "Genealogic Origins of Nurse-Midwifery Education Programs in the United States," *Journal of Midwifery and Women's Health* 48, no. 6 (November-December 2003): 464–72. Other works on the

history of nurse-midwifery are Hiestand, "Midwife to Nurse-Midwife"; Rooks, *Midwifery and Childbirth in America;* Rothman, *In Labor;* Litoff, *American Midwives;* Wertz and Wertz, *Lying-In;* Edwards and Waldorf, *Reclaiming Birth;* Dye, "Mary Breckinridge," 485–507; Campbell, "Mary Breckinridge," 257–76; Crowe-Carraco, "Mary Breckinridge," 179–91; and Harris, "Constructing Colonialism."

81. Dye, "Mary Breckinridge," 485–507, quotation on 507.

82. Morantz-Sanchez, *Sympathy and Science;* and More, *Restoring the Balance.*

83. The exhibition *Changing the Face of Medicine* also makes a similar argument. Fee, *Changing the Face of Medicine.*

84. Reverby, *Ordered to Care,* front matter; and Melosh, *"The Physician's Hand."*

85. Hine, *Black Women in White;* and Buhler-Wilkerson, *False Dawn.*

86. Buhler-Wilkerson, *False Dawn,* xi.

## Notes to Chapter 2

1. The information on Lester is from Betty Lester, interview by Jonathan Fried and other FNS couriers, 780H146, FNS 6, 3 March 1978, FNS Oral History Collection (online version), Archives and Special Collections, Margaret I. King Library, University of Kentucky, Lexington, kdl.kyvl.org/cgi/t/text/text-idx?c=oralhist&tpl =kukohfns. tpl (accessed 1 November 2003); Betty Lester, interview by Dale Deaton, 820H12, FNS 155, 27 July 1978, transcript, 2–3, 8–17, FNS Oral History Collection; Betty Lester, interview by Dale Deaton, 820H13, FNS 156, 3 August 1978, transcript, 11–17, 20, FNS Oral History Collection; and "Betty Lester Passes Away: Festival Spirit Will Be Dampened by Her Absence," *(Hyden, Ky.) Leslie County News,* 22, no. 32 (September 1988): 1.

2. "Resolutions," *Quarterly Bulletin of the Kentucky Committee for Mothers and Babies* 1, no. 1 (June 1925): 5–6.

3. Susan Ulrich, Chair of Midwifery and Women's Health, Frontier School of Midwifery and Family Nursing, telephone conversation with author, 10 November 2003; and Kitty Ernst (Mary Breckinridge Chair of Midwifery, Frontier School of Midwifery and Family Nursing), telephone conversation with author, 10 November 2003. According to Ulrich, in 2002, approximately 75 of the 326 women and men who took the licensing exam for certified nurse-midwives were graduates of the Frontier School's Community-Based Nurse-Midwifery Education Program (CNEP). Ulrich and Ernst both indicated that the percentage of CNEP graduates was much greater in the early 1990s. Ernst attributed the decrease to the doubling of nurse-midwifery schools between 1989, when CNEP first began, and today, along with the addition of several other distance-education programs.

4. See Dye, "Mary Breckinridge"; Campbell, "Mary Breckinridge"; and Crowe-Carraco, "Mary Breckinridge."

5. Marvin Breckinridge Patterson, "Foreword," in Breckinridge, *Wide Neighborhoods,* xiii.

6. Helen Browne, interview by Carol Crowe-Carraco, 790H173, FNS 74, 26 March 1979, transcript, 55, FNS Oral History Collection.

7. Lester interviews, 820H12, FNS 155, 27 July 1978, 35–36, and 820H13, FNS 156, 3 August 1978, 34–37.

8. For biographical information on Breckinridge, see Ettinger, "Mary Breckinridge," 462–63; Breckinridge, *Wide Neighborhoods*; Dye, "Mary Breckinridge"; Campbell, "Mary Breckinridge"; Crowe-Carraco, "Mary Breckinridge"; and Dammann, *Social History of the Frontier Nursing Service.*

9. Other Breckinridges were important political and social figures. Mary's cousin, Sophonisba Breckinridge, was part of the national progressive female reform network. The first woman to pass the Kentucky bar, Sophonisba was a Hull House resident, one of Chicago's most prominent reformers, and cofounder of the University of Chicago's School of Social Service Administration. In her autobiography, Mary Breckinridge explained how her mother used cousin "Nisba" to discourage her from going to college. Mary's family "disapproved of a college education for women. Years before [I was old enough to attend college], as a little girl in Washington, I listened to the family discussions when Cousin Willie Breckinridge's daughter, Sophonisba, elected to go to Wellesley. I recall my mother saying that college would not be detrimental in itself but that Nisba would not want to live at home afterward. When Nisba finished at Wellesley and started on her distinguished career, my mother said with disapproval, 'She refused to go back home to live.'" Breckinridge, *Wide Neighborhoods,* 32; and Muncy, *Creating a Female Dominion,* 68–87. For information on the Breckinridge family, see Klotter, *The Breckinridges of Kentucky.*

10. Breckinridge, *Wide Neighborhoods,* 48–50, 59, 60–74.

11. Breckinridge, *Wide Neighborhoods,* 111.

12. Breckinridge, "The Nurse-Midwife—A Pioneer," 1148.

13. Breckinridge, "The Nurse on Horseback," 7.

14. Mary Breckinridge to Josephine Hunt, 22 December 1941, box 345, folder 3, FNS Papers.

15. Mary Breckinridge, notes on Susan Stiddum, 1923, box 348, folder 2; and Mary Breckinridge, "Midwifery in the Kentucky Mountains: An Investigation," 1923, box 348, folder 1, both in FNS Papers.

16. Breckinridge, notes on Susan Stiddum, 1923.

17. Mary Breckinridge, notes on Nancy Brock, "Midwifery in the Kentucky Mountains: An Investigation," 1923, box 348, folder 2, FNS Papers.

18. Breckinridge, "Midwifery in the Mountains: An Investigation," 1923.

19. Of course, this community of native-born white Christians scored better on a test created for native-born white Christians than did mixed populations.

20. Mary Breckinridge, "Midwifery in the Kentucky Mountains, An Investigation in 1923," *Quarterly Bulletin of the Frontier Nursing Service, Inc.* 17, no. 4 (Spring 1942): 29–53. This is the published version of Breckinridge's investigation. Her earlier, unpublished version is cited above.

21. For Breckinridge's use of the phrase, "Mr. Ready-to-Halt," see Mary Breckinridge to Ella Phillips Crandall, 14 November 1923, box 348, folder 3, FNS Papers.

22. Dye, "Mary Breckinridge," 495–96. On the Commonwealth Fund, see Harvey and Abrams, *For the Welfare of Mankind.*

23. Annie S. Veech to Mary Breckinridge, 31 October 1923, box 348, folder 3, FNS Papers. Emphasis added.

24. Veech to Breckinridge, 31 October 1923.

25. Dye, "Mary Breckinridge," 496.

26. Veech to Breckinridge, 31 October 1923; and Altizer, "The Establishment of

the Frontier Nursing Service," 6–7.

Veech offered to print the report, only if Breckinridge agreed to send it "to those few who would understand and know how to help." Breckinridge declined the offer, telling Veech that she misunderstood Breckinridge's intentions, and did not publish the survey until almost twenty years later in *Quarterly Bulletin of the Frontier Nursing Service.* Veech to Breckinridge, 31 October 1923; Breckinridge to Veech, 14 November 1923, box 348, folder 3, FNS Papers; Alitzer, "Establishment of the Frontier Nursing Service," 7; and Breckinridge, "Midwifery in the Kentucky Mountains, An Investigation in 1923," 29–53.

27. Thompy [Mary Breckinridge] to Kitty [Jessie "Kit" Carson], 24 November 1926, 3–4, box 328, folder 1, FNS Papers.

28. Prior to 1965, the year of Breckinridge's death and passage of Medicare and Medicaid in Congress, FNS accepted government aid only once, during World War II. Breckinridge's successor, Helen E. Browne, explained, "I have been thankful so many times that Mrs. Breckinridge died when she did. Because the year after she died came the government. It would have killed her. They would have killed her. She would have tried to fight them." Breckinridge assumed government money would mean government interference in FNS. Over twenty-five years after founding FNS, she explained, "If we let government control the nursing and medical care we receive as *private* citizens, then government will become so paternalistic that we may expect officials to drop down from the heavens by parachute to tuck us in bed and hear our prayers." Breckinridge's distrust of public support set her apart from other progressive women reformers, who believed an active government could help to solve maternal and child health problems and who hoped government involvement in "women's issues" would lead to more women in government positions. Browne, interview by Deaton, 27 March 1979, 77; and Breckinridge, *Wide Neighborhoods*, 355.

29. Breckinridge, *Wide Neighborhoods,* 123–30. For further information on the history of British midwifery, see Towler and Bramall, *Midwives in History and Society;* and Bent, "The Growth and Development of Midwifery," 180–95.

30. Breckinridge, *Wide Neighborhoods,* 131–46.

31. Starting in 1948, if not before, FNS charged ten dollars for complete midwifery care; by 1949, the fee was fifteen dollars; and, by 1954, it was twenty dollars. FNS raised the general nursing fee from one to two dollars per year for each family in the early 1950s. Miles, "Heroines on Horseback," 29; "Frontier Nursing Service Aids Remote Areas in Hazard Section," *Hi-Power News* 5, no. 5 (May 1948): 2–3, box 36, folder 8, FNS Papers; Hyland, "The Fruitful Mountaineers," 65; Schupp, "Good Neighbor of 'Wide Neighborhoods,'" 14; and Haney, "Nursing by Jeep and Horseback," 140.

32. Breckinridge, *Wide Neighborhoods,* 202; Freda Caffin and Caroline Caffin, "Experiences of the Nurse-Midwife in the Kentucky Mountains," reprinted from *Nation's Health* 8, no. 12 (December 1926): 1–3, box 35, folder 1, FNS Papers; Agnes Lewis to Anne MacKinnon, 15 February 1939, box 339, folder 4, FNS Papers; Kooser, "Rural Obstetrics," 123–31; and Schupp, "Good Neighbor of 'Wide Neighborhoods,'" 14.

33. Willeford, *Income and Health in Remote Rural Areas,* 14, 18–24. Willeford, an FNS nurse-midwife, completed the study as her doctoral dissertation at Teachers College, Columbia University. As Willeford explained, "the total family income was determined from the following items: (a) wages from all members of the family (exclusive of

money both earned and spent elsewhere); (b) value of animal products, both sold and consumed, (sale of capital stock not included); (c) value of agricultural products, both sold and consumed; (d) value of cattle and poultry including number of animals bred, both sold and consumed; (e) value of natural products, sold; (f) value of handicraft products, sold; (g) moneys received from investments, from pensions and from relief, including Red Cross relief." Quotation is on page 14.

34. American Institute for Economic Research Cost-of-Living Calculator, www.aier.org/colcalc.html (accessed 27 March 2006) (hereafter AIER Cost-of-Living Calculator). Data source: U.S. Bureau of Labor Statistics.

35. Breckinridge stated: "There should, of course, be strong men on our [New York] Committee, but I am greatly opposed to committees exclusively of men or women for public work which concerns both sexes. I never liked the division of such committees into sexes, as I think that men and women both work better together and work is put over better which has combined ideas of the two, since it is meant to appeal both to men and women." T. [Mary Breckinridge] to Kit [Jessie Carson], 13 June 1927, 2, box 328, folder 1, FNS Papers.

36. Several of Breckinridge's letters explained the benefits of the courier system. See, for example, Breckinridge to Mrs. E. A. Codman, 10 April 1931, box 328, folder 6; and Breckinridge to Codman, 26 November 1935, box 328, folder 10, both in FNS Papers.

37. For an early example of Breckinridge's constant use of photographs, see Breckinridge to Mrs. Ernest Codman [FNS Boston Committee chair], 28 October 1929, box 328, folder 4, FNS Papers. At the end of the letter, Breckinridge wrote, "One thing more I have got wonderful stereopticon pictures in color. We have been trying them in Kentucky and they are extraordinarily good. They give me a new lease on life in speaking because they illustrate what I have to say; in fact, half of what I have to say now is said in pictures instead of words."

38. Many couriers wrote and directed films, books, and magazine and newspaper articles on FNS. See Gardner, *Clever Country;* Lansing, *Rider on the Mountains;* and Elisabeth Hubbard Lansing, "Rider on the Mountains," *Senior Prom: The Complete Magazine for Teens, Debs and Co-Eds* 10, no. 95 (March 1950): 68–78, box 36, folder 10, FNS Papers.

39. Quoted in Shapiro, *Appalachia on Our Mind,* 98–99. See also Batteau, *The Invention of Appalachia.*

40. Some key works on nativism in the 1920s include Higham, *Strangers in the Land;* Bennett, *The Party of Fear;* and Knobel, *'America for the Americans.'*

41. Caudill, *Night Comes to the Cumberlands.*

42. Whisnant, *All That Is Native and Fine,* 3–16.

43. Adelheid Mueller, "Frontier Nursing Service: Kentucky Contributes One of America's Noblest Ventures in Human Living," *Walther League Messenger* 56, no. 8 (April 1948): 16–17, 50–51, box 36, folder 7, FNS Papers.

44. Beth Burchenal Jones, interview by Dale Deaton, 820H39, FNS 182, 15 November 1978, transcript, 18–19, FNS Oral History Collection.

45. Breckinridge used nativism as more than a public relations tool; she truly believed in the importance of "old stock." For example, Breckinridge was delighted to hear that the daughter of one volunteer was getting married because, "personally, I love to see the old stock get married and have babies. It is almost a patriotic duty."

Breckinridge to Mrs. Gammell Cross [head of FNS Providence Committee], 3 December 1934, box 328, folder 9, FNS Papers.

46. Breckinridge, "The Nurse on Horseback," 7.

47. Frontier Nursing Service, Boston Committee pamphlet, c. early 1930s, box 329, folder 7, FNS Papers. The same language was also used in Frontier Nursing Service, Detroit Committee pamphlet, c. late 1920s–early 1930s, box 330, folder 7, FNS Papers.

48. Elizabeth Perkins, Letter to the Editor, *(Hyden, Ky.) Thousandsticks,* 16, no. 14 (7 April 1927), box 39, folder 1, FNS Papers.

49. Quotation is from "Frontier Nursing Service Brings Health to Kentucky Mountaineers," *Life* 33.

50. Fischer, *Albion's Seed,* 605–782.

51. Breckinridge, "Where the Frontier Lingers," 10.

52. Mary Breckinridge, "The Rural Family and Its Mother," reprinted from *The Mother*, April 1944, box 356, folder 15, FNS Papers.

53. For example, an introduction to Delphia Ramey's oral history explained that while she was growing up in eastern Kentucky in the 1910s and 1920s, "between men and women there was little separation of roles and both were expected to plant crops, hoe, gather fodder, split rails, and chop firewood." Shackelford and Weinberg, *Our Appalachia,* 123.

54. See, for example, Maggard, "Class and Gender," 100–113; and Maggard, "Will the Real Daisy Mae Please Stand Up?," 136–50.

55. On the concern about fertility rates and "race suicide," see McCann, *Birth Control Politics in the United States;* Pernick, "Eugenics and Public Health in American History," 1767–72; and Reed, *From Private Vice to Public Virtue.*

56. "Will Rogers Endorses the February 25th S/S Belgenland Cruise to the West Indies for the Benefit of the Frontier Nursing Service," 1933, box 329, folder 3, FNS Papers. Breckinridge's handwriting is on this letter, giving her approval.

57. Poole, "The Nurse on Horseback," 210.

58. Poole, "The Nurse on Horseback," 205.

59. Headlines from articles by Breckinridge, "Nurse on Horseback," 5–7, 38; and Breckinridge, "Saving Lives on the Last Frontier," 22.

60. Allen Batteau has argued that advanced capitalist societies destroy the myths and symbols necessary to create meaning and thus must turn to their "'folk' hinterland for cultural renewal." According to Batteau, middle- and upper-class Americans romanticized Appalachian people and Appalachia, the place, as exotic and primitive to fill a void in their own lives. Batteau, "Appalachia and the Concept of Culture," 153–69.

61. Miles, "Heroines on Horseback." This article is an example of the external press picking up on the romanticization perpetuated by FNS.

62. On automobile use in the United States, see Flink, *The Automobile Age.*

63. Mary Breckinridge, "An Adventure in Midwifery: The Nurse-on-Horseback Gets a 'Soon Start,'" reprinted from *Survey Graphic,* 1 October 1926, 1, box 356, folder 3, FNS Papers.

64. Marvin Breckinridge (later Marvin Breckinridge Patterson), *The Forgotten Frontier,* c. 1928, film. For more information about this film, see Marvin Breckinridge Patterson, speech, in *Presentation of the Frontier Nursing Service Collection,* 1985, video; and Breckinridge, *Wide Neighborhoods,* 277–79.

65. Dawley, "Campaign to Eliminate the Midwife," and Dawley, "Ideology and Self-Interest."

66. Pearl, "Distribution of Physicians in the United States," 1024–28.

67. Scott Breckinridge (Mary Breckinridge's cousin, Lexington physician, and member of FNS's medical advisory board) explained, the "raising of the standards of medical education and the increasing need of laboratory and hospital facilities for the satisfactory practice of medicine" created difficulties "persuad[ing] qualified practitioners to locate in isolated communities where those facilities are lacking and where the returns for the services rendered are, at best, most meager." He argued that FNS solved this problem: nurse-midwives provided necessary services; FNS created a small hospital for the most serious cases; and the presence of nurse-midwives and a hospital prompted a few qualified physicians to locate in the area. Scott D. Breckinridge, Letter to the Editor, *Lexington Herald,* 24 July 1931, 1, box 344, folder 2, FNS Papers.

68. As Mary Breckinridge explained to a medical audience, she found the local midwives, who attended the majority of births in Leslie County, "unimprovable," and many of the local doctors, some of whom were not licensed by the state, "grossly unfit." Mary Breckinridge, "A Frontier Nursing Service," reprinted from *American Journal of Obstetrics and Gynecology* 15, no. 6 (June 1928): 4–5, box 356, folder 6, FNS Papers.

69. Mary Brewer, interview by Dale Deaton, 78OH150, FNS 10, 10 August 1978, transcript, 3–4, FNS Oral History Collection; and Harris, "Constructing Colonialism," 64–65.

70. M. C. Roark, "The New York Women Missed the Trail," *(Hyden, Ky.) Thousandsticks* 16, no. 3 (20 January 1927), box 39, folder 1, FNS Papers.

71. Breckinridge, *Wide Neighborhoods,* 165; and Altizer, "Establishment of the Frontier Nursing Service," 33.

72. Betty Lester, "The Clinic the Neighbors Built," *Quarterly Bulletin of the Frontier Nursing Service, Inc.* 6, no. 1 (Summer 1930): 63–66.

73. Frank Bowling, interview by Dale Deaton, 78OH147, FNS 7, 31 July 1978, FNS Oral History Collection (online version, kdl.kyvl.org/cgi/t/text/textidx?c=oralhist&tpl=kukohfns.tpl, accessed 2 November 2003); and Altizer, "Establishment of the Frontier Nursing Service," 33.

74. Hallie Maggard, interview by Dale Deaton, 79OH81, FNS 37, 20 November 1978, transcript, 13–14, FNS Oral History Collection; and Altizer, "Establishment of the Frontier Nursing Service," 33.

75. Grace Reeder, interview by Carol Crowe-Carraco, 79OH144, FNS 51, 25 January 1979, transcript, 39, FNS Oral History Collection.

76. Lester, interview by Fried et al., 3 March 1978; and Altizer, "The Establishment of the Frontier Nursing Service," 35.

77. Ruth Huston, interview by Dale Deaton, 79OH80, FNS 36, 18 November 1978, transcript, 9, FNS Oral History Collection; and Altizer, "Establishment of the Frontier Nursing Service," 35.

78. Lester, interview by Fried et al., 3 March 1978.

79. Huston, interview by Deaton, 18 November 1978, 9.

80. Report of the Executive Committee of the Frontier Nursing Service, 1932, box 3, folder 8; and Report of the Director of the Frontier Nursing Service to the Executive Committee, 11 May 1933, box 3, folder 13, both in FNS Papers. On back payments owed to staff, see Minnie Grove to Mary Breckinridge, 27 January 1947; Breckinridge

to Grove, [2?] February 1947; Grove to Breckinridge, 6 February 1947; Breckinridge to W. A. Hifner, 24 February 1947; and Breckinridge to Hifner, 10 March 1947, all in box 317, folder 1, FNS Papers.

81. "Staff Notes," *Quarterly Bulletin of the Frontier Nursing Service, Inc.* 6, no. 3 (Winter 1931): 14; and "Sixth Annual Report," *Quarterly Bulletin of the Frontier Nursing Service, Inc.* 7, no. 1 (Summer 1931): 4–5.

82. Helen Marie Fedde explained that Willeford's dissertation originally outlined this plan. FNS published the dissertation the year Willeford finished it. Fedde, "A Study of Midwifery," 70–71; and Willeford, *Income and Health in Remote Rural Areas.*

83. Breckinridge, *Wide Neighborhoods,* 323–24.

84. Frontier Nursing Service, Inc., Executive Committee Meeting, 2 October 1935, 2, box 3, folder 25; Report of the Director of Frontier Nursing Service Given to the Executive Committee, 25 April 1936, 1–2, box 4, folder 3; Report of the Director of Frontier Nursing Service Given to the Executive Committee, 18 October 1937, 1, box 4, folder 15; Report of the Director of Frontier Nursing Service Given to the Executive Committee, 4 March 1938, 1, box 4, folder 17; and Report of the Director of the Frontier Nursing Service Given to the Executive Committee, 12 January 1939, 4–5, box 4, folder 22, all in FNS Papers.

85. Dorothy F. Buck, *The Frontier Graduate School of Midwifery* (Hyden, Ky.: Frontier Nursing Service, 1943), 1–2, box 323, folder 1, FNS Papers.

86. "Training Frontier Nurse-Midwives," *Quarterly Bulletin of the Frontier Nursing Service, Inc.* 15, no. 2 (Autumn 1939): 23–25.

87. "Annual Report of the Frontier Nursing Service, Inc., 1 May 1939 to 30 April 1940," *Quarterly Bulletin of the Frontier Nursing Service, Inc.* 16, no. 1 (Summer 1940): 4–15.

88. Buck, *Frontier Graduate School of Midwifery,* 2; Report of the Director of Frontier Nursing Service Given to the Executive Committee, 26 November 1940, 6, box 4, folder 33; and Report of the Director of Frontier Nursing Service Given to the Executive Committee, 7 November 1941, 2, box 5, folder 7, both in FNS Papers.

Between 1943 and 1945, most students of the Frontier Graduate School of Midwifery received money under the terms of the Bolton Act, providing federal dollars for expanding the pool of nurses to meet war-time needs. After the war, the school trained some veterans, whose expenses were met by the federal government. Report of the Director of the Frontier Nursing Service at the Executive Meeting, 2 December 1945, 8, box 5, folder 24; and Report of the Director of the Frontier Nursing Service at the Executive Committee Meeting, 2 December 1946, 5, box 6, folder 5, both in FNS Papers.

89. Report of the Director of Frontier Nursing Service Given to the Executive Committee, 31 October 1939, 3, box 4, folder 26, FNS Papers; [No title—part of Report of the Director of Frontier Nursing Service Given to the Executive Committee, probably from 1940], 2, box 4, folder 27, FNS Papers; Director's Report at the Annual Meeting of Trustees, Members, and Friends, 28 May 1941, 1, box 5, folder 5, FNS Papers; and Dorothy F. Buck, "The Training of Frontier Nurse-Midwives," *Quarterly Bulletin of the Frontier Nursing Service, Inc.* 15, no. 4 (Spring 1940): 18–20.

90. Buck, *Frontier Graduate School of Midwifery,* 2, 4–5.

91. Reeder, interview by Crowe-Carraco, 25 January 1979, 4–5, 10–11, 14–16, 35–37.

92. Lester, interview by Fried et al., 3 March 1978.

93. Lester, interview by Deaton, 27 July 1978, 4.

94. Edna C. Rockstroh, "Enter,—the Nurse-Midwife," reprinted from *American Journal of Nursing* (March 1927): 4–5, box 35, folder 2, FNS Papers; and Mary B. Willeford and Marion S. Ross, "How the Frontier Nurse Spends Her Time," *Quarterly Bulletin of the Frontier Nursing Service, Inc.* 12, no. 4 (Spring 1937): 5–9.

95. Rockstroh, "Enter,—the Nurse-Midwife," 4–5; and Louis I. Dublin, "Summary of Study of Second 1000 Maternity Cases of the Frontier Nursing Service," *Quarterly Bulletin of the Frontier Nursing Service, Inc.* 11, no. 1 (Summer 1935): 13–21.

96. Elizabeth J. Steele and Louis I. Dublin, "Report on the Third Thousand Confinements of The Frontier Nursing Service, Inc." *Quarterly Bulletin of the Frontier Nursing Service, Inc.* 14, no. 3 (Winter 1939): 23–32.

97. Rockstroh, "Enter,—the Nurse-Midwife," 4–5; and Lester, interview by Fried et al., 3 March 1978.

98. FNS Medical Advisory Committee, *Routine for the Use of the Frontier Nursing Service,* 1928, 20, box 27, folder 1, FNS Papers.

99. On rural mothers receiving the least food in the family, see John H. Kooser, "Rural Obstetrics: A Report of the Work of the Frontier Nursing Service," reprinted from *Southern Medical Journal* 35, no. 2 (February 1942): 3, box 36, folder 2, and John H. Kooser, "Dietary Deficiencies, A Review of Vitamin B Deficiencies," reprinted from *Kentucky Medical Journal* (June 1943): 5, box 36, folder 4, both in FNS Papers.

100. Vanda Summers, "Saddle-bag and Log Cabin Technic: The Frontier Nursing Service, Inc.," reprinted from *American Journal of Nursing* 38, no. 11 (November 1938): 5, box 35, folder 19, FNS Papers.

101. Willeford and Ross, "How the Frontier Nurse Spends Her Time," 5.

102. Reeder, interview by Crowe-Carraco, 25 January 1979, 12–13.

103. Among obstetricians, who served only the most elite women in the United States, prenatal care became accepted during the first few decades of the twentieth century. Certainly, by the 1930s, obstetricians provided regular prenatal care. Longo and Thomsen, "Prenatal Care and its Evolution in America," 29–70.

104. Dorothy Buck, "How Does the Frontier Nursing Service Handle Obstetrical Complications?" *Quarterly Bulletin of the Frontier Nursing Service, Inc.* 11, no. 3 (Winter 1936): 7–14.

105. Dorothy Buck to Anne Winslow (?), January 1932, box 338, folder 7, FNS Papers.

106. John H. Kooser, "Mountain Medicine," *Quarterly Bulletin of the Frontier Nursing Service, Inc.* 10, no. 4 (Spring 1935): 23–29.

107. Breckinridge used her connections to the Chicago North Shore Alumnae Chapter of Alpha Omicron Pi to get the sorority to form and support an FNS social-service department. Breckinridge, *Wide Neighborhoods,* 254, 341; Mary Dee Drummond, "The Frontier Nursing Service," *To Dragma* (October 1931): 32–43, box 39, folder 2, FNS Papers; Bland Morrow to Josephine Hunt, 7 February 1935, box 344, folder 8, FNS Papers; Morrow to Hunt, 14 January 1938, box 344, folder 11, FNS Papers; "Annual Report of the Frontier Nursing Service, 1 May 1936 to 30 April 1937," *Quarterly Bulletin of the Frontier Nursing Service, Inc.* 13, no. 1 (Summer 1937): 2–8; and "Annual Report of the Frontier Nursing Service, Inc., 1 May 1943 to 30 April 1944," *Quarterly Bulletin of the Frontier Nursing Service, Inc.* 20, no. 1 (Summer 1944): 3–15.

108. As Breckinridge explained, many mountaineers "emigrated to the railroad towns, lured by the prospect of cash wages and better opportunities for their families." These men and their families returned to their old homes when the jobs in the railroad and coal mining towns dried up. Mary Breckinridge, "The Corn-Bread Line," reprinted from *The Survey*, August 1930, box 356, folder 9, FNS Papers.

109. Breckinridge, "Corn-Bread Line," Mary Breckinridge, "What Price Famine?" *Quarterly Bulletin of the Frontier Nursing Service, Inc.* 6, no. 3 (Winter 1931): 1–4; and "Sixth Annual Report," *Quarterly Bulletin of the Frontier Nursing Service, Inc.* 7, no. 1 (Summer 1931): 1–5.

110. Ada Worcester, "The Making of a Home," *Quarterly Bulletin of the Frontier Nursing Service, Inc.* 10, no. 2 (Autumn 1934): 18–19.

111. Drummond, "Frontier Nursing Service," 37. On another FNS demonstration at a county fair, see "The County Fair," *Quarterly Bulletin of the Frontier Nursing Service, Inc.* 7, no. 2 (Autumn 1931): 19. I thank Ron Bryant, PhD, Kentucky History Specialist, Thomas D. Clark Library of the Kentucky Historical Society, Frankfort, Ky., for his information about privies.

112. "The Cleveland Clinic on Grassy Branch," *Quarterly Bulletin of the Frontier Nursing Service, Inc.* 9, no. 1 (Summer 1933): 13–14.

113. "Rounds," *Quarterly Bulletin of the Frontier Nursing Service, Inc.* 5, no. 2 (September 1929): 4–13. For a photograph of a mothers' club, see the cover of *Quarterly Bulletin of the Frontier Nursing Service, Inc.* 5, no. 3 (December 1929).

114. Lester, interview by Fried et al., 3 March 1978.

115. Davis-Floyd, *Birth as an American Rite of Passage,* 84–86. Today, even the most standard women's health texts explain: "You should challenge any hospital procedures that seem medically unnecessary, such as extensive shaving of your pubic area or administration of an enema. There is rarely any need for these outdated rituals, but though they have been eliminated in many birth centers, they persist in some institutions." "Medical Economics Data," *PDR Family Guide to Women's Health and Prescription Drugs,* Montvale, N.J., 2001, at infotrac.galegroup.com (accessed 15 June 2004).

116. Steele and Dublin, "Report on the Third Thousand Confinements," 23–32. Nurse-midwives delivered approximately the same proportion of cases in each series of one thousand midwifery cases. They obtained the services of a physician in fifty-two cases for the first series of one thousand cases, sixty-one for the second, and fifty-three for the third.

117. Breckinridge's cousins on the FNS medical advisory committee included Scott Breckinridge, Josephine Hunt, and Waller Bullock. Breckinridge, *Wide Neighborhoods,* 158–59; FNS Board of Governors (Executive Committee) meeting, 12 May 1926, 3, box 2, folder 13, FNS Papers.

118. The manuals always made clear that FNS nurse-midwives were not trying to compete with local physicians. Carl D. Fortune and Helen H. Fortune, interview by Dale Deaton, 790H25, FNS 26, 6 October 1978, transcript, 6, FNS Oral History Collection. See also *Routine for the Use of the Frontier Nursing Service, Authorized by Its Medical Advisory Committee Meeting August 27, 1928, in Lexington, Kentucky,* esp. 1, box 27, folder 1, FNS Papers; *Routine for the Use of the Frontier Nursing Service, Authorized by Its Medical Advisory Committee Meeting August 27, 1928, in Lexington, Kentucky, Revised September 23, 1930,* box 27, folder 2, FNS Papers; and *Medical Routine for the Use of the Nursing Staff of the Frontier Nursing Service, Fourth Edition, revised May 1948,*

esp. 3–4, box 27, folder 4, FNS Papers.

119. Breckinridge, *Wide Neighborhoods,* 243–44; "Annual Report of the Frontier Nursing Service, Inc., 1 May 1943 to 30 April 1944," 7. In the late 1940s, another surgeon from this mining town offered his services to FNS.

120. "Report of the Nursing Work of the Frontier Nursing Service, 1 May 1928–30 April 1929," *Quarterly Bulletin of the Frontier Nursing Service, Inc.* 5, no. 1 (June 1929): 47–49.

121. FNS had great difficulty retaining a medical director in the 1940s and 1950s. When John H. Kooser resigned in 1943 to join the Navy after twelve years of service to FNS, medical directors thereafter stayed no more than two years; many stayed for only a few months, and some periods had no medical director. Dammann, *Social History of the Frontier Nursing Service,* 87. For information on FNS's constant problems finding a medical director, see Mary Breckinridge to Josephine Hunt, 9 December 1937, box 344, folder 10; Director's Report to FNS Executive Committee, 28 November 1944, 2, box 5, folder 20; Breckinridge to Hunt, 4 September 1945, box 345, folder 7; Director's Report to FNS Executive Committee, 2 December 1945, box 5, folder 24; Breckinridge to Laura Ten Eyck, 22 March 1946, box 340, folder 3; Breckinridge to Members of the Executive Committee, 26 March 1946, box 345, folder 8; "Memorandum on the Post of Medical Director," 1946, box 345, folder 8; Director's Report to FNS Executive Committee, 28 February 1947, box 6, folder 7; and FNS Executive Committee, 30 November 1955, box 7, folder 15, all in FNS Papers.

122. Breckinridge, *Wide Neighborhoods,* 244–46.

123. Breckinridge, "The Nurse-Midwife—A Pioneer," 1149.

124. Medical Advisory Committee, *Medical Routine for the Use of the Frontier Nursing Service,* rev. ed., 1930, 22–23, box 27, folder 2; and Medical Director, Attending Surgeon, and the Medical Advisory Committee, *Medical Routine for the Use of the Frontier Nursing Service,* 3rd ed., rev. ed., 1936, 52–53, box 27, folder 3, both in FNS Papers.

125. Breckinridge, "Frontier Nursing Service," 6.

126. Breckinridge, "Frontier Nursing Service," 6.

127. Louis I. Dublin to Mary Breckinridge, letter, *Quarterly Bulletin of the Frontier Nursing Service, Inc.* 8, no. 1 (Summer 1932): 7–9; and Steele and Dublin, "Report on the Third Thousand Confinements," 32.

128. Breckinridge, *Wide Neighborhoods,* 306–7.

129. Steele and Dublin, "Report on the Third Thousand Confinements," 27, 32.

130. Breckinridge, "Frontier Nursing Service," 6.

131. FNS Medical Advisory Committee, *Medical Routine for the Use of the Frontier Nursing Service,* 1930, 24, 28–29. The reason for burning the placenta is unclear. In her study of African American traditional midwives in central Texas from 1920 to 1985, sociologist Ruth C. Schaffer noted these midwives "practiced with some magico-religious overtones, such as the eating of clay and the ritual disposition of the placenta. All placentas were burned or buried, and sometimes salt was applied before burning. The only explanation was that their grandmothers and great grandmothers had performed these actions." Perhaps FNS nurse-midwives continued some old birthing traditions, despite their interest in distinguishing their practices from those of traditional midwives. Schaffer, "The Health and Social Functions of Black Midwives," 95.

132. "Exceptional People," *Quarterly Bulletin of the Frontier Nursing Service, Inc.* 5, no. 4 (Spring 1930): 3–7.

133. Minnie Grove, "A Night Call," *Quarterly Bulletin of the Frontier Nursing Service, Inc.* 7, no. 3 (Winter 1932): 22–23.

134. FNS Medical Advisory Committee, *Medical Routine for the Use of the Frontier Nursing Service,* 2nd (revised) edition, 1930, 24; Breckinridge, "The Nurse-Midwife—A Pioneer," 1149. Breckinridge explained that once the patient was in labor, the nurse-midwives stayed with her for two days and nights in the home if necessary.

135. Lester, interview by Fried et al., 3 March 1978.

136. Apple, *Mothers and Medicine.* Apple explains that artificial infant feeding became widely accepted and breastfeeding decreased in the first half of the twentieth century, especially after 1920, for several interrelated reasons: 1) scientific theories suggested that many infants would benefit from infant formulas; 2) infant food companies used advertising to persuade physicians and mothers to use artificial formula; 3) artificial feeding helped physicians to gain status as scientific experts, control over their patients' lives, and money; and 4) women increasingly chose physician-directed bottle feeding because they put their faith in science and believed their babies would be healthier with "scientific" feeding.

137. Leavitt, *Brought to Bed,* 171–95; Leavitt, "'Strange Young Women on Errands,'" 3–24.

138. FNS Medical Advisory Committee, *Routine for the Use of the Frontier Nursing Service,* 1928, 17–20, FNS Papers, box 27, folder 1. Similar advice was given in the routines revised in 1930 and 1936.

139. Letter from Louis I. Dublin to Mary Breckinridge, *Quarterly Bulletin of the Frontier Nursing Service, Inc.* 8, no. 1 (Summer 1932): 7–9.

140. Frontier Nursing Service, Inc. Monthly Report, May 1—May 31, 1929, FNS Papers, box 10, folder 15.

141. Frontier Nursing Service, Inc. Monthly Report, November 1930, box 10, folder 19, FNS Papers.

142. Drummond, "Frontier Nursing Service," 34.

143. Ada Worcester, "Nancy's Baby," *Quarterly Bulletin of the Frontier Nursing Service, Inc.* 6, no. 3 (Winter 1931): 10–11.

144. Fannie Huff, interview by Sadie W. Stidham, 820H24, FNS 167, 16 March 1980, transcript, 14–15, FNS Oral History Collection.

145. Lester, interview by Fried et al., 3 March 1978.

146. Lester, interview by Fried et al., 3 March 1978.

147. From a 1926 letter, quoted in Breckinridge, *Wide Neighborhoods,* 242.

148. For a detailed description on the opening of each center, see Tirpak, "The Frontier Nursing Service," 55–87. Also see "In the Field—The Three Centers," *Quarterly Bulletin of the Kentucky Committee for Mothers and Babies, Inc.* 2, no. 2 (October 1926): 2–4; and "The Organization of the Frontier Nursing Service, Inc., 1946," *Quarterly Bulletin of the Frontier Nursing Service, Inc.* 22, no. 2 (Autumn 1946): 7–17.

149. "The First Centers of Nurse-Midwifery," *Quarterly Bulletin of the Kentucky Committee for Mothers and Babies, Inc.* 1, no. 2 (October 1925): 12–13.

150. "Frontier Nursing Service Primer," *Quarterly Bulletin of the Frontier Nursing Service, Inc.* 8, no. 1 (Summer 1932): 10–19.

151. "First Centers of Nurse-Midwifery," 12.

152. Kentucky Committee for Mothers and Babies Monthly Report, Hyden and Stinnett Centers, October 1925, box 10, folder 1, FNS Papers; and "In the Field—The

Three Centers," 2.

153. Loudon, *Death in Childbirth,* 320; and U. S. Bureau of the Census, *Historical Statistics of the United States,* 25. Loudon based his statistics on Dye, "Mary Breckinridge," 501, and on Browne and Isaacs, "The Frontier Nursing Service," 14–17; both studies use Louis I. Dublin's statistics on FNS.

Infant mortality rates at FNS were also low. However, the rates increased during the Depression. As Irvine Loudon explained regarding FNS in the 1930s: "Infant mortality rose, but maternal mortality did not, in line with the general principle that infant mortality is sensitive to social and economic change to a much greater extent than maternal mortality." Loudon, *Death in Childbirth,* 320.

154. "Biographical Note," Finding Aid to the Louis I. Dublin Papers, 1906–1968, Louis I. Dublin Papers, National Library of Medicine, Bethesda, Maryland; and Hamilton, "The Metropolitan Life Insurance Company Visiting Nursing Service," 41–42.

155. For Dublin's reports on the years 1925–1939, see Letter from Louis I. Dublin to Mary Breckinridge, *Quarterly Bulletin of The Frontier Nursing Service, Inc.* 7, no. 1 (Summer 1932): 7–9; Dublin, "Summary of Second 1000 Midwifery Records," 13–21; and Steele and Dublin, "Report on the Third Thousand Confinements," 23–32. Elizabeth Steele, who worked in the Statistical Bureau at Met Life, prepared the reports of the second and third 1,000 deliveries, and, at least with the second report, Dublin said that he went over Steele's work and vouched for its accuracy.

156. For articles showing Dublin's support of nurse-midwifery, see Louis I. Dublin, "The Hazards of Maternity," 1932, MCA (MCA) Archives, New York, New York, and Dublin, "The Problem of Maternity," 1205–14.

## Notes to Chapter 3

1. Unless otherwise noted in the endnotes, information in this chapter on McNaught is from Sally Austen Tom, "Rose McNaught: American Nurse-Midwifery's Own 'Sister-Tutor,'" *Journal of Nurse-Midwifery* 24, no. 2 (March/April 1979): 3–8.

2. Sally Austen Tom and *Quarterly Bulletin of the Frontier Nursing Service, Inc.* give slightly different years for the start of McNaught's employment at FNS and her midwifery education in Britain. I use the Bulletin's years because they were reported at the time, rather than long after the fact. "Staff Notes," *Quarterly Bulletin of The Kentucky Committee for Mothers and Babies, Inc.* 3, no. 3 (November 1927): 6; and "Staff Notes," *Quarterly Bulletin of the Frontier Nursing Service, Inc.* 4, no. 2 (September 1928): 12–13.

3. For the retirement date, see "Miss Rose McNaught, Nurse-Midwife Pioneer, Visits Former Students Here," undated article from a Santa Fe newspaper, container 11, file: Rose McNaught, n.d., American College of Nurse-Midwives (ACNM) Archives, National Library of Medicine, Bethesda, Maryland.

4. Cassells, "Manhattan Midwifery School." A few recent nurse-midwifery histories mention the Manhattan Midwifery School, citing Cassells's thesis. See Dawley and Burst, "American College of Nurse-Midwives and Its Antecedents," 16; and Varney et al., "Profession and History of Midwifery in the United States," 10.

5. MCA, *Maternity Center Association, 1918–1943,* 26.

6. MCA, *40th Annual Report of the Maternity Center Association,* 26.

7. MCA, *Maternity Center Association, 1918–1943,* 5–6.

8. Longo and Thomsen, "Prenatal Care and Its Evolution in America," 34–35.

9. Lubic, "Barriers and Conflict in Maternity Care Innovation," 12.

10. Louis Dublin and MCA director Hazel Corbin compiled statistics on this demonstration project for the years 1922 to 1929. See Dublin and Corbin, "A Preliminary Report of the Maternity Center Association," 877–81. For other information about MCA's early work in prenatal care and this demonstration project, see Louis I. Dublin, "The Risks of Childbirth," reprinted from *Forum and Century* (May 1932): 4, MCA Archives, New York, New York; Dublin, "The Problem of Maternity," 1205–14; and Longo and Thomsen, "Prenatal Care and Its Evolution in America," 36–37.

This chapter relies heavily on the MCA archives. Readers will note three different locations for these materials: MCA Archives, MCA Storage, and MCA Office. Until 1996, the archives were located in MCA's library; anything accessed until that time is listed as MCA Archives. In 1996, most of the archives were placed into storage; items accessed from storage are designated as MCA Storage. Some items remain in the MCA Office; those items are designated as such.

11. MCA, *Maternity Center Association, 1928,* 16, MCA Archives.

12. "The Effect of Prenatal Supervision on Maternal and Infant Welfare, A Report on the Work of the Maternity Center Association of New York City, May, 1919 to August, 1921," 1921, 9, MCA Archives.

13. Popular in the late-nineteenth and early-twentieth centuries, mothers' clubs held meetings where women discussed and received instruction on childrearing. MCA, *Routines for Maternity Nursing and Briefs for Mothers' Club Talks,* 37–71.

14. MCA, *Maternity Center Association, 1925,* n.p., MCA Archives; and MCA, *Maternity Center Association, 1928,* 16, 25.

15. On MCA's maternity institutes, see MCA, *Maternity Center Association, 1918–1943,* 61–62; "Institutes," 1929–1948, MCA Archives; and "Outline of Material Covered in Maternity Institute, Spring 1932," MCA Archives. On how an MCA maternity institute inspired one public-health nurse to begin classes for prenatal patients, see Thyrza R. Davies, "Expectant Mothers' Classes," *Public Health Nursing* 27 (1935): 336–37.

16. Kosmak, "The Trained Nurse and Midwife," 423.

17. MCA Minutes, 1924–1942, Meeting of the Board of Directors, 10 April 1930, MCA Office.

18. MCA Minutes, 1924–1942, Meeting of the Board of Directors, 12 March 1925, MCA Office.

19. Frederick W. Rice, "Regarding Recent Efforts to Reduce Mortality in Childbirth," reprinted from *American Journal of Obstetrics and Gynecology* 4, no. 3 (September 1922): 9, MCA Archives. For information on Rice, see "Frederick W. Rice," *Columbia Alumni News* 39 (May 1948): 32.

20. Ralph W. Lobenstine to Barbara Quinn, 31 October 1930, container 515655 (Reports on MCA Clinics, Booth Joint Programs, FC 4 of 8, 1920–1978, box 79): folder: Association for the Promotion and Standardization of Midwifery, 1930–1939, MCA Storage.

21. Ralph W. Lobenstine, "Practical Means of Reducing Maternal Mortality," reprinted from *American Journal of Public Health* (January 1922): 3, MCA Archives.

22. Watson, "Can Our Methods of Obstetrics Practice Be Improved?," 656–57. For information on Watson, see "Benjamin Watson," *Physicians and Surgeons* 22 (Spring 1977): 24–26; and *P&S Quarterly* (1976–1977): 20.

23. "Preliminary Report, Committee on Midwives," 1923, container 515655 (Reports on MCA Clinics, Booth Joint Programs, FC 4 of 8, 1920–1978, box 79), folder: Reports (Miscellaneous), 1920–1929, MCA Storage.

24. Lobenstine to Quinn, 31 October 1930.

25. Lobenstine, "Practical Means of Reducing Maternal Mortality," 2.

26. Rice, "Regarding Recent Efforts to Reduce Mortality in Childbirth," 8.

27. "Conference," MCA, 11 May 1923 (hereafter MCA 1923 Conference), 7, container 515655 (Reports on MCA Clinics, Booth Joint Programs, FC 4 of 8, 1920–1978, box 79), folder: Maternity Center-Bellevue Project, 1923–1929, MCA Storage.

28. John Osborn Polak to Ralph W. Lobenstine, 3 February 1930, container 512591 (Admin Records, Lobenstine Clinic, H. Hemschemeyer 2 of 3, 1931–1971, box 108), folder: Medical Board of Directors Re: Lobenstine Clinic, MCA Storage. For information on Polak, see the former official website of Long Island College Hospital, last updated 22 April 1996, www.albany.net/~orchard/history/history.html (accessed 22 November 2003).

29. Watson, "Can Our Methods of Obstetrics Practice Be Improved?," 657.

30. Louise Zabriskie was MCA's assistant field director and later field director and author of *Nurses' Handbook of Obstetrics;* Nancy Cadmus was MCA's general director in the early 1920s; Corbin's position will be discussed further. MCA 1923 Conference, 1; and Minutes of Committee on Postgraduate Courses in Midwifery for Nurses, 6 October 1927, container 515655 (Reports on MCA Clinics, Booth Joint Programs, FC 4 of 8, 1920–1978, box 79), folder: National Organiz. For Public Health Nursing, 1920–1929, MCA Storage.

31. Hazel Corbin to George W. Kosmak, 5 January 1929, container 515655 (Reports on MCA Clinics, Booth Joint Programs, FC 4 of 8, 1920–1978, box 79), folder: Maternity Center-Bellevue Project, 1923–1929, MCA Storage.

32. Lobenstine to Quinn, 31 October 1930.

33. MCA, *Lobenstine,* 3, MCA Archives.

34. MCA 1923 Conference, 3; and MCA Minutes, 1924–1942, Meeting of the Board of Directors, 9 February 1928, 106, MCA Office.

35. MCA 1923 Conference, 2.

36. MCA 1923 Conference, 3.

37. On nurses supporting the plan, see especially MCA 1923 Conference, 20–22, 31.

38. "Suggestions for Improving Existing Maternity Services in New York City," with "Appendix: The Affiliation of the Maternity Center Association with the Bellevue Training School for Midwives," 6a, container 515655 (Reports on MCA Clinics, Booth Joint Programs, FC 4 of 8, 1920–1978, box 79), folder: Maternity Center-Bellevue Project, 1923–1929, MCA Storage.

39. MCA 1923 Conference, 16.

40. The chair of the 1923 conference, MCA's Nancy E. Cadmus, concluded that participants were considering "the attitude of the medical fraternity to the question of nurses taking the regular training in midwifery." MCA 1923 Conference, 33–34.

41. MCA 1923 Conference, 15–16. Emphasis added.

42. Elizabeth F. Miller to Isabel M. Stewart, 27 January 1927, and Stewart to Miller, 26 January 1927, both in container 515655 (Reports on MCA Clinics, Booth Joint Programs, FC 4 of 8, 1920–1978, box 79), folder: National Organiz. For Public Health Nursing, 1920–1929, MCA Storage.

43. MCA 1923 Conference, 15.

44. MCA, *Maternity Center Association, 1918–1943*, 25.

45. MCA, *Maternity Center Association, 1918–1943*, 26.

46. MCA Minutes, 1924–1942, Meeting of the Board of Directors, 4 October 1934, 275, MCA Office.

47. "By-Laws of The Association for the Promotion and Standardization of Midwifery, Inc.," container 515655 (Reports on MCA Clinics, Booth Joint Programs, FC 4 of 8, 1920–1978, box 79), folder: Association for the Promotion and Standardization of Midwifery, 1930–1939, MCA Storage; and MCA, *Twenty Years of Nurse-Midwifery, 1933–1953,* 17.

48. MCA, *Twenty Years of Nurse-Midwifery, 1933–1953,* 17–18.

49. MCA, *Twenty Years of Nurse-Midwifery, 1933–1953*, 18.

50. MCA, *40th Annual Report of the Maternity Center Association,* 32–33.

51. MCA Minutes, 1924–1942, Meeting of the Board of Directors, 12 March 1925, MCA Office; MCA Minutes, 1924–1942, Meeting of the Board of Directors, 10 April 1930, MCA Office; and Rice, "Regarding Recent Efforts to Reduce Mortality in Childbirth," 9.

52. According to Hattie Hemschemeyer, director of the Lobenstine Midwifery School and Clinic, the percentage of midwife-attended births in New York City was 30 percent in 1919, 12 percent in 1929, and 2 percent in 1939. Hemschemeyer, "Midwifery in the United States," 1182.

53. Lobenstine, "Practical Means of Reducing Maternal Mortality," 3; and Watson, "Can Our Methods of Obstetrics Practice Be Improved?," 656–57.

54. "Graduates of the Maternity Center Association School of Midwifery," 1957[?], container 7, folder: ACNM Membership Archives.

55. "The School for Midwives Conducted by the Association for the Promotion and Standardization of Midwifery, Inc. at The Lobenstine Midwifery Clinic," 1932, container 515655 (Reports on MCA Clinics, Booth Joint Programs, FC 4 of 8, 1920–1978, box 79), folder: Association for the Promotion and Standardization of Midwifery, 1930–1939, MCA Storage.

56. MCA, *Twenty Years of Nurse-Midwifery, 1933–1953,* 25.

57. MCA, *Twenty Years of Nurse-Midwifery, 1933–1953,* 18–19, 22–23.

58. MCA, *Lobenstine,* 4–5. On medical students' observation of deliveries, see MCA, *40th Annual Report of the Maternity Center Association,* 28.

59. Frederick F. Russell to Hattie Hemschemeyer, 11 April 1935, container 512591 (Admin. Records, Lobenstine Clinic, H. Hemschemeyer 2 of 3, 1931–1971, box 108), folder: Rockefeller Foundation, MCA Storage; MCA, *Twenty Years of Nurse-Midwifery, 1933–1953,* 25; and Hazel Corbin, "Historical Development of Nurse-Midwifery in this Country and Present Trends," *Bulletin of the American College of Nurse-Midwifery* 4, no. 1 (March 1959): 13–26.

60. MCA, *Twenty Years of Nurse-Midwifery, 1933–1953,* 24, 104. The elimination of the four months in public-health nursing took place some time during the 1930s as

seen in MCA, *Lobenstine,* 4.

61. Corbin, "Historical Development of Nurse-Midwifery," 18.

62. Adapted from table and text in Minutes, Medical Board Meetings, MCA, 1931–1965, 28 January 1936, 31, 32–1, 32–2, MCA Office.

63. MCA, *Twenty Years of Nurse-Midwifery, 1933–1953,* 54. On the Social Security Act funding, see MCA Minutes, 1924–1942, Meeting of the Board of Directors, 12 March 1936, 318; and Minutes, Medical Board Meetings, MCA, 1931–1965, 1 December 1936, 36, both in MCA Office.

64. "Suggestions for Improving Existing Maternity Services in New York City," with "Appendix: The Affiliation of the Maternity Center Association with the Bellevue Training School for Midwives," 5.

65. On the demonstration, see MCA, *Twenty Years of Nurse-Midwifery, 1933–1953,* 54–57; and Elizabeth Ferguson, "Midwifery Supervision," *Public Health Nursing* 30 (August 1938): 482–85. For comments by a Johns Hopkins Medical School obstetrician based on his experiences with the demonstration, see Peckham, "The Essentials of Adequate Maternal Care in Rural Areas," 119–24. According to a list from MCA, Ferguson graduated from Lobenstine in 1935 and Solotar in 1937. It is possible that Solotar worked in Maryland as a student, or did not begin her position until after she graduated, even though she was appointed in 1936. "Graduates of the Maternity Center Association School of Midwifery," 1957[?], container 7, folder: ACNM Membership, List of Graduates from American Midwifery Programs, ACNM Archives.

66. For comments on the demonstration's maternal morbidity and mortality rates, see Corbin, "Historical Development of Nurse-Midwifery," 18.

67. MCA Minutes, 1924–1942, Meeting of the Board of Directors, 13 October 1938, 384, MCA Office. This story was also told—without Ferguson's name—in MCA, *Lobenstine,* 9.

68. MCA Minutes, 1924–1942, Meeting of the Board of Directors, 4 October 1934, 275, MCA Office.

69. The names of those resigning are listed in Minutes, Medical Board Meetings, MCA, 1931–1965, 10 January 1935, 10, MCA Office. With understated glee, Corbin noted Stander's change of heart several years later: "There are two nurse midwives [graduates of the Lobenstine School] on the staff of the New York Hospital, one in charge of the maternity pavilion and one in charge of the maternity clinics. Considering that Dr. Stander resigned from the Maternity Center Association Board because of the Association's interest in midwives, it is of passing interest that he has a midwife in charge of his two major departments." MCA Minutes, 1924–1942, Meeting of the Board of Directors, 19 October 1939, 409, MCA Office.

70. James A. Harrar to Hattie Hemschemeyer, 27 November 1934, container 512591 (Admin. Records, Lobenstine Clinic, H. Hemschemeyer 2 of 3, 1931–1971, box 108), folder: Medical Board of Directors Re: Lobenstine Clinic, MCA Storage.

71. Minutes, Medical Board Meetings, MCA, 1931–1965, 10 January 1935, 10, MCA Office.

72. As Watson explained, "The policy of the clinic is not to accept patients who could afford the minimum fee of a private physician." Minutes, Medical Board Meetings, MCA, 1931–1965, 1 December 1936, 36, MCA Office.

73. George W. Kosmak to Doctor, 6 April 1932, container 515655 (Reports on

MCA Clinics, Booth Joint Programs, FC 4 of 8, 1920–1978, box 79), folder: Lobenstine Midwifery Clinic, 1930–1939, MCA Storage.

74. Quoted in Tom, "Rose McNaught," 6.

75. The information and quotations can be found in several inspection reports of the Lobenstine Midwifery Clinic by the New York State Department of Social Welfare. See container 512591 (Admin. Records, Lobenstine Clinic, H. Hemschemeyer 2 of 3, 1931–1971, box 108), folder: State Department of Social Welfare (Inspections), MCA Storage.

76. Minutes, Medical Board Meetings, MCA, 1931–1965, 1 December 1936, 36, MCA Office; and AIER, "Cost-of-Living Calculator." I used the year 1936 to convert patient incomes into 2006 dollars, and I used the greatest income patients could have possibly received—pay for fifty-two weeks per year—even though they probably received less.

77. Minutes, Medical Board Meetings, MCA, 1931–1965, 23 January 1940, 43, 43a, MCA Office. AIER, "Cost-of-Living Calculator." Once again, I used the year 1936 to convert patient incomes into 2006 dollars. Note that patient incomes were worth the same in 1936 as in 1939.

78. MCA, *Lobenstine,* 4, 5.

79. This can be seen in the inspection reports of the Lobenstine Midwifery Clinic by the New York State Department of Social Welfare, as well as the annual reports of the clinic to the New York State Board of Charities. See container 512591 (Admin. Records, Lobenstine Clinic, H. Hemschemeyer 2 of 3, 1931–1971, box 108), folder: State Department of Social Welfare (Inspections), MCA Storage.

80. State of New York, Department of Social Welfare, Report of General Inspection of the Maternity Center Association Clinic (Lobenstine Midwifery Clinic), 17 June 1936, container 512591 (Admin. Records, Lobenstine Clinic, H. Hemschemeyer 2 of 3, 1931–1971, box 108), folder: State Department of Social Welfare (Inspections), MCA Storage.

81. The information and quotation can be found in several inspection reports of the Lobenstine Midwifery Clinic by the New York State Department of Social Welfare. See Container 512591 (Admin. Records, Lobenstine Clinic, H. Hemschemeyer 2 of 3, 1931–1971, box 108), folder: State Department of Social Welfare (Inspections), MCA Storage.

82. MCA Minutes, 1924–1942, Meeting of the Board of Directors, 19 October 1939, 409, MCA Office.

83. Kosmak to Doctor, 6 April 1932.

84. The district's location also suggests that a few patients would have been immigrants from Cuba, the West Indies, Mexico, and Central and South America, other inhabitants of what was known as "Spanish Harlem." But these immigrant groups were all much smaller in number than the Puerto Ricans, who made up 85 percent of the area's population. Works Progress Administration, *The WPA Guide to New York City,* 265–66.

85. Minutes, Medical Board Meetings, MCA, 1931–1965, 1 December 1936, 36, MCA Office.

86. Works Progress Administration, *WPA Guide to New York City,* 267; and Chenault, *Puerto Rican Migrant in New York City.*

To complicate matters further, another set of clinic statistics (1932–1939) indicates that 1051 patients (51 percent) were "white," 998 (48 percent) "black," and 9 (less than 1 percent), "other." However, the total number of patients in this set of statistics adds up to 2058, while the total number of patients at the clinic was supposed to have been 1545. Thus, the statistics do not make sense. Was there an error in the reporting? Or were Puerto Rican patients counted twice—as both "white" and "black"? Minutes, Medical Board Meetings, MCA, 1931–1965, 23 January 1940, 43a, MCA Office.

87. Chenault, *Puerto Rican Migrant in New York City,* 79.

88. Hattie Hemschemeyer to Mary Beard, 23 November 1934, container 512591 (Admin. Records, Lobenstine Clinic, H. Hemschemeyer 2 of 3, 1931–1971, box 108), folder: Rockefeller Foundation, MCA Storage.

89. Binder and Reimers, *All the Nations Under Heaven,* 179; Sherrill D. Wilson and Larry A. Greene, "Blacks," in *The Encyclopedia of New York City,* ed. Jackson, 114; and Works Progress Administration, *WPA Guide to New York City,* 258.

90. McBride, *From TB to AIDS,* 85–86; and Wilson and Greene, "Blacks," in *Encyclopedia of New York City,* ed. Jackson, 114.

91. Binder and Reimers, *All the Nations Under Heaven,* 176.

92. Rodriguez, *Puerto Ricans,* 1, 3, 6–7, 11; and Perez y Gonzalez, *Puerto Ricans in the United States,* 34–36.

93. Fitzpatrick, *Puerto Rican Americans,* 53–55.

94. Perez, "A Community at Risk," 18.

95. Korrol, *From Colonia to Community,* 91–92.

96. Virginia Sanchez Korrol, "Puerto Ricans," in *The Encyclopedia of New York City,* ed. Jackson, 962–63.

97. Chenault, *Puerto Rican Migrant in New York City,* 111–12.

98. Carson, "And the Results Showed Promise," 49–50.

99. While the New York Academy of Medicine claimed that midwives attended 10 percent of New York City's births, obstetrician George Kosmak suggested that they attended over 8 percent (see note 16). New York Academy of Medicine Committee on Public Relations, *Maternal Mortality in New York City,* 190–95.

100. Carson, "And the Results Showed Promise," 49.

101. McBride, *From TB to AIDS,* 111.

102. McBride, *From TB to AIDS*, 111–12; Jones, *Labor of Love, Labor of Sorrow,* 192; and Osofsky, *Harlem,* 143–44.

103. Perez, "A Community at Risk," 22.

104. Perez, "A Community at Risk," 23; and Gosnell, "The Puerto Ricans in New York City," quotation on 422.

105. From 1933 to 1942, MCA antepartal home visits averaged 2.9 per person; from 1943–1952, they averaged 1.7 per person. MCA, *Twenty Years of Nurse-Midwifery,* 27–32; and Dublin, "Risks of Childbirth," 3–4.

106. Shoemaker, *History of Nurse-Midwifery in the United States,* 29–30.

107. Hemschemeyer, "The Nurse-Midwife Is Here to Stay," 914. In this quotation, Hemschemeyer is referring to the founding of the nurse-midwifery school and clinic.

108. MCA, *Lobenstine,* 5.

109. Tom, "Rose McNaught," 6.

110. MCA, *Maternity Center Association: Six Years in Review, 1930–1935,* n.p., MCA Archives.

111. At that exhibit, parents and other interested parties visited a sample nursery

and received MCA's pamphlets, "Advice for Mothers," "Advice for Fathers," and "A Message to Expectant Fathers and Mothers," explaining prenatal care and how parents could prepare for home delivery and the arrival of a baby.

112. MCA, *Maternity Center Association: Six Years in Review, 1930–1935,* n.p.

113. Dickinson and Belskie, *Birth Atlas.*

114. The sixth edition of *Birth Atlas* was published in 1981. Drawings of the sculptures are included in a recent edition of the U.S. Public Health Service's *Prenatal and Postnatal Care,* a book descended from the Children's Bureau's first edition of *Prenatal Care* in 1913, and currently distributed nationwide by nurse-midwives, obstetricians, general practitioners, and nurses—and even included as an insert with prenatal vitamins produced by pharmaceutical companies. See for example, U.S. Public Health Service, *Prenatal and Postnatal Care* (Rockville, Md.: U.S. Public Health Service, 1983), included as an insert in Solvay Pharmaceuticals' prenatal multivitamin/mineral supplement tablets.

115. MCA, *Twenty Years of Nurse-Midwifery, 1933–1953,* 39–41.

116. Laird, "Report of the Maternity Center Association Clinic," 182, 184. Because available information on MCA's nurse-midwifery clinic provides only aggregate statistics and information about the clinic between 1931 and 1951, it is difficult to discern exactly what an MCA labor and delivery was like in the 1930s, compared to later years.

117. Tom, "Rose McNaught," 6.

118. MCA, *Lobenstine,* 4–5.

119. Hazel Corbin, interview by Ruth Watson Lubic, 27.

120. Hemschemeyer, "Midwifery in the United States," 1186–87.

121. As above, see inspection reports of the Lobenstine Midwifery Clinic by the New York State Department of Social Welfare, container 512591 (Admin. Records, Lobenstine Clinic, H. Hemschemeyer 2 of 3, 1931–1971, box 108), folder: State Department of Social Welfare (Inspections), MCA Storage.

122. On the decline in breastfeeding in the 1930s, see Wolf, *Don't Kill Your Baby,* 187–97. As Wolf notes, though, most older physicians continued to push breastfeeding well after infant formula became the norm.

123. MCA, *Maternity Handbook for Pregnant Mothers and Expectant Fathers,* 2nd ed., 1945, 43.

124. MCA, *Public Health Nursing in Obstetrics; Part 4: Mothers' and Fathers' Classes,* 55, 81–84, 93.

125. MCA, *Twenty Years of Nurse-Midwifery, 1933–1953,* 39–41; and U.S. Bureau of the Census, *Historical Statistics of the United States,* 25.

Infant mortality rates at MCA were also low but increased during the Depression. See note 153, chapter 2.

126. "The Effect of Prenatal Supervision on Maternal and Infant Welfare," A Report on the Work of the Maternity Center Association of New York City, May 1919 to August 1921, MCA Archives; and Dublin and Corbin, "A Preliminary Report of the Maternity Center Association," 877–81. The first study showed only a slightly lower maternal mortality rate and much lower infant mortality rate as compared with Manhattan as a whole; the surprisingly high number of maternal deaths appeared to be caused by poor care at the hospitals during labor and delivery. The second study showed improved maternal mortality resulting from prenatal care, labor and delivery assistance, and postpartum care by MCA's public-health nurses.

127. MCA, *Twenty Years of Nurse-Midwifery, 1933–1953,* 39–41.

128. This phrase was used in MCA, *Maternity Center Association: Six Years in Review, 1930–1935,* n.p.

129. On the common belief that "it was bad taste to comment in public on pregnancy" and on newspapers' prohibition of the word "pregnancy," see MCA, *Maternity Center Association, 1918–1943,* 7–8. On the comment that the film, "The Birth of the Baby," and the pictures of it shown in *Life,* were "obscene," and on the banning of the film, see MCA Minutes, 1924–1942, Meeting of the Board of Directors, 13 January 1938, 365, MCA Office; MCA Minutes, 1924–1942, Meeting of the Board of Directors, 14 April 1938, 377, MCA Office; and "The Mystery of Life Goes to the New York World's Fair," *Life Begins,* 30 March 1940, 20, MCA Archives. Also see "This Announcement Was Sent to *Life*'s 650,000 Subscribers about the Picture-Article on Following Pages," *Life* 4, no. 15 (11 April 1938): 32; "'The Birth of a Baby,'" 33–36; and Adair, *The Country Doctor and the Specialist,* esp. chaps. 7 and 8.

## Notes to Chapter 4

1. The information on Hyder is from Kate Hyder, interview by Sara Lee Silberman; Silberman, "Pioneering in Family-Centered Maternity and Infant Care," 262–87; Kate Hyder, Response to Committee on Organization's Questionnaire, 1954, container 1, File: Pre-Organization Questionnaire, H-O, ACNM Archives; and Social Security Death Index, www.ancestry.com/search/rectype/vital/ssdi/main.htm (accessed 6 August 2004).

2. On the Chicago Maternity Center, see Leavitt, "Joseph B. DeLee and the Practice of Preventive Obstetrics," 1353–59.

3. Of course, there were a number of nurse-midwives educated abroad who worked in the United States (such as the many British nurse-midwives at Frontier Nursing Service), and there were many nurse-midwives educated in the United States who practiced abroad (such as the women who worked in foreign missions). Lucille Woodville et al., "Descriptive Data, Nurse Midwives—U.S.A., American College of Nurse-Midwifery," *Bulletin of the American College of Nurse-Midwifery* 8, no. 1 (Summer 1963): 30–37; and Shoemaker, *History of Nurse-Midwifery in the United States,* 37.

4. Speert, *Obstetrics and Gynecology in America,* 113.

5. Wertz and Wertz, *Lying-In,* 164–65.

6. On the introduction of sulfa drugs, see Stevens, *In Sickness and In Wealth,* 177.

7. Stevens, *In Sickness and In Wealth,* 201–2, 204, 220.

8. Starr, *Social Transformation of American Medicine,* 348–51; and Stevens, *In Sickness and In Wealth,* 218–20.

9. The Hill-Burton program distributed funds to voluntary and public hospitals, but not to proprietary hospitals. Hollingsworth and Hollingsworth, *Controversy about American Hospitals,* 49–50.

10. Starr, *Social Transformation of American Medicine,* 294–310.

11. Starr, *Social Transformation of American Medicine,* 310–11, 327–31.

12. Lynaugh and Brush, *American Nursing,* 3.

13. "EMIC Program Draws to an End," *American Journal of Nursing* 47, no. 9 (September 1947): 643; and Temkin, "Driving Through," 587–95.

14. Hazel Corbin, "Safe Maternity for All," *Public Health Nursing* 37 (June 1945): 289–93.

15. Sinai and Anderson, *EMIC (Emergency Maternity and Infant Care),* 127–28, 131, 134–35.

16. Other women mistook "the professional approach . . . for personal indifference to the mother's needs. She missed the reassuring presence of her relatives or friends. Her sense of modesty was infringed. And not least of all, there was an unfounded fear of surgery or death." Sister M. Michael Waters, "Culture in Relation to a Maternity Service," *Public Health Nursing* 42 (1950): 69–72. The study to which Waters was referring is Van der Eerden, *Maternity Care in a Spanish-American Community of New Mexico.*

17. On women's own desires for access to medical science, see Leavitt, *Brought to Bed,* 171–77.

18. Smith, *Sick and Tired of Being Sick and Tired,* 119, 146–48.

19. Corbin, "Teaching Women about Prenatal Care," 875.

20. Hemschemeyer, "The Nurse-Midwife Is Here to Stay," 913–14.

21. Lynaugh and Brush, *American Nursing,* 3–4.

22. MCA, *40th Annual Report of the Maternity Center Association,* 14–15.

23. George Brown Tindall and David Emory Shi, *America: A Narrative History,* Vol. 2, 5th ed. (New York: W.W. Norton and Company, 1999), 1426.

24. Leavitt, *Brought to Bed,* 194–95.

25. Corbin, "Natural Childbirth," 660.

26. Leavitt, "'Strange Young Women on Errands,'" 3–24.

27. See Rinker, "To Spread the 'Gospel of Good Obstetrics,'" 282–85, for examples of mothers' frustrations with obstetric nurses. I thank Rinker for sharing her dissertation with me.

28. Leavitt, "'Strange Young Women on Errands,'" 9–10.

29. See Smyth, "History of the Catholic Maternity Institute from 1943 to 1958," 21, on nurse-midwives assuming responsibilities in the intrapartal and postpartal phases of birth, while obstetric nurses did not assume such roles.

30. Vera Keane, "Why Nurse-Midwifery," *Bulletin of the American College of Nurse-Midwifery* 2, no. 4 (December 1957): 58–61.

31. MCA, *Twenty Years of Nurse-Midwifery, 1933–1953,* 115.

32. MCA, *Twenty Years of Nurse-Midwifery, 1933–1953,* 113.

33. Hazel Corbin, "Nurse Midwives: The Torch Bearers," *Public Health Nursing* 44, no. 9 (September 1952): 499–501.

34. See, for example, Corbin, "Emotional Aspects of Maternity Care," 20–22; Hazel Corbin, "Changing Maternity Service in a Changing World," *Public Health Nursing* 42 (August 1950): 427–34; and Corbin, "Maternity Care Today and Tomorrow," 201–4.

35. On the small percentage of nurse-midwives actually practicing their profession, see Thomas, *The Practice of Nurse-Midwifery in the United States;* Responses to Committee on Organization's Questionnaire, 1954, container 1, files: Pre-Organization Questionnaire, A-G, H-O, P-Z, Late respondents, ACNM Archives; *Nurse-Midwife Bulletin* 1, no. 3 (November 1954): container 2, folder: Pre-organization, N.O.P.H.N. + N.A.C.N.M., ACNM Archives; and *Nurse-Midwife Bulletin* 2, no. 1 (April 1955): container 2, folder: Pre-organization, N.O.P.H.N. +

N.A.C.N.M, ACNM Archives.

36. Knowledge about hospital nurses who had degrees in nurse-midwifery comes from their comments on questionnaires completed in the mid-1950s by graduates of nurse-midwifery schools, and from their articles in nursing journals that challenge contemporary approaches to maternity nursing.

37. Barbara Sklar Laster, Response to Committee on Organization's Questionnaire, 1954, container 1, file: Pre-Organization Questionnaire, H-O, ACNM Archives.

38. Mildred Disbrow, Response to Committee on Organization's Questionnaire, 1954, container 1, file: Pre-Organization Questionnaire, A-G, ACNM Archives.

39. Aileen I. Hogan, Response to Committee on Organization's Questionnaire, 1954, container 1, file: Pre-Organization Questionnaire, H-O, ACNM Archives.

40. Aileen Hogan, "The Scope of Maternity Nursing," *Briefs* 15, no. 3 (Summer 1951): 8–12.

41. Grantly Dick-Read was the author of *Natural Childbirth* and *Childbirth without Fear.*

42. "I Watched My Baby Born," as told to Selwyn, 5–13; and "Natural Childbirth: Young Mother Has Her Baby with No Fear, Little Pain," 71–76.

43. Leavitt, *Brought to Bed,* 194–95.

44. Chapters 2 and 3 offer examples of the value FNS and MCA nurse-midwives placed on spending time with maternity patients. Several early MCA writings point to a belief in the normality of pregnancy and labor, and to an emphasis on eliminating fear from patients' minds. In 1922, Ralph Lobenstine, after whom MCA's Lobenstine Midwifery School was named, explained that fear should have no place in the mind of prospective mothers: "*Fear* acts peculiarly on the progress of the labor. It adds to the feeling of pain and, at the same time, it is likely to delay the progress by causing the contractions of the womb (which cause the pain) to be less effectual." An MCA pamphlet from 1934 argued that "pregnancy is natural and should be normal." In the same year, George Kosmak, chairman of MCA's Medical Board, stated: "Parents must realize that labor is a normal process and that its successful termination is not dependent upon the unrestricted use of anesthetics or the operative dexterity of the attendant." Lobenstine, *The Expectant Mother and the New Baby,* 12; MCA, "A Mother's Day Message to Men, May 13th, 1934" (New York: MCA, 1934); and MCA, *The Story of the New Mother's Day* (New York: MCA, 1935), 17, all in MCA Archives.

45. Ernestine Wiedenbach, "Childbirth as Mothers Say They Like It," *Public Health Nursing* 41 (August 1949): 417–21. On the limits of Read's work, see Frederick W. Goodrich, "Experience with Natural Childbirth," *Public Health Nursing* 41 (March 1949): 122–25.

46. MCA, *Twenty Years of Nurse-Midwifery, 1933–1953*, 99.

47. MCA, *Twenty Years of Nurse-Midwifery, 1933–1953*, 91.

48. Ruth Watson Lubic states: "It is interesting that Dr. Dick-Read . . . was well received by the public, but greeted with distrust and ridicule by many of his obstetrical colleagues. Indeed, when MCA initiated a demonstration of Dick-Read's principles, it was done out of New York City at a nearby major medical center, not completely by preference. Nowhere in New York was the agency able to initiate a program despite the fact that there was interest on the part of some academic obstetricians. It appears that department chiefs could be effectively stopped from changing the status quo of practice by the pressure of the conservative members of their staffs." Lubic, "Barriers and

Conflict in Maternity Care Innovation," 17.

49. Goodrich, "Experience with Natural Childbirth," 123.

50. Hyder interview.

51. Silberman, "Pioneering in Family-Centered Maternity and Infant Care," 276–77.

52. Hyder interview.

53. Laird and Hogan, "An Elective Program on Preparation for Childbirth at the Sloane Hospital for Women," 641–47.

54. MCA, *Twenty Years of Nurse-Midwifery, 1933–1953*, 96.

55. One letter explained, "I remember that you asked us to send you a full description of our experiences during birth, and so I will try to give you the full details as well as I can recall them now." David, Bob, and Day Levin to Miss Strachan and Miss Janeway, n.d., Natural Childbirth Letters, c. 1947–1951, MCA Archives.

56. "A doctor's daughter," n.d., Natural Childbirth Letters, c. 1947–1951, MCA Archives.

57. "A graduate nurse whose husband is finishing his work for his M.D.," May 1947, Natural Childbirth Letters, c. 1947–1951, MCA Archives.

58. "The wife of a Yale student," 7 May 1947, Natural Childbirth Letters, c. 1947–1951, MCA Archives.

59. While praising their experiences, some of these women also criticized aspects of their hospital stays, revealing their desire for more control over their birthing processes, more support in the delivery room, and more contact with their newborns. These women wanted an even better emotional experience of childbirth than postwar natural childbirth could offer. The nurse whose husband was a medical student wished she had "not . . . had my hands tied," that she had been "allowed to touch the baby immediately," and "that my husband might have been present at delivery." The wife of a Yale student wished her husband had been at the delivery: "He was such a comfort all during the rest of labor. I felt rather sorry he couldn't be there when our son was born." Some women expressed disappointment with natural childbirth, and/or a belief that they did not live up to the requirements of the Read method. These women generally did not blame the method itself, pointing instead to their personalities or external circumstances which harmed chances for success with natural childbirth. One woman, who thanked MCA "for a happier, more intelligent pregnancy and approach to childbirth," explained that she was only "partially successful with natural childbirth" because of "certain things in my temperament and character which are deterrent to it": "a deep rooted mistrust of hospitals"; " a great fear of 'being torn to pieces' in childbirth"; the need for "more personal encouragement and attention than I should ask for, than could be given me in any hospital in the world!"; that "I am inhibited and afraid of 'letting go' and 'giving myself away'"; and that "I am foolishly perfectionist." "A graduate nurse whose husband is finishing his work for his M.D."; "The wife of a Yale student"; and Toni Schwed to Miss Stevens, 24 February 1950, Natural Childbirth Letters, c. 1947–1951, MCA Archives.

60. *Webster's II New Riverside University Dictionary*, s.v. "natural."

61. For a discussion of the expansion of natural childbirth and a list of health professionals' studies of natural childbirth between 1946 and 1960, see Sandelowski, *Pain, Pleasure, and American Childbirth,* 91–92, 102–3n38.

62. Kroska, *50th Celebration Reunion.*

63. "Educational Programs," *Bulletin of the American College of Nurse-Midwifery* 1, no. 3 and 4 (September 1956): 16–19.

64. American College of Nurse-Midwifery, *Education for Nurse-Midwifery,* 31.

65. MCA, *Twenty Years of Nurse-Midwifery*, 96.

66. ACNM, *Education for Nurse-Midwifery*, 31–32.

67. "Graduate Program in Maternity Nursing," Columbia University, Department of Nursing and the Faculty of Medicine, 1957–1958, 6, container 515651 (Administration, Joint Programs, Motion Pictures, Copyrights, Transla., Filing Cabinet, 1 of 8, 1920–1978, box 76), folder: Joint Program-Columbia-Presbyterian, 1950–1959, MCA Storage.

68. *Science* 22 (6 January 1956): 123, container 518801 (Admin Records, Lobenstine, Hemschemeyer, 3 of 3, 1931–1970, box 109), folder: Johns Hopkins, MCA Storage.

69. Sara E. Fetter, "Johns Hopkins Nurse-Midwife Program: Progress, Prospects after Five Years," reprinted from *Hospital Topics* (December 1961/January 1962), container 518801 (Admin Records, Lobenstine, Hemschemeyer, 3 of 3, 1931–1970, box 109), folder: Conference Reports, Booklets, Pamphlets, folder #2, MCA Storage.

70. Fetter, "Johns Hopkins Nurse-Midwife Program."

71. Nicholson J. Eastman, "Nurse-Midwifery at the Johns Hopkins Hospital," *Briefs* 17, no. 6 (Winter 1953–1954): 8–13.

72. *Briefs* 20, no. 6 (June 1956): 90.

73. Fetter, "Johns Hopkins Nurse-Midwife Program."

74. ACNM, *Education for Nurse-Midwifery,* 21–25.

75. Susan Nickel, Theresa Gesse, and Aileen MacLaren, "Ernestine Wiedenbach: Her Professional Legacy," *Journal of Nurse-Midwifery* 37, no. 3 (May/June 1992): 161–67.

76. Nickel, Gesse, and MacLaren, "Ernestine Wiedenbach," 164; and Ernestine Wiedenbach, "Growth and Development of the Nurse-Midwifery Program at Yale," *Bulletin of the American College of Nurse-Midwifery* 7, no. 1 (March 1962): 16–21, 27.

77. "Educational Programs," 19–21.

78. Wiedenbach, "Growth and Development," 16–18.

79. Wiedenbach, "Growth and Development," 18–21, and Ernestine Wiedenbach, "Developments at Yale School of Nursing in the Programs of Maternal and Newborn Health Nursing and Nurse-Midwifery," *Bulletin of the American College of Nurse-Midwifery* 6, no. 3 (September 1961): 22–25.

80. Lynaugh and Brush, *American Nursing,* 22.

81. Hazel Corbin, "Recent Program Changes at Maternity Center Association School of Nurse-Midwifery," *Bulletin of the American College of Nurse-Midwifery* 4, no. 1 (March 1959): 29–30.

82. Corbin interview, 34.

83. Dawley, "Leaving the Nest," 184–85; on substandard care at Kings County, see Corbin interview, 36.

84. Ruth Watson Lubic, "Nurse-Midwifery in Context," reprinted from *Briefs,* 1–12, container 512590 (H. Hemschemeyer, Ed materials, 1 of 3, 1930s–1960s, box 119), MCA Storage.

85. Dawley, "Leaving the Nest," 185–86.

86. Marion Strachan to Robert A. Moore, 14 March 1958, container 515651

(Administration, Joint Programs, Motion Pictures, Copyrights, Transla., Filing Cabinet, 1 of 8, 1920–1978, box 76), folder: Joint Program-Kings County Hospital-State University of New York, 1950–1959, MCA Storage. Hazel Corbin also noted, "we all regret the closing of our clinic and loss of the family-centered experience field it offered students." Corbin, "Recent Program Changes," 30.

87. Dawley, "Leaving the Nest," 186.

88. Ruth Coates, "The Nurse-Midwifery Service at the Kings County Hospital," *Bulletin of the American College of Nurse-Midwifery* 5, no. 4 (December 1960): 82–86.

89. Corbin, "Recent Program Changes," 29–30.

90. Dawley, "Leaving the Nest," 186–87.

91. Fetter, "Johns Hopkins Nurse-Midwife Program."

92. "A Family Has a Baby," *Briefs* 16, no. 5 (Autumn 1952): 2–3, 16.

93. Eastman, "Nurse-Midwifery at the Johns Hopkins Hospital," 13.

94. See, for example, Wolf, *Misconceptions;* and Mitford, *The American Way of Birth.*

95. Eastman, "Nurse-Midwifery at the Johns Hopkins Hospital," 13.

96. Louis Hellman, "Let's Use Midwives—To Save Babies," *Saturday Evening Post,* 1964, MCA Archives.

97. Hellman, "Paraobstetric personnel," 503–7.

98. Hattie Hemschemeyer, "What Is Ahead for Nurse-Midwifery in the Next Few Years?" *Bulletin of the American College of Nurse-Midwifery* 5, no. 2 (June 1960): 25–27.

## Notes to Chapter 5

1. Unless otherwise noted, the information on Hannah Mitchell is from Cannon, "Enduring Echoes: Hannah D. Mitchell," 12; Hannah D. Mitchell, interview by Rose B. Cannon; and Stoney, "*All My Babies:* Research," 79–96.

2. Mitchell, "Coordinating Maternity Care," 10–12, Hannah D. Mitchell, Response to Committee on Organization's Questionnaire, 1954, container 1, file: Pre-Organization Questionnaire, H-O, ACNM Archives.

3. Based on Cannon's interview with Mitchell (see note 1), the *School Health Guide* is likely Georgia Department of Education and Georgia Department of Public Health, *School Health Guide* (Atlanta, 1955), and the documentary film is likely Southern Educational Film Production Service, producer, and George C. Stoney, writer, *Birthright* (Atlanta: Georgia Department of Public Health, 1951).

4. George C. Stoney, writer, director, and producer, *All My Babies* (Chicago: Medical Audio-Visual Institute of the Association of American Medical Colleges, 1952).

5. "Tisch School's Kanbar Institute of Film & TV at NYU to Honor Professor George Stoney, Documentarian, Humanitarian, and Teacher," New York University press release, 5 July 1999, www.nyu.edu/publicaffairs/newsreleases/b_Tisch.shtml (accessed 22 June 2004).

6. "Alternative Media Festival 2004: Uniting to Take Back Our Media," Indianapolis, Ind., www.indyaccess.org/what_s_new/festival.htm (accessed 22 June 2004).

7. "Stoney Film Named to National Registry," *NYU Today on the Web* 16, no. 5, 6 February 2003, www.nyu.edu/nyutoday/archives/16/05/Stories/Stoney.html (accessed 22 June 2004).

8. Marian F. Cadwallader, "Midwife Training in Georgia: Needs and Problems," *Bulletin of the American College of Nurse-Midwifery* 2, no. 2 (April 1957): 18–23.

9. Walsh, *Midwife Means with Woman,* 11.

10. Smith, *Sick and Tired of Being Sick and Tired,* 119.

11. On the need to understand the experiences of black nurses, see Hine, *Black Women in White,* xi.

12. Schwartz, "Nurse-Midwives in the Mountains," 103.

13. Betty Lester, "Home Delivery Technique," *Quarterly Bulletin of the Frontier Nursing Service, Inc.* 27, no. 4 (Spring 1952): 17–19.

14. "A Cadet Nurse with the F.N.S.," *Quarterly Bulletin of the Frontier Nursing Service, Inc.* 22, no. 1 (Summer 1946): 45–46.

15. Metropolitan Life Insurance Company, "Summary of the Tenth Thousand Confinement Records of the Frontier Nursing Service," *Bulletin of the American College of Nurse-Midwifery* 5, no. 1 (March 1960): 1–9.

16. Chetwynd, "The Frontier Nursing Service of Kentucky," vi.

17. "Twenty-Seventh Annual Report of the Frontier Nursing Service, Inc., for the Fiscal Year, May 1, 1951 to April 30, 1952," *Quarterly Bulletin of the Frontier Nursing Service, Inc.* 28, no. 1 (Summer 1952): 3–16.

18. "Annual Report of the Frontier Nursing Service, Inc., May 1, 1939, to April 30, 1940," *Quarterly Bulletin of the Frontier Nursing Service, Inc.* 16, no. 1 (Summer 1940): 4–15.

19. "The Organization of the Frontier Nursing Service, Inc., 1946," *Quarterly Bulletin of the Frontier Nursing Service, Inc.* 22, no. 2 (Autumn 1946): 7–17; "Frontier Nursing Service Aids Remote Areas in Hazard Section," *Hi-Power News* 5, no. 5 (May 1948): 2–3, box 36, folder 8, FNS Papers; and Schupp, "Good Neighbor of 'Wide Neighborhoods,'" 12–15.

20. Mary Breckinridge to Margaret Gage, 11–12 March 1949, box 341, folder 5, FNS Papers.

21. Breckinridge, *Wide Neighborhoods,* 314–15. Interestingly, Breckinridge also had a different view of rooming-in than some of her nurse-midwife contemporaries. She believed in keeping newborns near their mothers; as one writer explained, even in Hyden Hospital, "the babies were kept in the ward with their mothers, in their own little cribs to be sure but placed alongside their mothers' beds." However, Breckinridge criticized the "rooming in" philosophy: "As to this business of 'rooming in,' as they call it now, I personally am of a doubtful mind. The mother should have her baby near her, but the mother should not have the responsibility or the care of her baby for at least a week after it is born, in my opinion. Childbirth is exhausting no matter how normal. It calls for hard exercise, not one bit like reducing exercises. I have borne two children and I know. The woman who has just gone through childbirth rates a rest, and she should get it. Give her her baby, yes, whenever she wants it, but not the care of it and not the responsibility for it." Hope McCown, "Hail to Hyden Hospital!" *Quarterly Bulletin of the Frontier Nursing Service, Inc.* 22, no. 4 (Spring 1947): 7–10; and Mary Breckinridge, "Beyond the Mountains," *Quarterly Bulletin of the Frontier Nursing Service, Inc.* 25, no. 3 (Winter 1950): 57.

22. Marks, *Sexual Chemistry,* 96–103; and Harris, "Constructing Colonialism," 79–83.

23. Harris, "Constructing Colonialism," 68. The trial began in October 1959 and

ended in March 1968. Inventory for the FNS Medical Surveys, Archives and Special Collections, Margaret I. King Library, University of Kentucky, Lexington.

24. Browne, interview by Deaton, 27 March 1979, 61–62.

25. Breckinridge, "Is Birth Control the Answer?," 159–60.

26. On birth control activists' compromises with and resistance to the medical profession's domination, see McCann, *Birth Control Politics,* 58–97.

27. At the same time that some women—poor, black, or "feebleminded," depending on the state—were forced to be sterilized, many others who wanted a tubal ligation found they could not get one. As Dorothy McBride Stetson explains, "until the late 1960s, many physicians adhered to the 'rule of 120' recommended by the American College of Obstetrics and Gynecology: they performed sterilizations on private women patients only if their age multiplied by the number of their living children equaled at least that number." Dorothy McBride Stetson, "Sterilization," in *Historical and Multicultural Encyclopedia of Women's Reproductive Rights in the United States,* ed. Judith A. Baer (Westport, Conn.: Greenwood Press, 2002), 194–95; Schoen, *Choice and Coercion.*

28. Harris, "Constructing Colonialism," 70–73.

29. Harris, "Constructing Colonialism," 83–84.

30. Harris, "Constructing Colonialism," 90–91.

31. Harris, "Constructing Colonialism," 97–99.

32. Helen Varney Burst, "History of Nurse-Midwifery in Reproductive Health Care," *Journal of Nurse-Midwifery* 43, no. 6 (November/December 1998): 526–29.

33. MCA, *40th Annual Report of the Maternity Center Association,* 38, 40.

34. Minutes, Medical Board Meetings, MCA, 1931–1965, 19 November 1943, 46, MCA Office.

35. MCA, *40th Annual Report of the Maternity Center Association,* 38, 40, 43–44; and *Maternity Center Association, Berwind Branch,* revised 1953, 1, MCA Archives.

36. MCA Minutes, 1943–1960, Meeting of the Board of Directors, 13 November 1947, MCA Office; and Minutes, Medical Board Meetings, MCA, 1931–1965, 26 March 1959, 186.

37. MCA, *Twenty Years of Nurse-Midwifery, 1933–1953*, 78, 82.

38. Laird, "Report of the Maternity Center Association Clinic, New York, 1931–1951"; and Faison, "Report of the Maternity Center Association Clinic, 1952–1958," 395–402.

39. Corbin, "Recent Program Changes," 29–30.

40. The information on these women is taken from Bergstrom et al., "Full Circle," 29–45.

41. Smith, *Sick and Tired of Being Sick and Tired,* 119–20; and Holmes, "African American Midwives in the South."

42. Smith and Holmes, *Listen to Me Good,* 64; and Smith, *Sick and Tired of Being Sick and Tired,* 126–27.

43. Smith and Holmes, *Listen to Me Good,* 37–39; and Holmes, "African American Midwives in the South," 277–78.

44. Smith and Holmes, *Listen to Me Good,* 82–84.

45. Smith, *Sick and Tired of Being Sick and Tired,* 120.

46. Smith and Holmes, *Listen to Me Good,* 42.

47. Smith, *Sick and Tired of Being Sick and Tired,* 124.

48. Hine, *Black Women in White,* 72–73.

49. On a 1944 roster of the Medical Association of the State of Alabama, Segre is listed as "colored." A 1937 graduate of Howard University Medical School, Segre worked at the Slossfield Clinic, a clinic for African Americans in a poor area of Birmingham, prior to taking the position at Flint-Goodridge. Tim Pennycuff, University Archivist, University of Alabama at Birmingham, telephone conversation with author, 6 January 2006.

50. Horch, "Flint-Goodridge School of Nurse-Midwifery," 43–44.

51. Hiestand, "Midwife to Nurse-Midwife," 172–73.

52. Horch, "Flint-Goodridge School," 45.

53. Horch, "Flint-Goodridge School," 42–43.

54. Ruth Doran to Hazel Corbin, 23 March 1953, MCA Archives; and MCA, *Twenty Years of Nurse-Midwifery, 1933–1953*, 58–61.

55. Canty, "Graduates of the Tuskegee School," 13–14.

56. Canty, "Graduates of the Tuskegee School," 23–25.

57. Walsh, "Midwife Means with Woman," 13–14.

58. Doran to Corbin, 23 March 1953; and MCA, *Twenty Years of Nurse-Midwifery, 1933–1953,* 59–61.

59. Canty, "Graduates of the Tuskegee School," 23, 25.

60. The information on Hale is from Bell, "'Making Do' with the Midwife," 155–69. The year of Hale's graduation from Tuskegee is from Canty, "Graduates of the Tuskegee School," 30.

61. The information on Callen is from Hill, "Maude E. Callen," 49–54, quotation on 52. The year of Callen's graduation from Tuskegee is from Canty, "Graduates of the Tuskegee School," 29.

62. Smith, "Nurse-Midwife: Maude Callen Eases Pain of Birth, Life, and Death," 134–44.

63. Of course, the tradition of attending births at home predated nurse-midwives by centuries.

64. This story comes from Pauline E. King, producer, *Nurse-Midwife,* film (Santa Fe: CMI, 1948), MMS Archives. The film shows this family and the birth of their baby.

65. Debates abound over the appropriate terminology to use for people of Mexican origin. I have chosen to use the broad term, Latino, when discussing Catholic Maternity Institute's patients.

According to Felipe Gonzales, Director of the Southwest Hispanic Research Institute and Associate Professor of Sociology, University of New Mexico, it is safe to assume that the Latino population in Santa Fe County and surrounding areas had roots going back to the nineteenth century. Although New Mexico is at the Mexican border, it has received the smallest amount of modern Mexican immigration out of any border state with a large Mexican immigrant and/or Mexican-American population. In addition, the fact that CMI nurse-midwives described their patients as "Spanish American" gives more credence to the argument that Mexican Americans, not Mexican immigrants, populated the area. Gonzales said that Anglos would have been even more likely than Latinos to distinguish between different Latino populations, and would have called their patients "Mexicans" if they had been Mexican immigrants. Felipe Gonzales, telephone conversation with author, 15 February 2001.

66. Some women did not receive prenatal care as often as the nurse-midwives rec-

ommended. However, all received much more care than they would have had otherwise.

67. King, *Nurse-Midwife,* film, 1948.

68. I thank Molly Ladd-Taylor for helping me think further about how this work contributes to broader issues in women's health history. Robert A. Orsi also argues that in the twentieth-century Catholic context, religion and science were not considered opposing values, and patients' and caregivers' religious devotion was not part of an "anti-modernist impulse." In his study of women's devotion to St. Jude, the patron saint of hopeless causes, Orsi contends that devotion to this saint allowed sick women to challenge their physicians' authority and to develop more helpful responses to illness than those suggested by either male physicians or male priests. Orsi, *Thank You, St. Jude,* 182–83.

69. See Wessel, *Natural Childbirth and the Christian Family,* for a popular discussion of the connections between "natural childbirth" and Christianity. Wessel's book is currently in its fifth edition (1994).

70. In 1944, the sisters took over Atlanta's Catholic Colored Clinic, a clinic originally established by "apostolic-minded lay people" three years earlier. Although they had planned to stay only for the duration of the war, the sisters continued their work in Atlanta, opening the Holy Family Hospital in 1964. The sisters withdrew from the hospital in 1973. "Catholic Colored Clinic, Atlanta, Ga.," *Medical Missionary Magazine* (September-October 1955): 115, MMS Archives; MMS, *History of the Society of Catholic Medical Missionaries, Pre-Foundation to 1968* (London: MMS, 1991), 182–84, MMS Archives; McInerney, "DeGive Family Colorful in City, Catholic History," 4–5.

71. "Many Mothers and Babies Saved by Medical Mission Sisters," *Santa Fe New Mexican,* 8 March 1945, MMS Archives.

72. "Great Progress Made by Maternity Institute Nuns," *(Santa Fe) Register,* 15 July 1945, MMS Archives.

73. The 1950 Latino population statistic is from census statistics included in City Planning Commission, City of Santa Fe, *General Characteristics, City of Santa Fe, New Mexico,* 21. The 1960 statistic is from census statistics included in Bureau of Business Research, Institute for Social Research and Development, *New Mexico Statistical Abstract, 1970* (Albuquerque: University of New Mexico, 1970), 1: 16. The statistic from both decades includes "white persons of Spanish surname."

74. Schackel, *Social Housekeepers,* 50.

75. Although CMI served mostly poor Latinos, it was open to anyone. Shortly before it closed in 1969, CMI served several Anglo women who came there specifically for an alternative to hospital care. Sister Catherine Shean, telephone interview by author, 18 August 2000; and Rita Kroska, telephone interview by author, 24 July 2000. Although located in an urban area, CMI served women in an area of 2827 square miles in a radius of thirty miles from Santa Fe. Miller, "Grand Multiparas," 419.

76. Deutsch, *No Separate Refuge;* Yohn, *A Contest of Faiths;* and Hinojosa, "Mexican-American Faith Communities in Texas and the Southwest," 26–45.

77. Sister Catherine Shean, a nurse-midwife who worked at CMI from 1945 until its closing in 1969, does not think the Protestant missionaries posed a problem for the MMS. She argued that the sisters always tried to work in cooperation with others helping their patient populations. She also explained that in the early 1960s, CMI had a short-lived arrangement with Presbyterian-Embudo Hospital, north of Santa Fe, to

provide nurse-midwifery students with hospital experience. St. Vincent's Hospital, a Catholic hospital in Santa Fe, refused to allow the nurse-midwifery students to deliver babies there. Shean, interview by author.

78. Recent legal decisions allowed MHC to distribute birth control. In 1873, the federal Comstock Act had outlawed the distribution of birth control information and devices through the mail or across state lines. In 1930, a federal court decision modified the Comstock Act, and in 1936, in *United States v. One Package,* the Supreme Court allowed physicians to obtain and prescribe contraceptives whenever they chose. McCann, *Birth Control Politics in the United States.*

79. Sullivan, "Walking the Line."

80. Article in *El Paso News*, 27 October 1947, MMS Archives.

81. Rose Gioiosa, "Life Begins in an Adobe: Home Maternity Service of the Medical Mission Sisters," *Child-Family Digest* (October 1953): 56 (reprinted from *The Grail*), MMS Archives.

82. Mary Zook, "Sister-Doctor," *Extension* (November 1955): 68, MMS Archives.

83. Deutsch, *No Separate Refuge,* 183.

84. Dengel, *Mission for Samaritans,* 113.

85. Quoted from the Sacred Congregation of Bishops and Regulars, 1901, in Beck, "Society of Catholic Medical Missionaries," 20.

86. See, for example, a photograph of nuns in an operating room at the turn of the twentieth century in Franklin, "'A Spirit of Mercy.'" I wish to thank Carol K. Coburn for her helping me rethink the issue of nuns' work in obstetrics and surgery. Coburn's research on nuns at the Troy Maternity Hospital in 1909 and 1910 indicates that Catholic sisters did do obstetric work. Carol K. Coburn, conversation with author, San Marino, California, 17 May 1998.

87. McNamara, *Sisters in Arms,* 622–26. For the statistic on nuns administering hospitals in the nineteenth century, see Ewens, "The Leadership of Nuns in Immigrant Catholicism," 102. On the prohibition of "*even assisting* at obstetrical cases," see "First Medical Mission Sisterhood," 6.

88. Zook, "Sister-Doctor," 32–33; MMS, *History of the Society of Catholic Medical Missionaries,* chaps. 1–3; and Beck, "Society of Catholic Medical Missionaries," 47–48.

89. Quoted from Instruction, Issued by the Sacred Congregation for the Propagation of the Faith to the Religious Institutes of Women, 11 February 1936, in Beck, "Society of Catholic Medical Missionaries," 145–46.

90. "First Medical Mission Sisterhood," 12.

91. Smyth, "History of the Catholic Maternity Institute," 44–53. Starting in 1947, CMI also offered a master's program with a major in maternity nursing, designed to "give a broad professional background to graduate nurses who intended to do administration, teaching, supervision, or consultation in the field of obstetric nursing." In 1954, CMI extended the work for the certificate program from six months to one year.

92. Dunn, "They Save the Baby," 8–9.

93. I interviewed several sister-nurse-midwives who trained at CMI. The work of Sister Paula D'Errico seems typical. After receiving her nurse-midwifery certificate in 1952, D'Errico went on to medical missions in Venezuela, Ghana, Kenya, South Africa, and Ethiopia. Sister Paula D'Errico, interview by author, Philadelphia, Pennsylvania, 6 September 1995.

94. "First Medical Mission Sisterhood," 5.

95. Wynen, "The Society of Catholic Medical Missionaries," 45–46.

96. Beck, "Society of Catholic Medical Missionaries," 6.

97. See Brown, "Public Health Programs in Imperialism," 897–903, for an argument about how philanthropies set up health-care programs as a way to create a wedge into the native cultures where the programs were established.

98. Sandelowski, *Pain, Pleasure, and American Childbirth,* chaps. 4 and 5.

99. Silberman, "Pioneering in Family-Centered Maternity and Infant Care." Leavitt describes women's alienating experiences of hospital births in *Brought to Bed,* 171–95.

100. Sally Green, "Lo! A Child is Born: The Ever-Wondrous Miracle of the Birth of a Baby," *The Rosary* (December 1957): 13, MMS Archives.

101. Jacques [Lowe] and Jillen Lowe, "Nurse-Midwives of Santa Fe," *The Sign* (April 1955): 52, MMS Archives.

102. Kroska, *50th Celebration Reunion.*

103. On Catholic sister-nurses and the struggles they faced between their profession and their vocation, see Kauffman, *Ministry and Meaning,* 154–81, 238–44.

104. Gioiosa, "Life Begins in an Adobe," 55.

105. Green, "Lo! A Child is Born," 11.

106. Devitt, "The Transition from Home to Hospital Birth in the United States, 1930–1960," 56.

107. Smyth, "History of the Catholic Maternity Institute," 27–29.

108. Shean, interview by author.

109. On Latina women's preference for female attendants, see Van der Eerden, *Maternity Care in a Spanish-American Community of New Mexico,* 54–55.

110. Van der Eerden, *Maternity Care in a Spanish-American Community of New Mexico,* 8–19; Buss, *La Partera,* 7, 65–66; Anne Fox, interview by Jake Spidle, 11; and Shean, interview by author.

111. Miller, "Grand Multiparas," 418–19; and Cecilia Buser, "How I Came to Become a Nurse-Midwife and Came to Love It," in *CMI Graduates and Faculty Remember Nurse-Midwifery in Santa Fe, New Mexico,* ed. Kroska and Shean, 12–17.

112. Shean, interview by author.

113. Catholic nurses and nuns also supported Catholic patients' emphasis on prayer and religious rituals in hospitals. In Catholic hospitals in the 1950s, for example, nuns distributed prayer cards, said rosaries, and maintained hospital shrines to saints. According to Orsi, when female caregivers called on saints for support, they provided female patients the space to challenge their physicians' decisions because the patients believed in the authority of the saints more than of the physicians. Orsi, *Thank You, St. Jude,* 166–67, 177–82.

114. Sister Catherine Shean, interview, in Kroska, executive producer, *CMI: In-Depth Interviews with the Foundresses,* video; Shean, interview by author; and Kroska interview.

115. Waters, "Culture in Relation to a Maternity Service," 70. Emphasis added.

116. Most patients who registered with CMI for maternity care ultimately delivered with CMI's nurse-midwives, or in the case of problems, with the help of CMI's medical director. However, a few CMI patients who registered with CMI delivered their babies with a traditional midwife or a private physician. See Book #1, Deliveries Records, December 1943—April 1963, CMI, MMS Archives.

117. U.S. Public Health Service Bureau of Health, "A Study to Determine the Need and Scope for Educational Programs in Nurse-Midwifery," 10.

118. Shean and Kroska, interviews by author.

119. U.S. Public Health Service Bureau of Health, "A Study to Determine the Need and Scope for Educational Programs in Nurse-Midwifery," 14–16.

## Notes to Chapter 6

1. Unless otherwise noted, general information on Aileen I. Hogan is from Sally Austen Tom, "Spokeswoman for Midwifery: Aileen Hogan," *Journal of Nurse-Midwifery* 26, no. 3 (May/June 1981): 7–11.

2. Tom's article states that Hogan was chair of maternity nursing at a "Midwestern University." Her response to a 1954 questionnaire indicates that she was at Case Western Reserve University. Aileen I. Hogan, Response to Committee on Organization's Questionnaire, 1954, container 1, file: Pre-Organization Questionnaire, H-O, ACNM Archives.

3. Scott, *Weapons of the Weak,* xv. I thank Daniel Bradburd for recommending Scott's work.

4. Scott acknowledged that subtle methods of resistance rarely change a society's power structure but they can effectively undermine its dominant forces. Scott, *Weapons of the Weak,* 29–30.

5. "Membership of the American College of Nurse-Midwifery," *Bulletin of the American College of Nurse-Midwifery* 1, no. 2 (March 1956): 7–12; "The Membership Committee Reports," *Bulletin of the American College of Nurse-Midwifery* 1, no. 3 and 4 (September 1956): 27–28; "Membership Committee Reports," *Bulletin of the American College of Nurse-Midwifery* 2, no. 2 (April 1957): 31; "Membership Committee Reports," *Bulletin of the American College of Nurse-Midwifery* 2, no. 4 (December 1957): 75–76; "Membership Committee Reports," *Bulletin of the American College of Nurse-Midwifery* 3, no. 4 (December 1958): 85–86; and Dawley, "Leaving the Nest," 132–33, 181.

6. Betty Ann Bradbury, Response to Committee on Organization's Questionnaire, 1954, container 1, file: Pre-Organization Questionnaire, A-G, ACNM Archives.

7. Sister Beatrice Gallant, Response to Committee on Organization's Questionnaire, 1954, container 1, file: Pre-Organization Questionnaire, P-Z, ACNM Archives.

8. Mabel Zapenas, Response to Committee on Organization's Questionnaire, 1954, container 1, file: Pre-Organization Questionnaire, P-Z, ACNM Archives.

9. Helen Callon, Response to Committee on Organization's Questionnaire, 1954, container 1, file: Pre-Organization Questionnaire, Late Respondents, ACNM Archives.

10. Virginia Lamb Chrestman, Response to Committee on Organization's Questionnaire, 1954, container 1, file: Pre-Organization Questionnaire, A-G, ACNM Archives.

11. Jane McAllaster Burr, Response to Committee on Organization's Questionnaire, 1954, container 1, file: Pre-Organization Questionnaire, A-G, ACNM Archives.

12. Virginia Frederick Bowling, Response to Committee on Organization's Questionnaire, 1954, container 1, file: Pre-Organization Questionnaire, A-G, ACNM Archives.

13. Isabella Dougall Marraine, Response to Committee on Organization's Questionnaire, 1954, container 1, file: Pre-Organization Questionnaire, H-O, ACNM Archives.

14. Burr response, 1954.

15. Fred J. Taussig, "The Nurse-Midwife," *Public Health Nursing Quarterly* 6 (October 1914): 36–37.

16. Breckinridge, "The Nurse-Midwife—A Pioneer," 1147.

17. Josephine Kinman to Dorothy Buck, 22 November 1943, box 231, folder 4, FNS Papers.

18. Eastman, "Nurse-Midwifery at the Johns Hopkins Hospital," 8.

19. Sister M. Theophane Shoemaker to Sister M. Olivia, 22 March 1954, container 2, folder: Correspondence—Sr. M. Theophane, 1954, ACNM Archives.

20. *Nurse-Midwife Bulletin*, 1, no. 1 (May 1954), container 2, folder: Pre-organization, N.O.P.H.N. + N.A.C.N.M, ACNM Archives.

21. *Nurse-Midwife Bulletin,* 1, no. 1 (May 1954).

22. Sister M. Theophane Shoemaker to Mary Breckinridge, 15 April 1954, container 2, folder: Correspondence—Sr. M. Theophane, 1954, ACNM Archives.

23. Sister M. Theophane Shoemaker to Elizabeth K. Porter, 22 March 1954, container 2, folder: Correspondence—Sr. M. Theophane, 1954, ACNM Archives.

24. In 1973, the ACNM surveyed nurse-midwives about the relationship of nurse-midwifery to nursing, and whether nurse-midwifery should remain a part of nursing. The first two points in the following letter from a nurse-midwife are similar to comments some nurse-midwives made in the mid-1950s regarding organizing within the national nursing organizations:

"I strongly believe that we are and should remain a part of nursing. While much of this is gut level reaction, I would make the following points:

a) nurse midwives are few in number. We need the political clout of the entire nursing profession behind us if we are to accomplish our goals.

b) separation from the larger body of nursing, to me, raises the specter of loss of control over our own destiny. Physicians would be glad to dictate to a group to [*sic*] small to fight back.

c) What would be the effect of separation from nursing on the prerequisite of an R.N. for entrance to a midwifery school?"

Vanessa A. Marshall, CNM, to Executive Board, American College of Nurse-Midwives, 13 September 1973, container 2, file: Survey [Relationship of Nursing to Midwifery], 1973, ACNM Archives.

25. Fitzpatrick, *The National Organization for Public Health Nursing, 1912–1952,* 147, 177. The NOPHN's Committee on Maternity and Child Health, formed in 1935, included one nurse-midwife and some discussion of nurse-midwives. See, for example, "Report of the N.O.P.H.N. Committee on Maternity and Child Health," *Public Health Nursing* 27 (June 1935): 349–50; and "Summaries of Round Tables, Midwifery Supervision," *Public Health Nursing* 30 (July 1938): 434.

26. The NOPHN merged with several other nursing organizations to form the National League for Nursing. The demise of the NOPHN reflected a general trend in public-health nursing by the early 1950s. Public-health nurses gained credibility by moving from rural clinics and settlement houses to hospitals, but forfeited their independence and special role.

27. *Nurse-Midwife Bulletin,* 2, no. 1 (April 1955), container 2, folder: Pre-organization, N.O.P.H.N. + N.A.C.N.M., ACNM Archives.

28. Quoted in Sally Austen Tom, "The Evolution of Nurse-Midwifery, 1900–1960," *Journal of Nurse-Midwifery* 27, no. 4 (July/August 1982): 4–13. Quotation is on page 12.

29. *Nurse-Midwife Bulletin* 1, no. 3 (November 1954), container 2, folder: Pre-organization, N.O.P.H.N. + N.A.C.N.M., ACNM Archives.

30. The majority of respondents agreed with the definition from the Committee on Organization; however, the changes nurse-midwives offered to the definition suggest some of the issues and controversies surrounding the name "nurse-midwife." *Nurse-Midwife Bulletin* 2, no. 1 (April 1955): 2, container 2, folder: Pre-Organization, N.O.P.H.N. + N.A.C.N.M, ACNM Archives.

31. Helen Marie Fedde, Response to Committee on Organization's Questionnaire, 1954, including letter to Sister M. Theophane Shoemaker, 19 September 1954, container 1, file: Pre-Organization Questionnaire, A-G, ACNM Archives.

32. Emma Lois Shaffer, Response to Committee on Organization's Questionnaire, 1954, container 1, file: Pre-Organization Questionnaire, P-Z, ACNM Archives.

33. Sara Elizabeth Fetter, Response to Committee on Organization's Questionnaire, 1954, container 1, file: Pre-Organization Questionnaire, A-G, ACNM Archives.

34. Rachel Pierce Schottin, Response to Committee on Organization's Questionnaire, 1954, container 1, file: Pre-Organization Questionnaire, P-Z, ACNM Archives.

35. Reva Rubin, Response to Committee on Organization's Questionnaire, 1954, container 1, file: Pre-Organization Questionnaire, P-Z, ACNM Archives.

36. Peggy Helen Brown, Response to Committee on Organization's Questionnaire, 1954, container 1, file: Pre-Organization Questionnaire, A-G, ACNM Archives.

37. Anne Fox, Response to Committee on Organization's Questionnaire, 1954, container 1, file: Pre-Organization Questionnaire, A-G, ACNM Archives.

38. M. Elizabeth Dunbaden Hosford, Response to Committee on Organization's Questionnaire, 1954, container 1, file: Pre-Organization Questionnaire, H-O, ACNM Archives.

39. Betty Ann Bradbury, Response to Committee on Organization's Questionnaire, 1954, container 1, file: Pre-Organization Questionnaire, A-G; and Jean W. Dooley, Response to Committee on Organization's Questionnaire, 1954, container 1, file: Pre-Organization Questionnaire, A-G, both in ACNM Archives. Quotation is from Edith J. Galt, Response to Committee on Organization's Questionnaire, 1954, container 1, file: Pre-Organization Questionnaire, A-G, ACNM Archives.

40. Eunice LaRue, Response to Committee on Organization's Questionnaire, 1954, container 1, file: Pre-Organization Questionnaire, Late Respondents, ACNM Archives.

41. Fedde response.

42. "Kentucky State Association of Midwives, Inc.," *Quarterly Bulletin of the Frontier Nursing Service, Inc.* 14, no. 4 (Spring 1939): 19–21. The one nurse-midwife not affiliated with FNS was an American nurse who trained in London to be a midwife and worked in Asia.

43. "Members of American Association of Nurse Midwives, Inc., 11–25–43," box 227, folder 3, FNS Papers.

44. American Association of Nurse-Midwives pamphlet, January 1, 1959, box 228,

folder 1, FNS Papers.

45. Helen Browne to Sister M. Theophane Shoemaker and Hattie Hemschemeyer, 21 May 1954, container 2, folder: Correspondence—Sr. M. Theophane, 1954, ACNM Archives.

46. Sister M. Theophane Shoemaker to Mary Breckinridge, May 26, 1954, ACNM Archives, Container 2, folder: Correspondence—Sr. M. Theophane, 1954.

47. Ruth Boswell to Sister M. Theophane Shoemaker, 28 October 1954, container 2, folder: Correspondence—Sr. M. Theophane, 1954, ACNM Archives.

48. Shoemaker to Browne, 14 October 1954, box 232, folder 3, FNS Papers.

49. Louis Hellman, interview by Anne Campbell, 79OH273, FNS 124, 20 November 1979, transcript, 8, 16, Frontier Nursing Service (FNS) Oral History Collection, Archives and Special Collections, Margaret I. King Library, University of Kentucky, Lexington.

50. Minutes of meeting at MCA, 25 February 1944, 3, container 2, folder: Preorganization, N.O.P.H.N. + N.A.C.N.M, ACNM Archives.

51. As explained in chapter 5, thirty-one African American nurse-midwives graduated from Tuskegee and two graduated from Flint-Goodridge. Given that at least eight African Americans graduated from MCA, the total number of African American nurse-midwifery graduates would have been forty-one.

In 1942, leaders of the AANM and the director of the short-lived Tuskegee School of Nurse-Midwifery, F. Carrington Owen, suggested the AANM form an African American section of the association so that more African American nurse-midwives would join; they expected that the two associations would trade minutes. In 1943, Owen recommended a group of African American nurse-midwives for membership in the AANM, but, at its annual meeting, the association's board of directors decided not to issue memberships to African American nurse-midwives.

In 1944, the issue of African American members was revisited. This time, at the AANM annual meeting, two white nurse-midwives who supervised African American nurse-midwives asked whether qualified African Americans were eligible for AANM membership. According to the report of the annual meeting, AANM bylaws made no distinction between white and African American nurse-midwives, and several African Americans had been members, but virtually all had been dropped due to nonpayment of dues. The report carefully mentioned that some white nurse-midwives had been dropped for the same reason, and then quoted the bylaws regarding termination of members upon consistent nonpayment of dues. One suspects from this careful explanation that the AANM anticipated challenges to its actions. At the 1944 annual meeting, the AANM elected into membership several African American graduates of the Tuskegee School of Nurse-Midwifery. American Association of Nurse-Midwives, Inc., Annual Meeting, 20 November 1941, 3, box 229, folder 1; Dorothy F. Buck to F. Carrington Owen, 29 December 1943, box 231, folder 8; Owen to Buck, 2 January 1942 [actually 1943], box 231, folder 8; Owen to Buck, 6 April 1943, box 228, folder 6; American Association of Nurse-Midwives, Incorporated, First 1943 Meeting, Board of Directors, 7–15–43, box 228, folder 6; American Association of Nurse-Midwives, Inc., Annual Meeting, September 28, 1944, box 229, folder 1, all in FNS Papers.

52. For comments on Breckinridge's racial attitudes, see Browne, interview by Crowe-Carraco, 26 March 1979, 34–35; and Browne, interview by Deaton, 27 March 1979, 4–8.

53. Helen E. Browne to Sister M. Theophane Shoemaker, and attached memorandum, 5 October 1954, container 2, folder: Correspondence—Sr. M. Theophane, 1954, ACNM Archives.

54. Helen E. Browne to Sister M. Theophane Shoemaker, 3 November 1954, container 2, folder: Correspondence—Sr. M. Theophane, 1954, ACNM Archives.

55. Browne to Shoemaker, including memorandum, 5 October 1954; and Shoemaker to Browne, 14 October 1954, container 2, folder: Correspondence—Sr. M. Theophane, 1954, ACNM Archives.

56. Shoemaker to Browne, 14 October 1954; and Shoemaker to Ruth Doran et al. 16 October 1954, container 2, folder: Correspondence—Sr. M. Theophane, 1954, ACNM Archives. Sister M. Theophane was not the only frustrated committee member. Hattie Hemschemeyer told Helen Browne: "Frankly I had hoped for some indication [from Mary Breckinridge] of a more sympathetic understanding of the problems of the graduates of the three schools." Hemschemeyer felt that it would be very difficult to accomplish any goals under the AANM structure. Hemschemeyer to Browne, 12 October 1954, box 231, folder 2, FNS Papers.

57. Shoemaker to Hemschemeyer, 14 October 1954.

58. Fedde response.

59. Hattie Hemschemeyer, "Maternity Care within the Framework of the Public Health Service," *Bulletin of the American College of Nurse-Midwifery* 2, no. 3 (September 1957): 49–56.

60. Shoemaker, *History of Nurse-Midwifery,* 30.

61. Theoretically, FNS required medical supervision, but geographic isolation rendered this difficult and often impossible.

62. In reality, graduates and staff of all three schools and services often had little medical supervision. Both nurse-midwives and outsiders sensed that FNS graduates and staff practiced almost as private practitioners, while obstetricians directed the work of MCA and CMI graduates. Yet many MCA and CMI graduates went on to work in remote places where physicians often were inaccessible.

63. *Nurse-Midwife Bulletin* 2, no. 3 (October 1955), container 2, folder: Pre-Organization, N.O.P.H.N. + N.A.C.N.M., ACNM Archives; and "First Convention—Kansas City," *Bulletin of the American College of Nurse-Midwifery* 1, no. 1 (December 1955): 1–2.

64. The *Bulletin* explained, "nurse-midwives have originated, developed, and put into practice ideas that stand for the best in maternity care. But only to a small extent have these ideas been translated into the written word." The editors of the *Bulletin* hoped the journal would provide a venue in which the nurse-midwife could make "her unique contribution to professional literature." "Looking Ahead," *Bulletin of the American College of Nurse-Midwifery* 2, no. 1 (January 1957): 1–2. In 1968, the journal became the *Bulletin of the American College of Nurse-Midwives,* reflecting the ACNM's name change; in 1973, it switched to the *Journal of Nurse-Midwifery;* and in 2000, it became the *Journal of Midwifery and Women's Health,* its current title.

65. "First Slate of Officers," *Bulletin of the American College of Nurse-Midwifery* 1, no. 1 (December 1955): 2; "Membership of the American College of Nurse-Midwifery," *Bulletin of the American College of Nurse-Midwifery* 1, no. 2 (March 1956): 7–12; "Membership Committee Reports," *Bulletin of the American College of Nurse-Midwifery* 1, no. 3 and 4 (September 1956): 27–28; and "Membership Committee

Reports," *Bulletin of the American College of Nurse-Midwifery* 2, no. 2 (April 1957): 31.

66. Dawley, "Leaving the Nest," 132, 140–41, 152, 155–57.

67. Vera Keane (President, American College of Nurse-Midwifery) to Helen E. Browne (Secretary, American Association of Nurse-Midwives), 8 October 1965, container 2, folder: A.A.N.M., Correspondence [1959–1961, 1965, 1967–8], ACNM Archives; Agnes Shoemaker [formerly Sister M. Theophane Shoemaker] to Aileen Hogan (Executive Secretary, American College of Nurse-Midwifery), 8 September 1967, container 2, folder: A.A.N.M., Correspondence [1959–1961, 1965, 1967–8], ACNM Archives; Lucille Woodville to Barbara Walters, 25 July 1969, container 11, folder: Honor Roll, Lucille Woodville, ACNM Archives; and Elizabeth S. Sharp, "The Impossible Dreams Came True: Lucille Woodville (1904–1982)," *Journal of Nurse-Midwifery* 28, no. 5 (September/October 1983): 23–24.

## Notes to Epilogue

1. The state repealed the law and ended the project, despite evidence of improvements in maternal and infant morbidity. Rooks, *Midwifery and Childbirth in America,* 46–47.

2. Rooks, *Midwifery and Childbirth in America,* 52.

3. Rooks, *Midwifery and Childbirth in America,* 48–51.

4. Rooks, *Midwifery and Childbirth in America,* 51–53. For more information on the history of nurse practitioners and physician assistants, see Brush and Capezuti, "Revisiting 'A Nurse for All Settings,'" 5–11; Silver, Ford, Ripley, and Igoe, "Perspectives 20 Years Later," 15–22; and Holt, "'Confusion's Masterpiece,'" 246–78.

5. Rooks, *Midwifery and Childbirth in America,* 72–74.

6. Varney, *Varney's Midwifery,* 3rd ed., 13.

7. Rooks, *Midwifery and Childbirth in America,* 53–56.

8. Helen Varney Burst, "'Real' Midwifery," *Journal of Nurse-Midwifery* 35, no. 4 (July/August 1990): 189–91.

9. For a critique of nurse-midwives, see Arms, *Immaculate Deception.* See also Burst, "'Real' Midwifery," 190; and Rooks, *Midwifery and Childbirth in America,* 56.

10. Burst, "'Real' Midwifery," 189; and Rooks, *Midwifery and Childbirth in America,* 66–67.

11. Rooks, *Midwifery and Childbirth in America,* 67.

12. Rooks, *Midwifery and Childbirth in America,* 74–75.

13. Varney, *Varney's Midwifery,* 3rd ed., 14. The ACNM defines medical consultation, collaboration, and referral: "'*Consultation* is the process where by a CNM [certified nurse-midwife], who maintains primary management responsibility for the woman's care, seeks the advice or opinion of a physician or another member of the health care team. *Collaboration* is the process whereby a CNM and physician jointly manage the care of a woman or newborn who has become medically, gynecologically, or obstetrically complicated. The scope of the collaboration may encompass the physical care of the client, including delivery, by the CNM, according to a mutually agreed-upon plan of care. When the physician must assume a dominant role in the care of the client due to increased risk status, the CNM may continue to participate in physical care, counseling, guidance, teaching, and support. Effective communication between

the CNM and physician is essential for ongoing collaborative management. *Referral* is the process by which the CNM directs the client to a physician or another health care professional for management of a particular problem or aspect of the client's care.'" Deanne R. Williams, "Credentialing Certified Nurse-Midwives," *Journal of Nurse-Midwifery* 39, no. 4 (July/August 1994): 258–64.

14. Rooks, *Midwifery and Childbirth in America,* 182–84.

15. Rooks, *Midwifery and Childbirth in America,* 165, 167–70.

16. Varney, *Varney's Midwifery,* 3[rd] ed., 15.

17. Rooks, *Midwifery and Childbirth in America,* 186–89.

18. Mary Ann Shah, "The Nurse-Midwife as Primary Care Provider," *Journal of Nurse-Midwifery* 38, no. 4 (July/August 1993): 185–87.

19. Jane E. Brody, "Midwives Lead a Revolution in Quality Obstetric Care," *New York Times,* 28 April 1993, as quoted in Shah, "Nurse-Midwife as Primary Care Provider," 185.

20. Mary Ann Shah, "The Journal of Midwifery & Women's Health Celebrating Its Heritage—Forging Its Future," *Journal of Midwifery and Women's Health* 45, no. 1 (January/February 2000): 1–3.

21. Karen Burgin, "Into the Next Millennium with the American College of Nurse-Midwives," *Journal of Nurse-Midwifery* 44, no. 2 (March/April 1999): 87–88.

22. Judith Pence Rooks, "Unity in Midwifery? Realities and Alternatives," *Journal of Nurse-Midwifery* 43, no. 5 (September/October 1998): 315–19.

23. Julie A. Buenting, conversation with the author, June 1995, Rochester, New York. Buenting was director of the now defunct nurse-midwifery program at the University of Rochester School of Nursing.

24. Ernst, telephone conversation with author, 10 November 2003.

25. Burgin, "Into the Next Millennium," 87.

26. Rooks, "Unity in Midwifery?" 317.

27. For use of the statement, see, for example, Susan M. Jenkins, Letter to the Editor, *Journal of Midwifery and Women's Health* 47, no. 2 (March/April 2002): 118–19.

28. Joyce Roberts, "Revised 'Joint Statement' Clarifies Relationships between Midwives and Physician Collaborators," *Journal of Midwifery and Women's Health* 46, no. 5 (September/October 2001): 269–71.

29. The quotation is from Leanne B. Bedell, Letter to the Editor, *Journal of Midwifery and Women's Health* 47, no. 2 (March/April 2002): 117. The other letter is Jenkins, Letter to the Editor.

30. American College of Nurse-Midwives, "Basic Facts about Certified Nurse-Midwives," May 2004, www.midwife.org/prof/display.cfm?id=6 (accessed 22 December 2004); and Tim Clarke (Communications Manager, American College of Nurse-Midwives), e-mail to author, 4 January 2005.

31. ACNM, "Basic Facts about Certified Nurse-Midwives."

32. Rooks, *Midwifery and Childbirth in America,* 164–81; Katherine Camacho Carr, "Innovations in Midwifery Education," *Journal of Midwifery and Women's Health* 48, no. 6 (November/December 2003): 393–97; and ACNM, "Basic Facts about Certified Nurse-Midwives."

33. Rooks, *Midwifery and Childbirth in America,* 205.

34. In 1975, nurse-midwives attended less than 1.0 percent of all births in the United States. Martin et al., "Birth: Final Data for 2003," 15, 81.

35. Rooks, *Midwifery and Childbirth in America,* 145–51, 181, 190–91, 193–207, 464.

36. Williams, "Credentialing Certified Nurse-Midwives," 260.

37. Rooks, *Midwifery and Childbirth in America,* 161–63.

38. Alyson Reed and Joyce E. Roberts, "State Regulation of Midwives: Issues and Options," *Journal of Midwifery and Women's Health* 45, no. 2 (March/April 2000): 130–49.

39. On the United States' gross national product and health care, see Reinhardt, "Reforming the Health Care System," 29. On the United States' infant mortality rate, see Rooks, *Midwifery and Childbirth in America,* 394. On the United States' maternal mortality rate as compared to other countries, see World Health Organization, *Maternal Mortality in 2000.* On the number of Americans without health insurance, see Institute of Medicine, *Insuring America's Health: Principles and Recommendations.*

40. Criticism of obstetrical health-care personnel and hospital births can be found, for example, in Wolf, *Misconceptions;* Mitford, *American Way of Birth; Mothering* Magazine; and stories told by birthing women in Gaskin, *Ina May's Guide to Childbirth.*

41. Denise Grady, "What's Missing in Childbirth These Days? Often, the Pain," *New York Times,* 13 October 1999, A1; and C. J. Chivers, "Bearing With the Pain, and Fighting a Trend; Devotees of No-Drug Childbirth Frustrated by Rise in Use of Anesthesia," *New York Times,* 18 October 1999, B1. On the Caesarean section rate, see Martin et al., "Birth: Final Data for 2003," 2, 85–86.

In fact, some women, especially those of a higher socioeconomic status with access to many health-care options, feel as though the current cultural climate says that there is a "right way" to do childbirth—as naturally as possible—and that if they have medical interventions in childbirth they are failures. Roberts, "Push and Pull," 50; and Pan, "Not Mother Nature's Way," 106, 108.

42. Dower, Miller, O'Neil, and the Taskforce on Midwifery, *Charting a Course for the 21st Century: The Future of Midwifery.*

43. See Notes to Epilogue, notes 53 and 54.

44. In 2003, 1.1 percent of all nurse-midwife–attended births occurred at home; the percentage is 1.0 if "other" places of delivery (not hospital, freestanding birth center, clinic or doctor's office, or residence) are excluded. Martin et al. "Birth: Final Data for 2003," 81. On the safety of planned home births, see Murphy and Fullerton, "Outcomes of Intended Home Births in Nurse-Midwifery Practice," 461–70; Eugene R. Declercq, Lisa L. Paine, and Michael R. Winter, "Home Birth in the United States, 1989–1992: A Longitudinal Descriptive Report of National Birth Certificate Data," *Journal of Nurse-Midwifery* 40, no. 6 (November-December 1995): 474–82; and Rondi E. Anderson and Patricia Aikins Murphy, "Outcomes of 11,788 Planned Home Births Attended by Certified Nurse-Midwives: A Retrospective Descriptive Study," *Journal of Nurse-Midwifery* 40, no. 6 (November-December 1995): 483–92.

45. Holly Powell Kennedy, Maureen T. Shannon, Usa Chuahorm, and M. Kathryn Kravetz, "The Landscape of Caring for Women: A Narrative Study of Midwifery Practice," *Journal of Midwifery and Women's Health* 49, no. 1 (January/February 2004): 14–23.

46. Holly Powell Kennedy, "A Model of Exemplary Midwifery Practice: Results of a Delphi Study," *Journal of Midwifery and Women's Health* 45, no. 1 (January/February 2000): 4–19.

47. Bunny Adler, CNM, conversation with author, 13 April 1999, Massena, New York; "Massena Memorial Hospital, Hospital Policy and Procedure; Subject: Allied Health Professionals Caring for the Obstetrical Patient," 6 December 1995; Bunny Adler to Massena Memorial Hospital, 11 February 1999. I thank Adler for sharing these materials with me.

48. Heimlich, "Profile: Safety and Struggles of Midwifery."

49. See, for example, Joseph B. Treaster, "Rise in Insurance Forces Hospitals to Shutter Wards," *New York Times,* 25 August 2002, Section 1, 1.

50. American College of Nurse-Midwives, "ACNM Highlights Needs for Immediate Medical Malpractice Reform at Senate Press Committee," 19 February 2004, www.midwife.org/press/display.cfm?id=390 (accessed 20 February 2004).

51. Davis-Floyd, "Ups, Downs, and Interlinkages."

52. Davis-Floyd, "Ups, Downs, and Interlinkages."

53. L. G. Davis, G. L. Riedmann, M. Sapiro, J. P. Minogue, and R. P. Kazer, "Cesarean Section Rates in Low Risk Private Patients Managed by Certified Nurse-Midwives and Obstetricians," *Journal of Nurse-Midwifery* 39 (1994): 91–97; Brown and Grimes, "A Meta-Analysis of Nurse-Practitioners and Nurse-Midwives in Primary Care," 332–39; Hueston and Rudy, "A Comparison of Labor and Delivery Management," 449–54; Lisa C. Harrington, David A. Miller, Cindy J. McClain, and Richard H. Paul, "Vaginal Birth after Cesarean in a Hospital-Based Birth Center Staffed by Certified Nurse-Midwives," *Journal of Nurse-Midwifery* 42, no. 4 (July/August 1997): 304–7; Michele R. Davidson, "Outcomes of High-Risk Women Cared For by Certified Nurse-Midwives," *Journal of Midwifery and Women's Health* 47, no. 1 (January/February 2002): 46–49; and Rooks, *Midwifery and Childbirth in America,* 295–343.

54. MacDorman and Kingh, "Midwifery Care," 310–17.

55. Lisa M. Garceau, Lisa L. Paine, and Mary K. Barger, "Population-Based Primary Health Care for Women: An Overview for Midwives," *Journal of Nurse-Midwifery* 42, no. 6 (November/December 1997): 465–77. For a more recent study, see Eugene R. Declercq, Deanne R. Williams, Ann M. Koontz, Lisa L. Paine, Erica L. Streit, and Lois McCloskey, "Serving Women in Need: Nurse-Midwifery Practice in the United States," *Journal of Midwifery and Women's Health* 46, no. 1 (January/February 2001): 11–16.

56. Rooks, *Midwifery and Childbirth in America,* 386–89.

57. Rosenblatt, et al., "Interspecialty Differences in the Obstetric Care," 348–50.

58. Rooks, *Midwifery and Childbirth in America,* 386.

59. Barbara A. Petersen, "Nurse-Midwifery in a Managed Care Environment," *Journal of Nurse-Midwifery* 41, no. 4 (July/August 1996): 267–68.

60. McCloskey et al., "The Practice of Nurse-Midwifery in the Era of Managed Care," 127–36.

# BIBLIOGRAPHY

## Manuscript Collections

*American College of Nurse-Midwives:*

American College of Nurse-Midwives (ACNM) Archives, National Library of Medicine, Bethesda, Maryland.

*Catholic Maternity Institute:*

Catholic Maternity Institute (CMI) file, New Mexico Health Historical Collections, University of New Mexico Health Sciences Library and Informatics Center, Albuquerque, New Mexico.

Catholic Maternity Institute—Santa Fe file, Archives of the Archdiocese of Santa Fe, New Mexico.

Medical Mission Sisters (MMS) Archives, Philadelphia, Pennsylvania.

*Frontier Nursing Service:*

Audio-Visual Archives, Margaret I. King Library, University of Kentucky, Lexington.

Frontier Nursing Service (FNS) Oral History Collection, Archives and Special Collections, Margaret I. King Library, University of Kentucky, Lexington.

Frontier Nursing Service (FNS) Papers, Archives and Special Collections, Margaret I. King Library, University of Kentucky, Lexington.

Inventory for the FNS Medical Surveys, Archives and Special Collections, Margaret I. King Library, University of Kentucky, Lexington.

*Maternity Center Association:*

During the time that I did research for this book, the archives of the Maternity Center Association (MCA) in New York City had three different locations: MCA Archives, MCA Storage, and MCA Office. Until 1996, the archives were located in the MCA library; anything accessed until that time is listed as MCA Archives. In 1996, most of the archives were placed into storage; items accessed from storage are designated as MCA Storage. Some items remain in the MCA Office; those items are designated as such. The MCA archives will be housed at Archives and Special Collections, Augustus C. Long Health Sciences Library, Columbia University, starting in 2006.

## Interviews

Cauzillo, Sister Anne. Interview by author. Philadelphia, Pennsylvania. 7 September 1995.
Corbin, Hazel. Interview by Ruth Watson Lubic. Transcript. New York: Oral History Research Office, Columbia University, 1970.
D'Errico, Sister Paula. Interview by author. Philadelphia, Pennsylvania. 6 September 1995.
Fox, Anne. Interview by Jake Spidle. Transcript. Albuquerque: University of New Mexico Medical Center Library, 1986. Oral History Collection, New Mexico Medical History Project, University of New Mexico Health Sciences Center Library and Informatics Center, Albuquerque, New Mexico.
Gates, Sister Kathryn. Interview by author. Philadelphia, Pennsylvania. 23 February 1996.
Gavin, Sister Mary. Interview by author. Philadelphia, Pennsylvania. 23 February 1996.
Hyder, Kate. Interview by Sara Lee Silberman. Hamden, Connecticut. 6 March 1984. Personal collection of Sara Lee Silberman.
Kroska, Rita. Telephone interview by author. 24 July 2000.
McGinnis, Sister Sheila. Interview by author. Philadelphia, Pennsylvania. 8 September 1995.
Mitchell, Hannah D. Interview by Rose B. Cannon. Transcript. 16 May 1989. Georgia Public Health Nurses Oral History Collection, Special Collections and Archives, Robert W. Woodruff Library, Emory University, Atlanta, Georgia.
Shean, Sister Catherine. Telephone interview by author. 18 August 2000.

## Videos

Breckinridge, Marvin (later, Patterson, Marvin Breckinridge), director. *The Forgotten Frontier.* c. 1928. Audio-Visual Archives, Margaret I. King Library, University of Kentucky, Lexington. Film.
King, Pauline E., producer. *Nurse-Midwife.* Santa Fe, N.M.: Catholic Maternity Institute, 1948. Medical Missions Sisters (MMS) Archives, Philadelphia, Pennsylvania. Film.
Kroska, Rita A., executive producer. *CMI: In-Depth Interviews with the Foundresses.* Tucson: Medical Mission Sisters/Catholic Maternity Institute Historical Project, 1996. Video.
———, executive producer. *50th Celebration Reunion, Remembering CMI Santa Fe.* Tucson: Medical Mission Sisters/Catholic Maternity Institute Historical Project, 1994. Video.
Patterson, Marvin Breckinridge, speech. In *Presentation of the Frontier Nursing Service Collection.* 1985. Audio-Visual Archives, Margaret I. King Library, University of Kentucky, Lexington. Video.
Stoney, George, writer, director, and producer. *All My Babies.* Chicago: Medical Audio-

Visual Institute of the Association of American Medical Colleges, 1952.

## Journals, Reports, and Minutes of Meetings

*Briefs*, Maternity Center Association publication (1936–1966).

Inspection reports of the Lobenstine Midwifery Clinic by the New York State Department of Social Welfare, Container 512591 (Admin. Records, Lobenstine Clinic, H. Hemschemeyer 2 of 3, 1931–1971, Box 108), Folder: State Department of Social Welfare (Inspections), MCA Storage.

Minutes, Medical Board Meetings, MCA, 1931–1965, MCA Office.

Minutes, Meeting of the Board of Directors, MCA, 1924–1960, MCA Office.

*The Nurse-Midwife Bulletin* (1954–1955), *Bulletin of the American College of Nurse-Midwifery* (1955–1968), *Bulletin of the American College of Nurse-Midwives* (1969–1972), *Journal of Nurse-Midwifery* (1973–1999), and *Journal of Midwifery and Women's Health* (2000–present).

*Public Health Nursing Quarterly* (1913–1918), *Public Health Nurse* (1918–1931), and *Public Health Nursing* (1931–1952).

*Quarterly Bulletin of the Kentucky Committee for Mothers and Babies, Inc.* (1925–1928) and *Quarterly Bulletin of the Frontier Nursing Service, Inc.* (1928–1960).

## Primary Sources: Books and Articles

Adair, Fred Lyman. *The Country Doctor and the Specialist*. Maitland, Fla.: Adair Award Fund, 1968.

American College of Nurse-Midwifery. *Education for Nurse-Midwifery: The Report of the Work Conference on Nurse-Midwifery*. Santa Fe: American College of Nurse-Midwifery, 1958.

Arms, Suzanne. *Immaculate Deception*. Boston: Houghton-Mifflin, 1975.

Bailey, Harold. "Control of Midwives." *American Journal of Obstetrics and Gynecology* 6, no. 3 (September 1923): 293–98.

Baker, S. Josephine. "Schools for Midwives." In *The American Midwife Debate: A Sourcebook on Its Modern Origins,* ed. Judy Barrett Litoff, 153–66. New York: Greenwood Press, 1986. First published in *American Journal of Obstetrics and the Diseases of Women and Children* 65 (1912): 256–70.

———. "The Function of a Midwife." *Woman's Medical Journal* 23, no. 9 (1913): 196–97.

———. *Fighting for Life*. New York: The Macmillan Company, 1939.

"'The Birth of a Baby' Aims to Reduce Maternal and Infant Mortality Rates." *Life* 4, no. 15 (11 April 1938): 33–36.

Breckinridge, Mary. "The Nurse-Midwife—A Pioneer." *American Journal of Public Health* 17, no. 11 (November 1927): 1147–51.

———. "The Nurse on Horseback." *Women's Journal* 8, no. 2 (February 1928): 5–7, 38.

———. "Saving Lives on the Last Frontier." *Literary Digest* 119 (2 February 1935): 22.

———. "Where the Frontier Lingers." *The Rotarian* 157, no. 3 (September 1935): 9–12, 50.

———. "Is Birth Control the Answer?" *Harper's Magazine* 163, no. 974 (July 1931): 157–63.

Brown, S. A., and D. E. Grimes. "A Meta-analysis of Nurse-practitioners and Nurse-midwives in Primary Care." *Nurse Research* 44, no. 6 (November/December 1995): 332–39.

Browne, Helen E., and Gertrude Isaacs. "The Frontier Nursing Service: The Primary Care Nurse in the Community Hospital." *American Journal of Obstetrics and Gynecology* 121 (1976): 14–17.

Chenault, Lawrence R. *The Puerto Rican Migrant in New York City*. New York: Russell and Russell, 1938.

Chetwynd, Eve. "The Frontier Nursing Service of Kentucky." *Nursing Mirror and Midwives Journal* 100, no. 2598 (11 February 1955): v–vii.

City Planning Commission, City of Santa Fe. *General Characteristics, City of Santa Fe, New Mexico.* Santa Fe: Urban Planning Assistance Program of the New Mexico State Department of Finance and Administration, 1960.

Corbin, Hazel. "Teaching Women about Prenatal Care." *American Journal of Nursing* 42, no. 8 (August 1942): 873–76.

———. "Emotional Aspects of Maternity Care." *American Journal of Nursing* 48, no. 1 (January 1948): 20–22.

———. "Natural Childbirth." *American Journal of Nursing* 49, no. 10 (October 1949): 660–62.

———. "Maternity Care Today and Tomorrow." *American Journal of Nursing* 53, no. 2 (February 1953): 201–4.

Davis-Floyd, Robbie E. "The Ups, Downs, and Interlinkages of Nurse- and Direct-Entry Midwifery: Status, Practice, and Education." In *Pathways to Becoming a Midwife: Getting an Education*. Eugene, Ore.: Midwifery Today, 1998.

Dengel, Anna. *Mission for Samaritans: A Survey of Achievements and Opportunities in the Field of Catholic Medical Missions*. Milwaukee: The Bruce Publishing Company, 1945.

Dickinson, Robert Latou, and Abram Belskie. *Birth Atlas*. New York: Maternity Center Association, 1940.

Dick-Read, Grantly. *Natural Childbirth*. London: Heinemann, 1933.

———. *Childbirth without Fear*. New York: Harper and Brothers, 1944.

Dower, Catherine M., Janet E. Miller, Edward H. O'Neil, and the Taskforce on Midwifery. *Charting a Course for the 21st Century: The Future of Midwifery*. San Francisco: Pew Health Professions Commission and the UCSF Center for the Health Professions, April 1999.

Dublin, Louis I., and Hazel Corbin. "A Preliminary Report of the Maternity Center Association of New York." *American Journal of Obstetrics and Gynecology* 20 (December 1930): 877–81.

Dublin, Louis I. "The Problem of Maternity—A Survey and Forecast." *American Journal of Public Health* 29, no. 11 (November 1939): 1205–14.

Dunn, Rev. Daniel F. "They Save the Baby." *The Catholic Home Journal* 53, no. 6 (June 1953): 8–9.

Edgar, J. Clifton. "The Education, Licensing and Supervision of the Midwife." In *The American Midwife Debate: A Sourcebook on Its Modern Origins*, ed. Judy Barrett Litoff, 129–43. New York: Greenwood Press, 1986. First published in *American Journal of*

*Obstetrics and the Diseases of Women and Children* 73 (March 1916): 385–98.

Emery, Raymen. "Meddlesome Obstetrics." *The Pennsylvania Medical Journal* 41, no. 2 (November 1937): 88–91.

"EMIC Program Draws to an End." *American Journal of Nursing* 47, no. 9 (September 1947): 643.

Faison, Jere B. "Report of the Maternity Center Association Clinic, 1952–1958." *American Journal of Obstetrics and Gynecology* 81, no. 2 (February 1961): 395–402.

"First Medical Mission Sisterhood." *Catholic Missions* 27, no. 6 (August–September 1950): 5–7, 10–13.

Flexner, Abraham. *Medical Education in the United States and Canada: A Report to the Carnegie Foundation for the Advancement of Teaching*, Bulletin #4. New York: Carnegie Foundation, 1910.

"Frontier Nursing Service Brings Health to Kentucky Mountaineers." *Life* 2, no. 24 (14 June 1937): 32–35.

Gardner, Caroline. *Clever Country: Kentucky Mountain Trails.* New York: Fleming H. Revell Company, 1931.

Gaskin, Ina May. *Ina May's Guide to Childbirth.* New York: Bantam Books, 2003.

Gilbreth, Jr., Frank B., and Ernestine Gilbreth Carey. *Cheaper by the Dozen.* New York: Bantam Books, Inc., 1948.

Haney, Anne. "Nursing by Jeep and Horseback." *Progressive Farmer* 69, no. 9 (September 1954): 24–25, 140.

Heimlich, Janet. "Profile: Safety and Struggles of Midwifery." *Weekend Edition,* National Public Radio, 17 January 2004.

Hellman, Louis M. "Paraobstetric Personnel." *American Journal of Obstetrics and Gynecology* 83, no. 4 (15 February 1962): 503–7.

Hemschemeyer, Hattie. "Midwifery in the United States." *American Journal of Nursing* 39, no. 11 (November 1939): 1181–87.

———. "The Nurse-midwife Is Here to Stay." *American Journal of Nursing* 43, no. 10 (1943): 913–16.

Hueston, W. J., and M. Rudy. "A Comparison of Labor and Delivery Management between Nurse-midwives and Family Physicians." *Journal of Family Practice* 37 (1993): 449–54.

Hyland, T. S. "The Fruitful Mountaineers." *Life* (26 December 1949): 60–67.

Institute of Medicine. *Insuring America's Health: Principles and Recommendations.* Washington, D.C.: National Academies Press, 2004.

"I Watched My Baby Born." As told to Amy Selwyn. *Pageant* 4, no. 7 (January 1949): 5–13.

Kooser, John H. "Rural Obstetrics: A Report of the Work of the Frontier Nursing Service." *The Southern Medical Journal* 35, no. 2 (February 1942): 123–31.

Kosmak, George W. "Results of Supervised Midwife Practice in Certain European Countries: Can We Draw a Lesson from This for the United States?" *Journal of the American Medical Association* 89, no. 24 (10 December 1927): 2009–12.

———. "The Trained Nurse and Midwife." *American Journal of Nursing* 34, no. 5 (May 1934): 421–23.

Laird, Marion D. "Report of the Maternity Center Association Clinic, New York, 1931–1951." *American Journal of Obstetrics and Gynecology* 69, no. 1 (January 1955): 178–84.

———, and Margaret Hogan. "An Elective Program on Preparation for Childbirth at the Sloane Hospital for Women, May, 1951, to June, 1953." *American Journal of Obstetrics and Gynecology* 72, no. 3 (September 1956): 641–47.

Lansing, Elisabeth Hubbard. *Rider on the Mountains.* New York: Thomas Y. Cromwell Co., 1949.

Lobenstine, Ralph. *The Expectant Mother and the New Baby.* Child Health Series. Bulletin No. 1. New York: Butterick Publishing Company, 1922.

MacDorman, M. F., and G. K. Kingh. "Midwifery Care, Social and Medical Risk Factors, and Birth Outcomes in the USA." *Journal of Epidemiology and Community Health* 52, no. 5 (May 1998): 310–17.

Martin, Joyce A., Brady E. Hamilton, Paul D. Sutton, Stephanie J. Ventura, Fay Menacker, and Martha L. Munson. "Birth: Final Data for 2003." In *National Vital Statistics Reports* 54, no. 2. Hyattsville, Md.: National Center for Health Statistics, 2005.

Maternity Center Association. *Maternity Center Association, 1925.* New York: Maternity Center Association, 1926.

———. *Maternity Center Association, 1928.* New York: Maternity Center Association, 1929.

———. *Routines for Maternity Nursing and Briefs for Mothers' Club Talks,* 3rd ed. New York: Maternity Center Association, 1929.

———. *Maternity Handbook for Pregnant Mothers and Expectant Fathers.* New York: G. P. Putnam's Sons, 1932.

———. *Maternity Center Association: Six Years in Review, 1930–1935.* New York: Maternity Center Association, 1935.

———. *Lobenstine: The Only School for Nurse-Midwives in the United States.* New York: Maternity Center Association, [1939?].

———. *Maternity Center Association, 1918–1943.* New York: Maternity Center Association, 1943.

———. *Public Health Nursing in Obstetrics; Part IV: Mothers' and Fathers' Classes.* New York: Maternity Center Association, 1943.

———. *Maternity Handbook for Pregnant Mothers and Expectant Fathers,* 2nd ed. New York: G. P. Putnam's Sons, 1945.

———. *Twenty Years of Nurse-Midwifery, 1933–1953.* New York: Maternity Center Association, 1955.

———. *40th Annual Report of the Maternity Center Association.* New York: Maternity Center Association, 1959.

McCloskey, Lois, Holly Powell Kennedy, Eugene R. Declercq, and Deanne R. Williams. "The Practice of Nurse-Midwifery in the Era of Managed Care: Reports from the Field." *Maternal and Child Health Journal* 6, no. 2 (June 2002): 127–36.

Miles, Dorothy. "Heroines on Horseback." *Colliers Magazine* (31 August 1946): 24–26, 29.

Miller, Elinor. "Grand Multiparas: A Ten-Year Study." *Obstetrics and Gynecology* 4, no. 4 (October 1954): 418–25.

Mitchell, Hannah D. "Coordinating Maternity Care: The Role of Nursing." *American Journal of Public Health* 41, no. 11 (November 1951): 10–12.

Murphy, Patricia Aikins, and Judith Fullerton. "Outcomes of Intended Home Births in

Nurse-Midwifery Practice: A Prospective Descriptive Study." *Obstetrics and Gynecology* 92, no. 3 (September 1998): 461–70.

"Natural Childbirth: Young Mother Has Her Baby with No Fear, Little Pain." *Life* 28, no. 5 (30 January 1959): 71–76.

New York Academy of Medicine Committee on Public Health Relations. *Maternal Mortality in New York City: A Study of all Puerperal Deaths, 1930–1932*. New York: The Commonwealth Fund, 1933.

Noyes, Clara D. "Training School for Midwives at Bellevue and Allied Hospitals." *American Journal of Nursing* 12, no. 5 (February 1912): 417–18.

———. "The Midwifery Problem." *American Journal of Nursing* 12, no. 6 (March 1912): 466–71.

———. "The Training of Midwives in Relation to the Prevention of Infant Mortality." *American Journal of Obstetrics and Diseases of Women and Children* 66 (1912): 1051–59.

Pan, Esther. "Not Mother Nature's Way." *Newsweek* 134, no. 22 (29 November 1999): 106, 108.

Pearl, Raymond. "Distribution of Physicians in the United States." *Journal of the American Medical Association* 84, no. 14 (4 April 1925): 1024–28.

Peckham, Charles H. "The Essentials of Adequate Maternal Care in Rural Areas." *The Child* 4, no. 5 (November 1939): 119–24.

Philadelphia County Medical Society Committee on Maternal Welfare. *Maternal Mortality in Philadelphia, 1931–1933*. Philadelphia: Philadelphia County Medical Society, 1934.

Poole, Ernest. "The Nurse on Horseback, Has Brought New Life and Hope to the Kentucky Mountaineers." *Good Housekeeping* (June 1932): 38–39, 203–10.

Reinhardt, Uwe E. "Reforming the Health Care System: The Universal Dilemma." *American Journal of Law and Medicine* 19, nos. 1 and 2 (1993): 21–36.

Roberts, Hope. "Push and Pull." *New Republic* 225, no. 21 (19 November 2001): 50.

Rosenblatt, Roger A., Sharon A. Dobie, L. Gary Hart, Ronald Schneeweis, Debra Gould, Tina R. Raine, Thomas J. Benedetti, Michael J. Pirani, and Edward B. Perrin. "Interspecialty Differences in the Obstetric Care of Low-Risk Women." *American Journal of Public Health* 87, no. 3 (March 1997): 348–50.

Rude, Anna E. "The Midwife Problem in the United States." *Journal of the American Medical Association* 81, no. 12 (22 September 1923): 987–92.

Schupp, William E. "The Good Neighbor of 'Wide Neighborhoods.'" *In Kentucky* 17, no. 2 (Summer 1953): 12–15.

Schwartz, Doris. "Nurse-Midwives in the Mountains." *American Journal of Nursing* 51, no. 2 (February 1951): 102–3.

Shoemaker, Sister M. Theophane. *History of Nurse-Midwifery in the United States*. 1947; reprint, New York: Garland, 1984.

Sinai, Nathan, and Odin W. Anderson. *EMIC (Emergency Maternity and Infant Care): A Study of Administrative Experience*. 1948; reprint, New York: Arno Press, 1974.

Smith, Betty. *A Tree Grows in Brooklyn*. Philadelphia: The Blakiston Company, 1943.

Smith, W. Eugene. "Nurse-Midwife: Maude Callen Eases Pain of Birth, Life, and Death." *Life* 31 (3 December 1951): 134–44.

Stoney, George C. "*All My Babies*: Research." In *Film: Book 1, The Audience and the Filmmaker*, ed. Robert Hughes, 79–96. New York: Grove Press, 1959.

Thomas, Margaret. *The Practice of Nurse-Midwifery in the United States.* Washington, D.C.: U.S. Department of Health, Education, and Welfare, 1965.

U.S. Public Health Service Bureau of Health, Manpower Education, Division of Nursing. "A Study to Determine the Need and Scope for Educational Programs in Nurse-Midwifery and/or Continuing Education for Maternity Nursing in New Mexico and the Direction Each Should Take." Final Report, 1 October 1970 to 31 December 1971. From the personal files of Ruth Watson Lubic.

Van Blarcom, Carolyn Conant. *The Midwife in England.* Philadelphia: The Press of William F. Fell, 1913.

———. "Midwives in America." *American Journal of Public Health* 4 (March 1914): 197–207.

Van der Eerden, Sister M. Lucia. *Maternity Care in a Spanish-American Community of New Mexico.* Catholic University of America Anthropological Series, No. 13. Washington, D.C.: Catholic University of America Press, 1948.

Varney, Helen. *Varney's Midwifery.* 3rd ed. Boston: Jones and Bartlett Publishers, 1997.

Watson, B. P. "Can Our Methods of Obstetrics Practice Be Improved?" *Bulletin of the New York Academy of Medicine* 6, no. 10 (October 1930): 647–63.

Wessel, Helen. *Natural Childbirth and the Christian Family.* New York: Harper and Row, 1963.

White House Conference on Child Health and Protection. *Fetal, Newborn, and Maternal Mortality and Morbidity.* New York: The Century Company, 1933.

Willeford, Mary B. *Income and Health in Remote Rural Areas: A Study of 400 Families in Leslie County, Kentucky.* New York: Frontier Nursing Service, Inc., 1932.

Wolf, Naomi. *Misconceptions: Truth, Lies, and the Unexpected on the Journey to Motherhood.* New York: Doubleday, 2001.

Works Progress Administration. *The WPA Guide to New York City.* 1939; reprint, New York: Pantheon Books, 1982.

World Health Organization. *Maternal Mortality in 2000: Estimates Developed by WHO, UNICEF and UNFPA.* Geneva: World Health Organization, 2004.

Wynen, Sister M. Elise. "The Society of Catholic Medical Missionaries." *Catholic Medical Quarterly* 2 (20), no. 2 (January 1949): 45–52.

## Secondary Sources: Books, Exhibitions, and Articles

Antler, Joyce, and Daniel M. Fox. "The Movement toward a Safe Maternity: Physician Accountability in New York City, 1915–1940." In *Sickness and Health in America: Readings in the History of Medicine and Public Health,* Rev. Ed., ed. Judith Walzer Leavitt and Ronald L. Numbers, 490–506. Madison: University of Wisconsin Press, 1985. First published in the *Bulletin of the History of Medicine* 50, no. 4 (Winter 1976): 569–95.

Apple, Rima D. *Mothers and Medicine: A Social History of Infant Feeding, 1890–1950.* Madison: University of Wisconsin Press, 1987.

———. "Constructing Mothers: Scientific Motherhood in the Nineteenth and Twentieth Centuries." *Social History of Medicine* 8, no. 2 (1995): 161–78.

Batteau, Allen W. *The Invention of Appalachia.* Tucson: University of Arizona Press, 1990.

Batteau, Allen. "Appalachia and the Concept of Culture: A Theory of Shared Misunderstandings." In *Appalachia: Social Context, Past and Present,* 3rd ed., ed. Bruce Ergood and Bruce E. Kuhre, 153–69. Dubuque, Iowa: Kendall/Hunt Publishing Company, 1991.

Bell, Pegge L. "'Making Do' with the Midwife: Arkansas's Mamie O. Hale in the 1940s." *Nursing History Review* 1 (1993): 155–69.

Bennett, David H. *The Party of Fear: From Nativist Movement to the New Right in American History*. Chapel Hill, N.C.: University of North Carolina Press, 1988.

Bent, E.A. "The Growth and Development of Midwifery." In *Nursing, Midwifery and Health Visiting Since 1900,* ed. Peta Allen and Moya Jolley, 180–95. London: Faber and Faber Limited, 1982.

Bergstrom, Linda, Marie E. Pokorny, Margaret B. Davis, and Terrell O. Wootten. "Full Circle: The Nurse-Midwifery Careers of Elizabeth Berryhill and Gabriela Olivera." *Nursing History Review* 7 (1999): 29–45.

Binder, Frederick M., and David M. Reimers. *All the Nations Under Heaven: An Ethnic and Racial History of New York* City. New York: Columbia University Press, 1995.

Bonner, Thomas Neville. *Becoming a Physician: Medical Education in Britain, France, Germany, and the United States, 1750–1945*. New York: Oxford University Press, 1995.

Borst, Charlotte G. *Catching Babies: The Professionalization of Childbirth, 1870–1920*. Cambridge, Mass.: Harvard University Press, 1995.

Breckinridge, Mary. *Wide Neighborhoods: A Story of the Frontier Nursing Service*. 1952; reprint, Lexington, KY: University Press of Kentucky, 1981.

Brown, E. Richard. "Public Health Programs in Imperialism: Early Rockefeller Programs at Home and Abroad." *American Journal of Public Health* 66, no. 9 (September 1976): 897–903.

Brush, Barbara L., and Elizabeth A. Capezuti. "Revisiting 'A Nurse for All Settings': The Nurse Practitioner Movement, 1965–1995." *Journal of the American Academy of Nurse Practitioners* 8, no. 1 (January 1996): 5–11.

Buhler-Wilkerson, Karen. *False Dawn: The Rise and Decline of Public Health Nursing, 1900–1930*. New York: Garland, 1989.

Buss, Fran Leeper. *La Partera: Story of a Midwife*. Ann Arbor: University of Michigan Press, 1980.

Campbell, Anne G. "Mary Breckinridge and the American Committee for Devastated France: The Foundations of the Frontier Nursing Service." *Register of the Kentucky Historical Society* 82, no. 3 (Summer 1984): 257–76.

Cannon, Rose B. "Enduring Echoes: Hannah D. Mitchell." *Georgia Nursing* 60, no. 3 (August–October 2000): 12.

Carson, Carolyn Leonard. "And the Results Showed Promise . . . Physicians, Childbirth, and Southern Black Migrant Women, 1916–1930; Pittsburgh as a Case Study." *Journal of American Ethnic History* 14, no. 1 (Fall 1994): 32–64.

Cassedy, James. *Medicine in America: A Short History*. Baltimore, Md.: The Johns Hopkins University Press, 1991.

Caudill, Harry M. *Night Comes to the Cumberlands: A Biography of a Depressed Area*. Boston: Little, Brown, 1962.

Crowe-Carraco, Carol. "Mary Breckinridge and the Frontier Nursing Service." *Register of the Kentucky Historical Society* 76, no. 3 (July 1978): 179–91.

Crunden, Robert M. *Ministers of Reform: The Progressives' Achievement in American Civilization, 1889–1920.* New York: Basic Books, 1982.

Dammann, Nancy. *A Social History of the Frontier Nursing Service.* Sun City, Ariz.: Social Change Press, 1982.

Davis-Floyd, Robbie E. *Birth as an American Rite of Passage.* Berkeley and Los Angeles: University of California Press, 1992.

Dawley, Katy. "The Campaign to Eliminate the Midwife." *American Journal of Nursing* 100, no. 10 (October 2000): 50–56.

———. "Ideology and Self-Interest: Nursing, Medicine, and the Elimination of the Midwife." *Nursing History Review* 9 (2001): 99–126.

———. "Perspectives on the Past, View of the Present: Relationship between Nurse-midwifery and Nursing in the United States." *Nursing Clinics of North America* 37, no. 4 (December 2002): 747–55.

———. "American Nurse-Midwifery: A Hyphenated Profession with a Conflicted Identity." *Nursing History Review* 13 (2005): 147–70.

Deutsch, Sarah. *No Separate Refuge: Culture, Class, and Gender on the Anglo-Hispanic Frontier in the American Southwest, 1880–1940.* New York: Oxford University Press, 1987.

Devitt, Neal. "The Transition from Home to Hospital Birth in the United States, 1930–1960." *Birth and the Family Journal* 4, no. 2 (Summer 1977): 47–58.

De Vries, Raymond. *A Pleasing Birth: Midwives and Maternity Care in the Netherlands.* Philadelphia: Temple University Press, 2004.

Donnison, Jean. *Midwives and Medical Men: A History of Inter-Professional Rivalries and Women's Rights.* New York: Schocken Books, 1977.

Dye, Nancy Schrom. "Mary Breckinridge, the Frontier Nursing Service and the Introduction of Nurse-Midwifery in the United States." *Bulletin of the History of Medicine* 57 (1983): 485–507.

———. "The Medicalization of Birth." In *The American Way of Birth,* ed. Pamela S. Eakins, 17–46. Philadelphia: Temple University Press, 1986.

Edwards, Margot, and Mary Waldorf. *Reclaiming Birth: History and Heroines of American Childbirth Reform.* Trumansburg, N.Y.: The Crossing Press, 1984.

Ettinger, Laura E. "Nurse-Midwives, the Mass Media, and the Politics of Maternal Health Care in the United States, 1925–1955." *Nursing History Review* 7 (1999): 47–66.

———. "Mary Breckinridge." In *American National Biography,* Vol. 3, ed. John A. Garraty and Mark C. Carnes, 462–63. New York: Oxford University Press, 1999.

———. "Mission to Mothers: Nuns, Latino Families, and the Founding of Santa Fe's Catholic Maternity Institute." In *Women, Health, and Nation: Canada and the United States Since 1945,* ed. Georgina Feldberg, Molly Ladd-Taylor, Alison Li, and Kathryn McPherson, 144–60. Montreal: McGill-Queen's University Press, 2003.

Ewens, Mary. "The Leadership of Nuns in Immigrant Catholicism." In *Women and Religion in America,* Volume I: *The Nineteenth Century,* ed. Rosemary Radford Ruether and Rosemary Skinner Keller, 101–7. San Francisco: Harper and Row, 1981.

Fee, Elizabeth. *Changing the Face of Medicine: Celebrating America's Women Physicians.* National Library of Medicine Exhibition, Bethesda, Md. 14 October 2003 to 18

November 2005.

Fischer, David Hackett. *Albion's Seed: Four British Folkways in America.* New York: Oxford University Press, 1989.

Fitzpatrick, Joseph P. *Puerto Rican Americans: The Meaning of Migration to the Mainland.* Englewood Cliffs, N.J.: Prentice-Hall, 1971.

Fitzpatrick, M. Louise. *The National Organization for Public Health Nursing, 1912–1952: Development of a Practice Field.* New York: National League for Nursing, 1975.

Flink, James J. *The Automobile Age.* Cambridge, Mass.: Massachusetts Institute of Technology Press, 1988.

Harvey, A. McGehee, and Susan Abrams. *For the Welfare of Mankind: The Commonwealth Fund and American Medicine.* Baltimore, Md.: The Johns Hopkins University Press, 1986.

Higham, John. *Strangers in the Land: Patterns of American Nativism, 1860–1925*, 2[nd] ed. New Brunswick, N.J.: Rutgers University Press, 1988.

Hill, Patricia Evridge. "Maude E. Callen." In *Doctors, Nurses, and Medical Practitioners: A Bio-Bibliographical Sourcebook,* ed. Lois N. Magner, 49–54. Westport, Conn.: Greenwood Press, 1997.

Hine, Darlene Clark. *Black Women in White: Racial Conflict and Cooperation in the Nursing Profession, 1890–1950.* Bloomington: Indiana University Press, 1989.

Hinojosa, Gilberto M. "Mexican-American Faith Communities in Texas and the Southwest." In *Mexican Americans and the Catholic Church, 1900–1965,* ed. Jay P. Dolan and Gilberto M. Hinojosa, 26–45. Notre Dame, Ind.: University of Notre Dame Press, 1994.

Hollingsworth, J. Rogers, and Ellen Jane Hollingsworth. *Controversy about American Hospitals: Funding, Ownership, and Performance.* Washington, D.C.: American Enterprise Institute for Public Policy Research, 1987.

Holmes, Linda Janet. "African American Midwives in the South." In *The American Way of Birth,* ed. Pamela Eakins, 275–81. Philadelphia: Temple University Press, 1986.

Holt, Natalie. "'Confusion's Masterpiece': The Development of the Physician Assistant Profession." *Bulletin of the History of Medicine* 72, no. 2 (Summer 1998): 246–78.

Jackson, Kenneth T., ed. *The Encyclopedia of New York City.* New Haven, Conn.: Yale University Press, 1995.

Jones, Jacqueline. *Labor of Love, Labor of Sorrow: Black Women, Work, and the Family, From Slavery to the Present.* New York: Vintage Books, 1986.

Kauffman, Christopher J. *Ministry and Meaning: A Religious History of Catholic Health Care in the United States.* New York: The Crossroad Publishing Company, 1995.

Klaus, Alisa. *Every Child a Lion: The Origins of Maternal and Infant Health Policy in the United States and France, 1890–1920.* Ithaca, N.Y.: Cornell University Press, 1993.

Klotter, James C. *The Breckinridges of Kentucky, 1760–1981.* Lexington, Ky.: University Press of Kentucky, 1986.

Knobel, Dale T. *'America for the Americans': The Nativist Movement in the United States.* New York: Twayne Publishers, 1996.

Kobrin, Frances E. "The American Midwife Controversy: A Crisis of Professionalization." In *Women and Health in America: Historical Readings,* ed. Judith Walzer Leavitt, 318–26. Madison: University of Wisconsin Press, 1984. First published in the *Bulletin of the History of Medicine* 40 (1966): 350–63.

Korrol, Virginia E. Sanchez. *From Colonia to Community: The History of Puerto Ricans in New York City*. Berkeley and Los Angeles: University of California Press, 1993.

Kroska, Rita A., and Catherine Shean, eds. *CMI Graduates and Faculty Remember Nurse-Midwifery in Santa Fe, New Mexico*. Tucson: Medical Mission Sisters/Catholic Maternity Institute Historical Project, 1996.

Ladd-Taylor, Molly. *Mother-Work: Women, Child Welfare, and the State, 1890–1930*. Urbana: University of Illinois Press, 1994.

Leavitt, Judith Walzer. *Brought to Bed: Childbearing in America, 1750–1950*. New York: Oxford University Press, 1986.

———. "Joseph B. DeLee and the Practice of Preventive Obstetrics." *American Journal of Public Health* 78, no. 10 (October 1988): 1353–59.

———. "The Medicalization of Childbirth in the Twentieth Century." *Transactions and Studies of the College of Physicians of Philadelphia* Series 5, vol. 11, no. 4 (1989): 299–319.

———. "'Strange Young Women on Errands': Obstetric Nurses between Two Worlds." *Nursing History Review* 6 (1998): 3–24.

Lindenmeyer, Kriste. *"A Right to Childhood": The U.S. Children's Bureau and Child Welfare, 1912–46*. Urbana: University of Illinois Press, 1997.

Litoff, Judy Barrett. *American Midwives, 1860 to the Present*. Westport, Conn.: Greenwood Press, 1978.

Longo, Lawrence D., and Christina M. Thomsen. "Prenatal Care and its Evolution in America." *Second Motherhood Symposium, Childbirth: The Beginning of Motherhood*, Proceedings of the Second Motherhood Symposium of the Women's Studies Research Center, 9-10 April 1981, 29–70. Madison: University of Wisconsin, Madison, 1981.

Loudon, Irvine. *Death in Childbirth: An International Study of Maternal Care and Maternal Mortality, 1800–1950*. Oxford: Clarendon Press, 1992.

Lynaugh, Joan E., and Barbara L. Brush. *American Nursing: From Hospitals to Health Systems*. Cambridge, Mass.: Blackwell Publishers, 1996.

Maggard, Sally Ward. "Class and Gender: New Theoretical Priorities in Appalachian Studies." In *The Impact of Institutions in Appalachia, Proceedings of the Eight Annual Appalachian Studies Conference*, ed. Jim Lloyd and Anne G. Campbell, 100–13. Boone, N.C.: Appalachian Consortium Press, 1986.

———. "Will the Real Daisy Mae Please Stand Up? A Methodological Essay on Gender Analysis in Appalachian Research." *Appalachian Journal: A Regional Studies Review* 21, no. 2 (Winter 1994): 136–50.

Marks, Lara V. *Sexual Chemistry: A History of the Contraceptive Pill*. New Haven, Conn.: Yale University Press, 2001.

Marland, Hilary, and Anne Marie Rafferty, eds. *Midwives, Society, and Childbirth: Debates and Controversies in the Modern Period*. London: Routledge, 1997.

McBride, David. *From TB to AIDS: Epidemics among Urban Blacks since 1900*. Albany: State University of New York Press, 1991.

McCann, Carole R. *Birth Control Politics in the United States, 1916–1945*. Ithaca, N.Y.: Cornell University Press, 1994.

McInerney, Rita. "DeGive Family Colorful in City, Catholic History." *Georgia Bulletin: The Official Newspaper of the Archdiocese of Atlanta* 31, no. 20 (20 May 1993): 4–5.

McNamara, Jo Ann Kay. *Sisters in Arms: Catholic Nuns through Two Millennia*. Cambridge, Mass.: Harvard University Press, 1996.

Meckel, Richard A. *Save the Babies: American Public Health Reform and the Prevention of Infant Mortality, 1850–1929*. Baltimore, Md.: The Johns Hopkins University Press, 1990.

Medical Mission Sisters. *History of the Society of Catholic Medical Missionaries, Pre-Foundation to 1968*. London: Medical Mission Sisters, 1991.

Melosh, Barbara. *"The Physician's Hand": Work Culture and Conflict in American Nursing*. Philadelphia: Temple University Press, 1982.

Mitford, Jessica. The *American Way of Birth*. New York: Dutton, 1992.

Morantz-Sanchez, Regina Markell. *Sympathy and Science: Women Physicians in American Medicine*. New York: Oxford University Press, 1985.

More, Ellen S. *Restoring the Balance: Women Physicians and the Profession of Medicine, 1850–1995*. Cambridge, Mass.: Harvard University Press, 1999.

Muncy, Robyn. *Creating a Female Dominion in American Reform, 1890–1935*. New York: Oxford University Press, 1991.

Orsi, Robert A. *Thank You, St. Jude: Women's Devotion to the Patron Saint of Hopeless Causes*. New Haven, Conn.: Yale University Press, 1996.

Osofsky, Gilbert. *Harlem: The Making of a Ghetto, Negro New York, 1890–1930*. New York: Harper and Row, 1963.

Perez y Gonzalez, Maria E. *Puerto Ricans in the United States*. Westport, Conn.: Greenwood Press, 2000.

Perez, Nelida. "A Community at Risk: Puerto Ricans and Health, East Harlem, 1929–1940." *CENTRO: Journal of the Center for Puerto Rican Studies* 2, no. 4 (Fall 1988): 16–27.

Pernick, Martin S. "Eugenics and Public Health in American History." *American Journal of Public Health* 87, no. 11 (November 1997): 1767–72.

Reed, James. *From Private Vice to Public Virtue: The Birth Control Movement and American Society Since 1830*. New York: Basic Books, 1978.

Reverby, Susan M. *Ordered to Care: The Dilemma of American Nursing, 1850–1945*. New York: Cambridge University Press, 1987.

Rodriguez, Clara E. *Puerto Ricans: Born in the U.S.A*. Boston: Unwin Hyman, 1989.

Rooks, Judith Pence. *Midwifery and Childbirth in America*. Philadelphia: Temple University Press, 1997.

Rothman, Barbara Katz. *In Labor: Women and Power in the Birthplace*. 1982; reprint, New York: W. W. Norton, 1991.

Sandelowski, Margarete. *Pain, Pleasure, and American Childbirth: From the Twilight Sleep to the Read Method, 1914–1960*. Westport, Conn.: Greenwood Press, 1984.

Schackel, Sandra. *Social Housekeepers: Women Shaping Public Policy in New Mexico, 1920–1940*. Albuquerque: University of New Mexico Press, 1992.

Schaffer, Ruth C. "The Health and Social Functions of Black Midwives on the Texas Brazos Bottom, 1920–1985." *Rural Sociology* 56, no. 1 (1991): 89–105.

Schoen, Johanna. *Choice and Coercion: Birth Control, Sterilization, and Abortion in Public Health and Welfare*. Chapel Hill, N.C.: University of North Carolina Press, 2005.

Scott, James C. *Weapons of the Weak: Everyday Forms of Peasant Resistance*. New Haven, Conn.: Yale University Press, 1985.

Shackelford, Laurel, and Bill Weinberg. *Our Appalachia*. New York: Hill and Wang, 1977.

Shapiro, Henry D. *Appalachia on Our Mind: The Southern Mountains and Mountaineers in the American Consciousness, 1870–1920*. Chapel Hill: University of North Carolina Press, 1978.

Shorter, Edward. *A History of Women's Bodies*. New York: Basic Books, 1982.

Silberman, Sara Lee. "Pioneering in Family-Centered Maternity and Infant Care: Edith B. Jackson and the Yale Rooming-In Research Project." *Bulletin of the History of Medicine* 64, no. 2 (Summer 1990): 262–87.

Silver, Henry K., Loretta C. Ford, Susan S. Ripley, and Judith Igoe. "Perspectives 20 Years Later: From the Pioneers of the NP Movement." *Nurse Practitioner* 10, no. 1 (January 1985): 15–22.

Smith, Margaret Charles, and Linda Janet Holmes. *Listen to Me Good: The Life Story of an Alabama Midwife*. Columbus: The Ohio State University Press, 1996.

Smith, Susan L. *Sick and Tired of Being Sick and Tired: Black Women's Health Activism in America, 1890–1950*. Philadelphia: University of Pennsylvania Press, 1995.

Speert, Harold. *Obstetrics and Gynecology in America: A History*. Chicago: American College of Obstetricians and Gynecologists, 1980.

Starr, Paul. *The Social Transformation of American Medicine: The Rise of a Sovereign Profession and the Making of a Vast Industry*. New York: Basic Books, 1982.

Stevens, Rosemary. *In Sickness and In Wealth: American Hospitals in the Twentieth Century*. New York: Basic Books, 1989.

Temkin, Elizabeth. "Driving Through: Postpartum Care during World War II." *American Journal of Public Health* 89, no. 4 (April 1999): 587–95.

Towler, Jean, and Joan Bramall. *Midwives in History and Society*. London: Croom Helm, 1986.

Ulrich, Laurel Thatcher. *A Midwife's Tale: The Life of Martha Ballard, Based on Her Diary, 1785–1812*. New York: Vintage Books, 1990.

U.S. Bureau of the Census. *Historical Statistics of the United States, Colonial Times to 1957*. Washington, D.C.: U.S. Government Printing Office, 1960.

Varney, Helen, Jan M. Kriebs, and Carolyn L. Gegor. "The Profession and History of Midwifery in the United States." In *Varney's Midwifery*, 4th ed., 3–27. Sudbury, Mass.: Jones and Barlett Publishers, 2004.

Walsh, Linda V. *Midwife Means With Woman: An Exhibit at the National Library of Medicine, 16 September 1991–15 January 1992*. Exhibition catalog. Bethesda, Md.: National Institutes of Health, 1991.

Wertz, Richard W., and Dorothy C. Wertz. *Lying-In: A History of Childbirth in America*. New York: Free Press, 1977.

Whisnant, David E. *All That Is Native and Fine: The Politics of Culture in an American Region*. Chapel Hill: University of North Carolina Press, 1983.

Wolf, Jacqueline H. *Don't Kill Your Baby: Public Health and the Decline of Breastfeeding in the Nineteenth and Twentieth Centuries*. Columbus: The Ohio State University Press, 2001.

Yohn, Susan M. *A Contest of Faiths: Missionary Women and Pluralism in the American Southwest*. Ithaca, N.Y.: Cornell University Press, 1995.

## Theses and Unpublished Manuscripts

Altizer, Anna L. "The Establishment of the Frontier Nursing Service: A Resource Mobilization Approach." Master's thesis, University of Kentucky, 1990.

Beck, Sister M. Bonaventure. "The Society of Catholic Medical Missionaries: Origin and Development." Master's thesis, Catholic University of America, 1955.

Canty, Lucinda. "The Graduates of the Tuskegee School of Nurse-Midwifery." Master's thesis, Yale University School of Nursing, 1994.

Cassells, Jill. "The Manhattan Midwifery School." Master's thesis, Yale University School of Nursing, 2000.

Dawley, Katherine Louise. "Leaving the Nest: Nurse-Midwifery in the United States 1940–1980." PhD diss., University of Pennsylvania School of Nursing, 2001.

Fedde, Helen Marie. "A Study of Midwifery with Special Reference to its Historical Background, its Present Status, and a Consideration of its Future in the United States." Master's thesis, University of Kentucky, 1950.

Franklin, Kathy Smith. "'A Spirit of Mercy': The Sisters of Mercy and the Founding of Saint Joseph's Hospital, Phoenix, 1892–1912." Paper presented at the twenty-ninth annual conference of the Western Association of Women Historians, San Marino, California, 17 May 1998.

Gosnell, Patria Aran. "The Puerto Ricans in New York City." PhD diss., New York University, 1945.

Hamilton, Diane Bronkema. "The Metropolitan Life Insurance Company Visiting Nursing Service (1909–1953)." PhD diss., University of Virginia, 1987.

Harris, Heather. "Constructing Colonialism: Medicine, Technology, and the Frontier Nursing Service." Master's thesis, Virginia Polytechnic Institute and State University, 1995.

Hiestand, Wanda Caroline. "Midwife to Nurse-Midwife: A History. The Development of Nurse-Midwifery Education in the Continental United States to 1965." EdD diss., Teachers College, Columbia University, 1977.

Horch, Jennifer. "The Flint-Goodridge School of Nurse-Midwifery." Master's thesis, Yale University School of Nursing, 2002.

Lubic, Ruth Watson. "Barriers and Conflict in Maternity Care Innovation." EdD diss., Teachers College, Columbia University, 1979.

Rinker, Sylvia Diane. "To Spread the 'Gospel of Good Obstetrics': The Evolution of Obstetric Nursing: 1890–1940." PhD diss., University of Virginia School of Nursing, 1995.

Smyth, Sister Rosemary. "History of the Catholic Maternity Institute from 1943 to 1958." Master's thesis, Catholic University of America, 1960.

Sullivan, Michael Anne. "Walking the Line: Birth Control and Women's Health at the Santa Fe Maternal Health Center, 1937–1970." Master's thesis, University of New Mexico, 1995.

Tirpak, Helen. "The Frontier Nursing Service: An Adventure in the Delivery of Health Care." PhD diss., University of Pittsburgh, 1972.

Tyndall, Rose Mary Murphy. "A History of the Bellevue School for Midwives: 1911–1936." EdD diss., Teachers College, Columbia University, 1978.

# INDEX